MAKING SENSE OF INTERSEX

MAKING SENSE
OF INTERSEX
Changing Ethical Perspectives in Biomedicine

Ellen K. Feder

Indiana University Press

Bloomington and Indianapolis

This book is a publication of

Indiana University Press
Office of Scholarly Publishing
Herman B Wells Library 350
1320 East 10th Street
Bloomington, Indiana 47405 USA

iupress.indiana.edu

Telephone   800-842-6796
Fax   812-855-7931

© 2014 by Ellen K. Feder

Manufactured in the United States of America

Cataloging information is available from the Library of Congress.
ISBN 978-0-253-01224-1 (cloth)
ISBN 978-0-253-01228-9 (paperback)
ISBN 978-0-253-01232-6 (ebook)

1 2 3 4 5 19 18 17 16 15 14

This is for Zoey and for Enza
(as Nic said)

All knowledge and every intention desire some good . . . Most people are almost agreed as to its name; for both ordinary and cultivated people call it "happiness."

—Aristotle, *Nicomachean Ethics*

Contents

Acknowledgments

Among the virtues that Aristotle discusses in the *Nicomachean Ethics* is generosity. Its practice is essential for the promotion of happiness—or human flourishing—that Aristotle took to be the purpose of a good life. I am grateful to so many whose sustained, and sustaining, generosity made this project possible.

Most of the central chapters have their origins in invitations that took my thinking to unexpected places. My thanks first to Eva Kittay, whose insistence that I keep my promises resulted in the research that became chapter 2. This chapter no doubt would have been the last I wrote on the ethical questions raised by the standard of care were it not for Erik Parens's invitation to participate in the Hastings Center project on Surgically Shaping Children (2002–2004). In retrospect, I see that participation in this two-year project marked the beginning of this book; I have continued to rely on the insight of those involved in the project and am glad to have had the opportunity to work with and among the committed group Erik assembled.

I would also not know until sometime later how influential Lewis Gordon's 2006 invitation to present in Philadelphia at Heretical Nietzsche Studies would become in my thinking about the place of shame and disgust in the standard of care. His admonition to reconsider my criticism of normalization also shaped my thinking about the new nomenclature. Subsequent presentations of the work that became chapter 3 benefited from the criticism of those attending the Workshop on Sexual Difference and Embodiment at McGill University later that year, as well as the McDowell Conference on Philosophy and Social Policy on "Philosophy and the Emotions" at American University in 2008. My thanks to Alia Al-Saji, Marguerite Deslauriers, and Cressida Heyes for their invitation to McGill, and to Jeffrey Reiman for his invitation to present this work at the McDowell conference. It was there that I was fortunate to meet Jane Flax, whose advice that I address the question of envy in the context of this analysis was especially productive in leading me to the questions I pursue over the rest of the project. The chapter that resulted benefited immensely from the encouragement and criticism of Gail Weiss and Debra Bergoffen in developing the shorter version of chapter 3 that appeared in *Hypatia*.

The invitation from Lisa Käll and Kristin Zeiler to the conference on Feminist and Phenomenology and Medicine at Uppsala University in 2011 resulted in my beginning chapters 5 and 6 and working out the substance of chapter 4, which appears in the edited collection resulting from that conference. Comments from the conference participants, especially the prepared response of Kristin Zeiler and

Lisa Guntram, helped further clarify my analysis. I am grateful for Gail Weiss's always spirited, and generously critical, presence through developing the last section of this book, usually on the road, but also at home, where I depend on her steadfast presence.

Janice McLaughlin's timely invitation to present at the Policy Ethics and Life Sciences Center symposium at the University of Newcastle in 2012 was the impetus for the central arguments in chapters 7 and 8. It is fitting that Eva Kittay was instrumental at both the beginning and end of this project, for it was her work that got it started and to which I returned.

I am fortunate to have received significant institutional support. I prepared the paper that I describe in the introduction very soon after I started teaching at American University, and I was awarded a research grant that allowed me in 2000 to undertake the first interviews that resulted in chapter 2. The flexible time granted by the dean of the College of Arts and Sciences allowed me to complete a first draft of the manuscript. I am especially grateful to my colleagues in the Department of Philosophy and Religion who have encouraged the direction of my research. Particular thanks are owed to Gershon Greenberg, Jeff Reiman, and Andrea Tschemplik, who so willingly provided guidance in their areas of expertise, and to Amy Oliver, whose persistently helpful comments were second only to her tireless support as chair of our department. Debra Bergoffen's arrival at American University coincided with the publication of her book, which shaped my thinking about the meaning of human rights. I have relied on Shelley Harshe's wide-ranging expertise and her assistance, which is characteristically above and beyond. I thank my students with whom I have grappled over many of the problems in these pages, particularly those in the graduate seminar in Modern Moral Problems. I hope their influence and the depth of my gratitude are clear to my colleagues and students alike. I thank the American Association of University Women for their award of an American Fellowship at a crucial moment in the development of this project.

My department has afforded me the opportunity to work with a number of students over the years I have worked on this book. These include Kiersten Batzli, John Fantuzzo, Martina Ferrari, Abigail Goliber, Elizabeth McDermott, Amy McKiernan, and Lauren Zahn. I had the privilege of working with Amy, Lauren, and Martina at the point when the research and writing for the project was at its most intense, and their efforts were essential for maintaining the momentum necessary for its completion.

Several individuals provided assistance with special areas. The afternoon I spent with Wilfried Ver Eeke discussing Jacques Lacan made me wish I were fortunate enough to have taken a class with him. On genetic counseling, I'm indebted to Caroline Lieber and Taylor Sale, both of whom provided insight and helpful direction. I hope to pay forward David Brodzinsky's immediate willingness to answer my questions about adoption. Carol Bakkhos provided help with my understanding of Halakha, as did Kenneth Prager, who provided insight into its employment in bioethics. Faye Ginsburg and Rayna Rapp helped me think more clearly about the responsibilities of researchers whose scholarship relies on the experiences of individuals. My discussions with Fuambai Ahmadu not only provided a corrective education but also deepened my understanding of questions concerning culture and violation.

The substantial beginnings of a project that began and ended with thinking about ethics and parenting took place before I was a parent myself. Among the gifts of the parents I interviewed were early lessons in the hard and rewarding work of parenting as well as keener appreciation of the ethical reflection it requires. Friendships with other parents—including those that began before any of us had children—have provided occasions for developing the thinking that became the focus of the last part of this book. For their interest and their expertise—in law, medicine, and philosophy, as well as in parenting—I am grateful to Susanna Baruch, Jeanie Bhuller, Sally Bloom-Feshbach, Barbara Butterworth, Bill Ecenbarger, Jeremiah Gallay, Elysa Gordon, Bridgette Kaiser, Matt Kaiser, Meri Kohlbrener, Pei Jen Wang, Jeff Weaver, and Steven Wexler. I am especially grateful for the consistent moral and material support provided by members of the Feder and Di Toro families.

There are, in addition, many whose input and careful readings have been invaluable over the course of this project. Arlene Baratz, Carolyn Betensky, Deborah Cohen, Katrina Karkazis, Rory Kraft, Bo Laurent, Kimberly Leighton, Hilde Lindemann, Sharon Meagher, Iain Morland, Uma Narayan, Mary Rawlinson, Falguni Sheth, Jim Stam, Dianna Taylor, Roberto Toledo, and Cynthia Willett have provided insight, encouragement, and good advice at key junctures over the course of this project.

Dee Mortensen's enthusiasm and support at Indiana University Press were invaluable, and I am grateful for the ready and capable assistance of Sarah Jacobi, June Silay, and Jill R. Hughes throughout the book's production. I thank Michael Wyeztner for his vision of the cover art, Laura Szumowski and Mary Blizzard for their support in making it all work, and Liz Connor for her good advice. Special thanks to DEFD for his contribution and the inspiration it provided.

Some of the support and participation in this project cannot adequately be described in terms of generosity. Aristotle describes a particular kind of generosity that only those with great means can offer, what he calls "munificence." The generosity demonstrated by those whose lives have been profoundly affected by the medical treatment of atypical sex who have shared their experiences is of this order. I have encountered the munificence of those who have been willing to think about that experience in ways that may have been unfamiliar. I hope my discussions of their accounts have done some justice to their gifts.

The sustained intellectual and moral support I have received is also a generosity of this order. Alice Dreger's invitation to collaborate with her and others to oppose the practices associated with the administration of prenatal dexamethasone provided new insight into the ethical challenges posed by the medical management of atypical sex anatomies of children. Her careful readings at various points have been essential for shaping the final work. Eileen Findlay has been a close reader and patient instructor in history. Karmen MacKendrick has cheerfully and willingly served as first reader, seemingly effortlessly discerning my intentions. Without Andrea Tschemplik's repeated readings and her insistent and kind questions, I would not have been able to complete many of the arguments. Alison Flaum did me the honor of reading the completed manuscript from beginning to end. For love and forbearance in equal measure, I thank Jennifer Di Toro. And a lifetime of gratitude, too, to Dominic, Zoey, and Enza Feder Di Toro, who have taught me a thing or two about the dignity of vulnerability.

Earlier versions of chapter 2 were published as "'Doctor's Orders': Parents and Intersexed Children" in *The Subject of Care: Feminist Perspectives on Dependency,* edited by Eva Feder Kittay and Ellen K. Feder (Lanham, MD: Rowman and Littlefield, 2002), and "'In Their Best Interests': Parents' Experience of Atypical Genitalia" in *Surgically Shaping Children: Technology, Ethics, and the Pursuit of Normality,* edited by Erik Parens (Baltimore: Johns Hopkins University Press, 2006). A shorter version of chapter 3 was published in "Tilting the Ethical Lens: Shame, Disgust, and the Body in Question," *Hypatia,* special issue "Ethics and Embodiment" 26:3 (2011). A shorter version of chapter 4 is in the collection *Feminist Phenomenology and Medicine,* edited by Kristin Zeiler and Lisa Folkmarson Käll (Albany: SUNY Press, 2013)

MAKING SENSE OF INTERSEX

Introduction

Disciplinary Limits: Philosophy, Bioethics, and the Medical Management of Atypical Sex

"THE BIRTH OF a child with ambiguous genitalia constitutes a social emergency."
So begins the statement published in 2000 by the American Academy of Pediatrics
(AAP) titled "Evaluation of Newborn with Developmental Anomalies of the External Genitalia." What the AAP means by "social emergency" appears to concern
the emotional confusion and distress that parents may immediately experience
upon learning they have a newborn with atypical sex, meaning a sex anatomy that
is neither clearly male nor clearly female. "Words spoken in the delivery room,"
the statement continues, "may have a lasting impact on parents and the relationship with their infant." It is especially important that medical personnel take care
in discussions of "the infant [who] should be referred to as 'your baby,' or 'your
child'—not 'it,' 'he,' or 'she'" (2000, 138). As damaging as a mistaken assignment
of gender would be for the parents and the child is the kind of treatment that de-
nies the infant's personhood. We may readily appreciate the difficulty parents and
medical professionals face when they are so challenged by an infant's anatomy
that they risk causing harm to the child and to the relationship between the child
and those charged with caring for the child.

The term "social emergency" conveys the urgency of a situation that can effect considerable damage to the vulnerable child and to the fragile—for newly
forming—bonds between parents and children. Without saying so outright, the
AAP's description of the birth of children with ambiguous genitalia as a social
emergency expresses the apparent, and apparently obvious, discomfort that atypical sex generally provokes. But the term also raises the question of the place of
medicine in addressing a matter not of medical urgency, but of social urgency. In
seeking a response to this question, perhaps we may be guided by the AAP's statement itself, which goes on to detail the variety of diagnostic and surgical tools
that may "fix" the problem of sex that bodies with ambiguous genitalia present.

Contemporary French philosopher Luce Irigaray famously opens her book
An Ethics of Sexual Difference with the claim that "sexual difference is one of the
major philosophical issues, if not the issue, of our age" (1993 [1984], 5). While I
think many people believe that the urgent status attributed to the birth of a child

1

with atypical sex gives truth to, or perhaps exemplifies, Irigaray's claim that sexual difference is the problem of our time, each of the chapters that make up this project treats the medical management of atypical sex not as a problem of sexual difference, but as a problem of ethics.

There is no mention of ethics or ethical treatment in the 2000 AAP statement concerning the treatment of newborns with ambiguous genitalia. This is hardly remarkable, since there is little explicit discussion of ethics in medical literature concerning treatment of most any other condition. It appears that, for many, it goes without saying that good medical care is "always already" ethical medical care. But perhaps the identification of "good" care with "ethical" care is too quick. However skilled or nuanced, a fair amount of medical practice could be described in mechanistic or technical terms, something we may hesitate to describe in ethical terms at all (the language of "compliance" seems more apt). Describing something as "not ethical" may confuse matters, however, for we tend to think that such a characterization somehow implies that something is *un*ethical— in other words, that it violates accepted ethical principles. It is probably fair to say that most physicians are like the rest of us with respect to the conduct of our professional and personal lives. We do not, as John Stuart Mill pointed out, actively and continuously question our motives and scrutinize our behavior; instead, we rely on habituated tendencies—for example, in treating others with respect. We tend to believe that we know what is right and that we will act in ways that conform to what Immanuel Kant called "the moral law."

But because of the confidence that most of us have, and on which we rely, it can be difficult to appreciate where we might go wrong ethically, especially when our actions—and the understandings that ground those actions—are thoroughly embedded in what we might describe as a "social sense" of what is right and good. As perhaps no era more than our own has taught us, it is precisely in the failure to identify an ethical problem *as* an ethical problem that grave violations may occur and be allowed to persist. In the case of atypical sex, serious ethical violations have occurred in the course of the development of the "standard of care," which has functioned to treat a social problem as a medical issue. Accepted medical practice in the care of individuals with atypical sex anatomy is intended to conceal the variation of sex anatomies—something that occurs far more often than most of us have been led to believe.[1] Over the last sixty to seventy years, physicians have recommended and performed genital surgery and gonadectomy and prescribed hormone replacement specifically to normalize the bodies of infants, older children, and young adults with atypical sex. The concealment of atypical sex anatomies that these interventions aim to achieve, I argue, makes of the bodies of those with atypical sex "the problem" when we should better see the problem, not as one concerned with gender and genitalia, but as an ethical problem—that is to say, a problem located with those who find intolerable the variation that those with atypical sex anatomies embody.

*   *   *

Those working in the humanities or social sciences are often asked—sometimes repeatedly—how it is that they came to be working on whatever comprises the subject of their research. Given the range and sometimes obscurity of the areas of our work, the question is not unexpected. I too want to know, for example, how someone decided to write her dissertation in anthropology on the experiences of Guatemalan foster mothers of children who will be adopted in the United States, or why another became interested in the mid-twentieth-century history of Puerto Rican beet farmers in Michigan. Why the fascination with "bourgeois compassion" in Victorian novels? The question may be merely polite or may express genuine interest; it may also be a way of asking why anyone but the author should be interested in someone's research. Why is it important or interesting or significant? What's to be gained from it? For those of us who have worked in various ways on the ethical problems of the medical management of atypical sex, the question may also be prompted by a baser sort of curiosity concerning our own embodiment, or perhaps that of someone close to us—a sibling, a partner, a friend. It may also be a question provoked by suspicions or worries about what could motivate someone's interest in such bodies, especially when the person asking is someone with an atypical sex anatomy or the parent of a child with atypical sex anatomy.

I understand these suspicions. When Margaret McLaren, a senior colleague and friend I had admired for years, called me in the spring of 1999 to ask that I participate in the first panel on intersex at the American Philosophical Association, it took me only a moment to say no. It wasn't that her invitation was unwelcome or inappropriate somehow. She knew I had worked for some time on the development of the diagnosis of gender identity disorder in children. It is also possible that we had spoken years earlier about my teaching of social psychologist Suzanne Kessler's groundbreaking 1990 article, "The Medical Construction of Gender: Case Management of Intersexed Infants." Like almost every other feminist I knew, I regularly included this article in the courses in feminist theory and women's studies I taught as a graduate student in the early 1990s.

Drawing on interviews with physicians she conducted in the late 1980s, Kessler brought to light the rationale guiding decisions about sex assignment in the cases of children with ambiguous genitalia, an area of medical practice that was almost entirely unknown outside of medicine at that time. The prevailing standard of care meant that nearly every child born with atypical sex anatomy—including 46,XY (that is, chromosomally typical) males whose penises fell short of the standard of one inch—would be reassigned female. It meant that a girl with complete androgen insensitivity syndrome would be told by her endocrinologist that her "ovaries weren't normal and had been removed . . . [he] told her that she could marry and have normal sexual relations . . . [that her] uterus won't develop but [she] could adopt children" (S. J. Kessler 1990, 230). She would not be told that she was genetically male, but because her body lacked androgen receptors, her physical development took a path that made her look, and (probably) feel, like a girl. Instead of a uterus and ovaries, she was born with testes that, absent those androgen receptors, had not descended. Doctors make treatment decisions, Kessler wrote in her 1998 book, *Lessons from the Intersexed*, "on the basis of shared cultural values that are unstated, perhaps even unconscious, and therefore considered objective rather than subjective" (18).

Many of us spent a lot of time through the early 1990s arguing about the "construction" of gender and asking what it meant to see gender as constructed. Judith Butler's *Gender Trouble* (1990)—published the same year as Kessler's article—was a frequent topic of our reading groups. We taught Kessler's article not only because it was so accessible to our students but also because it upset the distinction that had taken hold of feminist thinking by that time, namely, the distinction between gender as "social construction" and sex as a product of "nature." It was even this difference, we instructed our students (and ourselves), that required "problematization": We trained students to critically examine this concept that functioned as an unspoken foundation for action and understanding. Instead, they should see this seeing this taken-for-granted thing as a question meriting exploration and interrogation. Kessler's analysis of the doctors' belief that sex was something they could manipulate demonstrated how it was not only gender that was affected by social thinking; in "the case management of intersexed infants" it became evident that even sex—supposedly natural, stable, fixed—could be a matter that was "decided." Historian Thomas Laqueur's *Making Sex: Body and Gender from the Greeks to Freud* (1990), also published in what was evidently a critical year in thinking about sex, showed us and our students that thinking about the putative "immutability" of sex had a much longer history.

My research project—what eventually became *Family Bonds: Genealogies of Race and Gender* (2007)—took shape in the context of this discussion. My interest in gender identity disorder was motivated by my effort to understand the kind of power that "produced gender," that made gender make sense as a category of difference. The production of gender was different from the production of race, I argued, and if we were to appreciate how gender and race worked together as categories of difference, as they were in fact experienced in people's lives—another focus of the thinking of the early 1990s—it was important to see how they functioned differently, how they were the products of different kinds of power. If our bodies were the place where those expressions of power came together in individuals' and communities' experiences, a more finely tuned understanding of how these expressions of power differed could provide a means of talking about gender or race (or gendered or raced experience) in ways that did not promote exclusion of one category at the expense of the other.

My project was a theoretical one. It sought to make a case for how the work of twentieth-century French philosopher Michel Foucault could be used to understand the workings of these different kinds of power and their effects. The project applied Foucault's method in recounting histories intended to illuminate these different operations of power. Between the stories of the founding of the first middle-class suburb of Levittown, New York, and the story of a federally financed effort to coordinate genetic and biological research into the causes of "violent behavior" was the story of the development of the psychiatric diagnosis of gender identity disorder (GID) in children. GID is a diagnosis that, starting in the 1970s, began to be treated, first primarily in little boys who acted like little girls and soon thereafter to little girls who acted like little boys.[2] But while the application of Foucault's concept of power was helpful in understanding the operation of GID, it seemed to me that the normalizing practices involved in the medical management of intersex conditions could not be so neatly described in these terms.[3]

All this is to say that I didn't refuse Margaret's invitation because I didn't know anything about the medical management of intersex, or because I didn't care about it. In fact, Kessler's long-awaited *Lessons from the Intersexed*—which remains, fifteen years later, a landmark book—had just been published, and I had eagerly read it. I refused Margaret's invitation because I didn't think the work I had been doing on the question of power and the production of gender was of any use in thinking about what was going on at that moment in people's lives. The fact that Margaret prefaced her request by telling me that the impetus for the panel had been a conversation with Cheryl Chase, the founder of the Intersex Society of North America, who would also participate, only confirmed for me that I had no place speaking on such a panel, which I immediately understood would need to address current practices as they affected those with atypical sex and to make criticism of those practices central to the analysis. The work that I had done focused on historical cases for the purposes of making theoretical points; it might be—and like most people working in social and political philosophy, I hoped it could be—relevant and useful for social and political thinking and action. My primary aim in examining the cases described in the emerging literature on gender identity disorder was not to expose or criticize practices associated with the creation of the diagnosis (though there was no doubt that I found that aspect of the work gratifying); these cases served the purpose of clarifying or arguing for theoretical points; they were instrumental to my analysis, not the focus of it. But in the case of the treatment of intersex, the relationship between theory and what was going on at that moment in people's lives needed to be reversed: rather than the cases serving the theory, the theory needed to serve the cases. And besides, I didn't see what I could add to what Kessler—and to what Alice Dreger, the historian who had published the year before an excellent ethical analysis in the *Hastings Center Report* (1998a)—had already done so well.

That's a long way of explaining why I declined Margaret's invitation. She understood, she told me, and we said good-bye.

A few weeks later Margaret called back and told me, "You have to be on the panel; I can't find anyone else." Well, all right, then, I thought. I still didn't think that any of my previous work was really useful for thinking about intersex, and I knew that I couldn't treat intersex as another "case." So if I was going to think about what philosophy could contribute to critical thinking about the medical management of intersex, I had to start from scratch. But Margaret told me I would have nearly a year to prepare my paper. Because this was a panel at the American Philosophical Association, it struck me that figuring out what—or maybe whether—philosophy had something to say had to be the task.

This book is the result of my trying to answer that question of what philosophy has to offer, a task that has occupied me—and with which, many can attest, I have been preoccupied—for almost fifteen years. I began by asking what I thought philosophers working in medicine, biomedical ethicists, had had to say about the medical management of intersex, and I was surprised to find that the answer was, nothing. I found this silence especially surprising in light of what began to seem like routine violations of some of the most thoroughly investigated problems in medical ethics, especially the question of deceiving patients. But the reason—or reasons—why bioethics had had nothing to say surprised me even more. I soon learned that my assumptions about biomedical ethics, as well as the role of philosophy within the field, were not well informed. I did not sufficiently understand the contemporary history of my own profession, which included the "confinement" of philosophy in the wake of the McCarthy era that John McCumber discusses in his article "Time in the Ditch: American Philosophy and the McCarthy Era" (1996), and I was completely ignorant of the history of the formation of bioethics.[4]

Philosophy in the History of Bioethics

Beginning in the 1950s, philosophy would be restricted, McCumber writes, to "second-order inquiry . . . [that] also carried through in ethics. Philosophers of the day were not to take ethical stands or give moral advice but simply to reflect on the meaning of ethical terms" (2001, 38).[5] Contemporary work in applied ethics might appear to constitute an important departure, and indeed its entrance into the field coincides with some significant changes. Rather than seeking "truth," the initial aim of applied philosophers generally, and bioethicists in particular, was to put the tools of philosophical analysis to work. Their goal, in the parlance of the sixties, was to give new "relevance" to philosophy. Albert Jonsen's account of *The*

Birth of Bioethics (1998) traces the shift from the strictly metaethical analysis that counted as "ethical philosophy," to the "new vitality" of applied ethical interrogation, to the "public agony" provoked by the Vietnam War. Jonsen relates that consternation over the war and its implications peaked during the years 1968–1969 and "swarmed," as he writes,

> into the ordinarily sedate annual meeting of the Western Division of the American Philosophical Association . . . [L]inguist Noam Chomsky . . . had been invited to open a symposium entitled, "Philosophers and Public Policy." After delivering a stinging attack on the American government for its pursuit of the war and for its imperialism, and on the general dominance of a power elite wielding technological mastery that it proclaimed to be "value-free," Chomsky challenged the audience of philosophers: "These are the typical questions of philosophy . . . philosophers must take the lead in this effort." (1998, 75)

Jonsen rightly observes that "only a non-philosopher could believe that such issues had been 'typical questions of philosophy,' at least during its recent history." It is not surprising that Chomsky's exhortation met with strong resistance from the philosophers present. John Silber pointed out the error of Chomsky's characterization of his discipline. "As philosophers," he said, "we can assist in the formation of sound public policy by distinguishing appropriately different kinds of ethical theories and kinds of moral and political obligation" (quoted in Jonsen 1998, 76).

But some philosophers would embark on a new beginning in the early 1970s. No longer could the kinds of ethical violations marked by the Holocaust, Hiroshima, and the McCarthy purges themselves go all but completely ignored by philosophers.[6] Questions of human rights brought to a head by Vietnam and the civil rights and women's liberation movements (the latter of which is almost never acknowledged in histories of bioethics) would come to the fore, and new questions would be raised by the growing technologies of the life sciences. At the same time that philosophy was seeing a kind of revival, bioethics as a discipline began to take shape. And yet it is not entirely clear to what extent the changes in philosophy bear upon, or are themselves influenced by, the development of bioethics.

Most historical accounts of bioethics trace its origins to the public revelations, beginning around 1965, of unpalatable practices that were common in human experimentation after the Second World War; some involved injections of live cancer cells or "artificial induction of hepatitis" into unsuspecting patients; a good deal of research involved experimentation on the senile and elderly, as well as mentally retarded adults and children.[7] The disclosure in 1972 of the forty-year-long Tuskegee syphilis experiment, examining the effects of untreated syphilis in nearly four hundred poor black men to determine the long-term effects of the disease (Jones 1993; Reverby 2009), also spurred federal regulation.[8] That same year saw news reports of radiation experiments in Cincinnati that over the previous twelve years had exposed more than eighty mostly indigent, black cancer patients to radiation—not for therapeutic purposes, but in the interest of national defense (Stephens 2002). In the utilitarian terms in which doctors were then schooled, the practices were justified by the extraordinary understanding and array of therapeutic products that resulted from these studies (D. Rothman 1991, 79). In the wake of increasing revelations of the questionable use of human subjects, the National Institutes of Health (NIH), which was funding much of the work, and the U.S. Food and Drug Administration (FDA), with a mandate of "consumer protection," grappled with what sort of standards to apply to human research, making distinctions between therapeutic and nontherapeutic research, invigorating peer review, and providing the first standards concerning consent (91–92). Toward the end of the decade, Princeton philosopher Paul Ramsey began to study the problem of human experimentation. Experimentation involving human subjects, as David Rothman puts it in *Strangers in the Bedside,* "presented an unavoidable conflict of interest. The goals of the researcher did not coincide with the well-being of the subject; human experimentation pitted the interests of society against the interests of the individual. In essence, the utilitarian calculus put every human (subject) at risk" (1991, 96).

Doctors came under increasing scrutiny not only because of questions of human experimentation but also because of scarcities created by the limited availability of new technologies. In 1960 a Dr. Scribner in Seattle, Washington, developed a "permanent indwelling shunt" that would permit patients with advanced kidney disease to be connected to a dialysis machine. With far fewer machines available than eligible patients, Seattle doctors were faced with the dilemma of who would live and who would die. Daunted by the prospect of making such decisions—and finding themselves in a position where a doctor's imperative to "do everything possible to enhance the well-being" of his patient might be impossible (D. Rothman 1991, 151)—a committee of what were described as "quite ordinary people" was appointed by a county medical society and charged with making the decisions the doctors declined to make. Reflecting on the ethical problems posed by the committee's own decisions (which involved preferences for churchgoers and married men with children over single women, for example), a public lesson in the need for "principles or guidelines" was learned (152).

Philosophers began to be summoned to help doctors respond to these questions posed by fast-expanding research programs, new technologies, and the scarcities and liabilities they engendered. This call culminated in the founding of the Hastings Center, located in Garrison, New York, in 1969 (Stevens 2000, 48). The center (originally called the "Center for the Study of Value and the Sciences of Man") was the first organization dedicated to the advancement of bioethics. Its decision to stand independent of and unaffiliated with any university or professional school was motivated by a view that such an organization must remain "outside" the institutions whose practices it would examine. The vision of its founder and until 1996 its president, Daniel Callahan, was a grand one, infused with the critiques of technology associated with thinkers such as Herbert Marcuse. It would confront the problems emerging from "advances in the life sciences [that] pose social and ethical questions touching the fate of individuals and societies, now and in the future. The common phrases 'biological revolution,' 'population explosion,' and 'environmental crisis' only hint at the terrible complexity of these advances and the problems that follow in their wake" (Callahan 1970, cited in Stevens 2000, 51). Despite the lofty vision of the Hastings Center's leading light, accounts of bioethics' origins make clear that even if the new field was not precisely intended to function at the pleasure of medical practitioners and to respond to fast-multiplying queries from "legislators, educational institutions, parties to pending litigation, and others seeking advice and assistance" (Stevens 2000, 56), satisfying the new demand for answers would nevertheless come to function as the center's mainstay and as its most important source of ongoing financial support (65).

In the inaugural issue of the *Hastings Center Studies,* Callahan published the first effort to define the emerging field. In "Bioethics as a Discipline," he writes, "The discipline of bioethics should be so designed, and its practitioners trained, that it will directly . . . serve those physicians and biologists whose positions demand that they make practical decisions" (Callahan 1973, cited in Jonsen 1998, 326). Certainly, applied ethical theory should serve practitioners. But in the case of bioethics, and clearly as the example of the medical management of atypical sex indicates, the specific nature of that service—to supply guidelines and to seek answers to questions framed by practitioners rather than pose independently formulated questions (see also Jonsen 1998, 333)—bears scrutiny.

One of the forms that these "answers" has taken is the adumbration of principles that would guide practices; early discussions of bioethics focused on the positing of these principles. These would famously take shape in *The Belmont Report,* produced at the end of the National Commission for the Protection of Human Subjects of Biomedical and Behavioral Research (begun in 1976 and appearing in final form in the *Federal Register* in 1979), as respect for persons (autonomy), beneficence (and non-malificence), and justice (see Jonsen 1998, 333, 103–104).[9] Where Chomsky exhorted philosophers to ask questions, then, bioethicists have, in the years since the field's first emergence, largely limited themselves to providing answers to questions that they are not permitted to pose themselves. Instead of promoting a critical stance toward the scientific enterprise, bioethicists have been required to occupy a supporting role, to become, as Callahan glumly characterized bioethics' role in a 1996 article, "good team players" (Callahan 1996, cited in Stevens 2000, 73).[10]

Examining the history of bioethics helped me to better understand how it was that bioethicists had not intervened in the unethical treatment of children with atypical sex. But it was not at all clear to me that there was anything I could do about it. At the same time, as I had remarked in my panel presentation, much of what makes intersex conditions threatening is not a matter of scientific understanding or careful reflection, but issues from that unreflected realm of knowing, of what is taken for granted, that has been the object of the work of philosophy since Socrates. When at the end of the session at the American Philosophical Association, intersex activist Chase leaned closer to me and said, "You need to do more. It's time that philosophers say something about what's happening," I thought she was right, but I also thought, "What could that be?"

Telling Stories: History and Method

It would make for a better story if I could report that I experienced some sense of personal mission from that moment, but what occurred between that panel and today probably looks a lot like how many other book projects come about, in fits and starts (and a number of stops along the way). What would make this work different for me was my understanding that however much theoretical analysis this thinking demanded, I wasn't working on a theoretical issue, but on practices that affected people who had experienced violation of their bodies and senses of self. Children and adults had endured a kind of suffering that was obviously wrong. But if history is any indication, that suffering would be repeated and would spread as more specialists were trained in the United States, Europe, and all over the world. So Chase was right that philosophers needed to say something about what was happening. I am not sure it will make any difference, but I began to feel, and have felt ever more strongly since, an obligation to try to say something, to use the tools of philosophy to make sense of what is happening, to make arguments about what I think is wrong and why, and to try to envision a way forward. This project is my effort to do just that.

Unlike much work in philosophy that examines ethical problems in medical practice, my work makes use of the tools of philosophy in the continental tradition—that is, philosophy that works from thinkers from France and Germany—as well as from thinkers in the more extended history of Western philosophy. It also makes use of empirical research that I conducted myself. The former stems from my graduate training and to the teaching I do now, but the latter came about as a result of the limits on the primary source material that would help me understand the ethical problems the management of atypical sex anatomies poses.

Just at the time I was writing that first presentation for the APA panel in 1999–2000, I was working with Eva Kittay, who had been my mentor as a graduate student, on a project on the ethics of care and questions of dependency, particularly what Kittay describes as the "secondary" or "derivative" dependency of one whose caring for a dependent other renders the caregiver vulnerable. It was the coincidence of what initially seemed entirely separate projects that led me to ask how we might better understand the extraordinary character of the medical management of intersex by attending to the situation of those charged with making decisions on behalf of their infants and young children: the parents. Parents have a critical and complex role in their children's experience of normalization, one that is explicitly recognized in the standard of care. And yet we knew little about how physicians were treating the parents of children with atypical sex. There was at that time only some material from Kessler's 1998 book, as well as an article from 1970 by psychologists Elizabeth Bing and Esselyn Rudikoff, that considered the role cultural differences may play in persuading parents that it would be in their children's "best interests" to undergo normalizing genital surgery. Existing empirical literature could not serve as the basis of my analysis. I would need to talk to parents themselves.

This prospect was not a little daunting. Talking to people had played no significant role in my training in philosophy. Furthermore, I had scant knowledge of social scientific method, and I would be faced for the first time with submitting my research plan for review, a process that was at that time, and arguably remains, ill-defined for those working in the humanities. I did not have particular questions to ask parents. I wanted them to describe their experiences as they themselves understood them. I asked Chase if she would provide some direction, and she suggested I begin with a Listserv that a technologically capable parent of a child with atypical sex had established shortly before, at a time when such Listservs were relatively new. Having received the institutional go-ahead, I posted the letter I had written. It explained that I was interested in speaking to parents of children with intersex conditions who wanted to share their stories for a project that sought to understand parents' vulnerability.

My efforts to be honest and clear about my project and its aims were soon eclipsed by what was received as an entirely unwelcome and offensive query. My posting erred in every way: I used the term "intersex": parents took this to mean that I intended to focus on their children's "abnormal sexuality," which had been effectively concealed by sensitive and compassionate doctors the parents trusted; I had attributed vulnerability to parents who saw themselves as their children's capable protectors. The Listserv lit up with vociferous criticism of my request and the questionable intentions parents read in it. There was also deep suspicion that my interest was not genuinely in the parents, but in the children for whom they rightly felt protective. Some misread my post entirely, believing that my interest was in their children's vulnerability, or even in their children's "disability," which they protested. I had committed a grave insult, most agreed, and I would not be permitted to post again.

I immediately extended my sincere and public apologies, but that didn't stop additional postings, including one suggesting that a careful reading of my request would reveal that I was "fishing for circus freaks" for my project on dependency. Not only this, but the poster also added that some internet investigation revealed that I had published feminist work that made obvious the "direction" my research would take.[11]

I felt terrible. However "honest" my mistake, it seemed to me that the ire I had provoked was a measure of the vulnerability that had motivated my question. Rather than a better understanding of that vulnerability, I had managed only to aggravate it, and with it the pain and distress these parents felt. I really didn't have any business doing this sort of work. But that anger, and perhaps also the repeated expression of fear in the posted threads—not so much for the health of the children, many of whom faced genuine medical challenges, but fear that their children might turn out to be gay—turned out to be the real beginning of the work I had proposed. Just when the members of the Listserv declared an end to the project before it had begun, one adult with atypical sex sent me a one-line e-mail message that read, "My mom will talk to you." That mother was the woman I call Ruby, in chapter 2. It was hearing her story that made me feel that I really needed to write that article, and it is her story to which I have returned most frequently over the years that I have been working on this project.

We initially spoke by phone, and I had intended to travel to meet her in person. However, having not spoken about the protracted ordeal she had experienced with her daughters, who had each been announced male at birth, she began to tell her story and didn't stop until it came out. I've never written so fast, and as the story spilled out of her, I worked to blink back my own tears. When we hung up I knew I had to write her story immediately, not only because I wanted to capture her voice, which I could still hear, but also because I knew I might not be able to read my own barely legible writing the next day. I sent her what I wrote and she made minor corrections, adding details about long car rides with her two young children.

A couple of years later we finally met face-to-face, along with her two adult daughters, and we have maintained sporadic contact over the years since. I spoke with other parents that year, mostly in person but also by phone. I recorded our conversations with their permission and transcribed our conversations using pseudonyms. Three of the families who did not participate in that Listserv contacted me after being alerted of my request by friends or acquaintances who had seen my posting; other families were parents of adults I had gotten to know.

It would be a few years after publication of the work on parents and dependency that I decided to go forward with completing a book. However, I had no intention of pursuing additional interviews for the project I then envisioned. I had sought the opportunity to speak with parents when I did, because I could find no other means of pursuing the questions I was asking with respect to dependency and care. Since completing that first essay, a wealth of first-person narratives and new scholarship in anthropology and sociology would, I believed, make any forays I might make into social scientific research unnecessary.

It wasn't until 2010–2011—more than two years after I had planned to complete the book I thought I was writing—when I was trying to find out to what extent the new recommendations that came in the 2006 "Consensus Statement on Management of Intersex Conditions" (hereafter referred to as the Consensus Statement) by the U.S. and European endocrinological societies (Lawson Wilkins Pediatric Endocrine Society and the European Society for Paediatric Endocrinology, respectively) had actually changed the standard of care, that I would again find it necessary to seek permission to talk to people as part of my research. I spoke with pediatric specialists in urology, endocrinology, gynecology, psychiatry, as well as psychology—twelve in all—who treated children with atypical sex anatomies and who could tell me more about whether any changes had been made in related clinical practice since 2006.[12] These conversations told me a great deal about how care had—and had not—changed; they also yielded a number of surprising insights into the conditions of the possibility of changes in practice that significantly shaped my arguments in chapters 5 and 6.

It was while talking to physicians about their experiences with parents faced with making decisions about the care of their children that I began to have questions regarding the nature of the potential harms brought about by surgeries that physicians recommend and perform. Published narratives of individuals who have had normalizing genital surgery, as well as accounts collected by social scientists, provide evidence that both physical and emotional harm has occurred as a result of these surgeries. But these accounts provide little detail concerning the specific nature of that harm or what have been characterized as multiple harms. It seemed to me that the failure to investigate these harms had implications for efforts to secure truly informed consent from parents regarding normalizing genital surgeries for their children. I needed to talk not only to those who had experienced this harm but also to some of them who would share with me the work of thinking about it.

Since that first panel at the American Philosophical Association, I had worked in nonacademic settings with individuals who identify themselves as intersex activists. The informal conversations I had had over those years suggested something of the nature of the harm that is not recorded in current research. I asked two of those individuals—Jim and Andie—whom I first met separately more than ten years ago, if they would be willing to think about what is meant when we talk about harm resulting from the medical management of atypical sex. Each of these conversations was in some respects a lot like the initial conversation I had had with Ruby, but they also differed in that I was asking these individuals not only to recount their stories but also to try to identify what they meant when they talked about harm. These were difficult conversations. The thinking that is reflected in the chapters in which their stories appear (chapters 4 and 5) is a result of their analysis, together with mine, and like so much of the work of this project, it moved in directions I could not have anticipated when we began these conversations.

I also did not expect to have the conversations I did with the mother whose story appears in chapter 7. She and her husband reached out to me and to Alice Dreger following the publication in *Bioethics Forum* of short essays we had written. The first essay criticized questionable research practices involving the administration of dexamethasone to women at risk of giving birth to girls with congenital adrenal hyperplasia (Lindemann, Feder, and Dreger 2010). The second described the work of a pediatric urologist who was conducting genital sensitivity exams on young girls after surgical reduction of their clitorises in infancy, usually those with the same condition (Dreger and Feder 2010). Sonja and her husband wanted to tell their story in part because they wanted to record for their daughter the decisions they had made and the reasons for those decisions. When I spoke with them, I did not anticipate that our conversations would provoke yet more questions for me—concerning the ethics of parenting, autonomy, dignity, and human rights—which would result in the addition of what would become chapters 7 and 8.

Over the course of this project I came to understand that the conversations that I had had over these years constituted fragments of oral history. It wasn't that I was trying to write history or conduct a sociological study, but in order to understand what questions philosophers should be asking, I needed insight into the meanings of decisions that had been made, to understand the assumptions that guided the practices of physicians and the parents they advised, and to learn more directly than the literature provided the consequences of these practices. At the same time, following Foucault, I saw that the questions I posed should be informed by what he called a "history of the present" (1979 [1975], 31). My research into the history of bioethics had already revealed my misunderstanding of the work of bioethics. A similar history lesson could help make sense of what was meant by hermaphroditism, intersex, or "disorders of sex development," and how these meanings had changed over time. In addition to the personal narratives I had gathered, I needed a broader understanding of the history of medical practices regarding people with atypical sex anatomies and the medical thinking about these individuals.

* * *

We know that terrible violations of ethics are often recognized only in retrospect; for that reason, ethicists must take history seriously. Attending to the historical development of the standard of care that sought to make individuals' sex of assignment consistent with their body's appearance is essential for understanding the ethical questions that standard poses today. Chapter 1, "The Trouble with Intersex," traces the changing views of the stories of "the problem" of atypical sex anatomies. Although through much of the nineteenth century atypical sex anatomies were taken to be a social danger rather than a medical danger, "hermaphroditism" was figured as a problem for medicine. In the early twentieth century physicians recognized that the most frequent cause of atypical sex in females, congenital adrenal hyperplasia, poses a genuine health risk—and in many cases a mortal danger—to an individual. This recognition may appear to have displaced the preceding view of atypical sex as a social threat; however, the standard of care crafted at mid-century suggests instead that this standard responds to a problem figured as a risk both to an affected individual and to the society in which that individual lives. In other words, the early twentieth-century advances may appear in many respects to have displaced the Victorian treatment of what was called "doubtful sex," but the standard of care crafted in the 1950s suggests that what actually occurred was a revitalization of a nineteenth-century fascination with or curiosity about those with atypical sex constituted as a social danger. Rather than adults found to be occupying a social role that was discordant with their anatomies, this threat came in the form of infants most often identified at birth or soon after. It was this convergence of social and medical danger, I argue, that made of these conditions "extraordinary" cases, or "disorders like no other," and has apparently justified the routine violations of well-established ethical principles through the end of the twentieth century, a period when what we might have expected to be the keenest moral sensitivities were awakened and regulation of ethical practice was institutionalized. The chapters that follow "The Trouble with Intersex" proceed chronologically and trace the changes to the contemporary standard of care that have occurred as this project was underway from their proximate origins in the mid-1950s till today.

The first conversations I had with parents became the primary sources for the second chapter, "'In Their Best Interests': Parents' Experience of Atypical Sex Anatomy in Children." The chapter joins the work of a feminist ethics of care and the analysis of *habitus* provided by social theorist Pierre Bourdieu in an effort to understand the operation and consequences of a singular norm of gender formation in the lives of people with atypical sex anatomies and their families. "Habitus" is a term that describes that understanding we take to be "common sense," of what goes without saying. The fact of sexual difference has functioned as that background of intelligibility that orders our social world and the sense we make of it. Although this common sense has indubitably shaped the standard of care, Cheryl Chase (2003) famously challenged the understandings steadfastly maintained by proponents and critics of the imperative of normality and claimed that "the problem" of intersex is one of "stigma and trauma, not gender."

Chapter 3 is my effort to take seriously Chase's characterization of the problem of intersex and to emphasize the moral significance of this characterization. I argue that in Friedrich Nietzsche's *Genealogy of Morality* (1998 [1887]), we may find a framework that allows us a transformative view that directs us to shift our focus from the bodies of those born with atypical sex anatomies, which have been the privileged objects of attention both in medical practice and in criticisms of it, and moves us to consider instead the bodies of those whose responses constitute the motivating force for normalizing practices in the first place. This chapter is at the center of the text because the question it seeks to address is what I take to be the most confounding question posed by the medical management of atypical sex: what can account for the urgency "to fix" children in ways that have been demonstrated to promote harm rather than flourishing? This question becomes more confounding still, I propose, when we take into account the fact that we know there are individuals whose atypical sex anatomies have not been medicalized.[13] And yet the sort of criticism that Nietzsche offers does not suggest a simple response, or, put another way, it doesn't provide direction in a manner that can be readily articulated within the terms of the discussion of the medical treatment of atypical sex anatomies today. That is to say, there is not an obvious way of tackling the issue of *ressentiment* head-on. Thinking practically (as is ultimately my goal), one may reasonably ask how to combat (an unconscious) ressentiment in parents, doctors, even society? The inability to do so may lead one to conclude that if the philosophical analysis Nietzsche offers cannot lend itself to a direct response, what good is it?

It was not my principal aim to respond to the question of what good theory in the continental tradition could do. Nevertheless, I found that the work of Bourdieu and Nietzsche offered tools for understanding how the standard of care that made surgical and hormonal "normalization" of children's atypical sex anatomies come to be regarded as necessary, and why, in the face of compelling arguments for change, these beliefs persisted. The work of these thinkers did not, however, offer obvious resources for shaping that change. What might be characterized as the defensive tackling of "the problem" of intersex—what I suggest we see in terms of Nietzsche's concept of ressentiment—has not proved as successful as intersex activists once hoped. I propose that what is required is a kind of offensive end run of the sort I develop in the final chapters of the book, which focus on the ethical construction of meaningful change. Before moving to the possibilities for change, however, we must understand the nature of the harm effected by that standard, to consider more carefully the role of culture in the development of both the standard of care and challenges to that standard, and to know more about the clinical practices that continue to promote a medical treatment that has resulted in harm.

The harm effected by the medical management of atypical sex anatomies has now been documented at considerable length. Physicians, parents, and patients agree that physical and psychological injury has resulted from castration and sex reassignment in boys with micropenis, as well as from clitorectomy or clitoral recession in girls with a clitoris determined to be "too big." Uncomfortable or painful vaginal dilation in young children following vaginoplasty or the construction of a neovagina, repeated genital exams, and medical photography have produced trauma. There is also emotional harm caused by the intentional misrepresentation of a condition or procedure and the insistence that parents maintain the secrecy of a child's atypical sex from the child and extended family. But the enumeration of harms may have proved insufficient to convey the nature of the injury.

In chapter 4 I propose that French phenomenologist Maurice Merleau-Ponty's concept of "the body schema" offers a resource for a deeper appreciation of the violation that normalizing interventions for atypical sex anatomies effect. This concept encompasses the ground for Merleau-Ponty's understanding of who and what we are as embodied subjects, which is neither reducible to nor separable from our somatic being. Merleau-Ponty (1962 [1945]) makes much of what he calls the "ambiguity" of our human being as subject and object, perceiver and perceived. In his view, human consciousness cannot be understood purely as a function of cognition, of "I think that," but should be conceived instead as an embodied consciousness, of "I can"—that is, what I am able to effect—in order to engage in the world and with others. For Merleau-Ponty, thinking and understanding are never separable from our being in the world, in culture and society, and among embodied others. If this phenomenological approach helps us to better appreciate the experience of Jim, who had been born male and was reassigned female as an infant, and that of his sister, Mary Katherine, who was not informed of Jim's history until she was an adult, I think it is because Merleau-Ponty's thinking about our embodied consciousness provides a means of thinking about harms that are inadequately described in the limited—and limiting—terms of "the physical" or "psychological" to which we usually resort.

Although I had initially spoken with Andie to gain better understanding of harm, our conversation led me to consider more carefully the way that "ethics" may be understood to figure in the care of children with atypical sex anatomies. The extent to which a conception of ethics is continuous with the rules of "culture" was something I had begun to explore in chapter 2, but Andie's account provided the impetus to reflect in a more considered way how cultural rules or expectations may conflict with ethical imperatives. In the bioethical literature, questions about the role that cultural difference may play are more frequently discussed with respect to intercultural difference—for example, when the cultural expectations governing patient care in a given context are at variance with expectations of a patient's culture of origin. Intracultural rules and expectations of the sort that Bourdieu discusses are more rarely a source of conflict or worry, as they proved to be in the case of atypical sex anatomies in children in the West at least since the 1950s.[14]

This tension between the rules of culture and those of ethics may explain why physicians' accounts have come to increasingly portray parents as "demanding" or "insistent on" surgical intervention. I wondered how changes announced in the 2006 Consensus Statement had transformed care. Based on the conversations I had with physicians in 2010–2011, chapter 6 provides a good idea of the state of care at this time. Physicians' accounts of their discussions with parents of children born with atypical sex anatomies for which surgery is an option demonstrate changes consistent with the recommendations of the Consensus Statement. Rather than providing clear recommendations in favor of normalizing surgery, however, doctors now appear to provide what is known as "nondirective" counseling. Analysis of the apparently value-neutral options that involve what is presented as a choice between either aggressive and active medical intervention aimed at securing a child's well-being or "doing nothing," as one clinician has put it, may contribute to parents' experience of urgency or certainty with respect to decisions to pursue surgical intervention.

My discussions with doctors at this time coincided with my meeting of Sonja and her husband, Elias, whose careful thinking about parenting their daughter, Shai, evoked a tradition of moral reflection grounded in what philosophers call virtue ethics. Sonja and Elias's reasoning stands in stark contrast to what was in 2010 the most developed statement of an "ethical" approach to normalizing interventions for children with atypical sex anatomies, produced by the German Bioethics and Intersex Group. My criticism of the limits of this approach through the moral framework employed by Sonja and Elias forms the basis of chapter 7. Privileging the question of parental rights, the approach of the Bioethics and Intersex Group fails to promote both the well-being of children with atypical sex anatomies and the bonding that is in the best interests of parents and children alike.

Chapter 8 extends the analysis begun in chapter 7 to develop a more detailed philosophical ground for the concept of human rights implicit in the approach of Sonja and Elias. It makes central the ethical value of human vulnerability and investigates what duties are entailed in what contemporary philosopher Debra Bergoffen describes as the obligation to honor the "dignity of the vulnerable body." The conclusion of this project is dedicated to the stories of those physicians whose reflection on their medical practice is a moving demonstration of the recognition of this obligation and what we may hope is the promise of change already under way.

1 The Trouble with Intersex
History Lessons

In a short talk he delivered in 2000 at the American Association for the History of Medicine, pediatric endocrinologist Jorge Daaboul reflected on the revelatory character of history in his own practice. He recounts that he had begun to have serious doubts about the standard of care that made imperative the surgical normalization of atypical genitalia in children. Though this was the standard in which he had been trained—in the tradition of Lawson Wilkins, the founder of pediatric endocrinology, and John Money, the preeminent psychologist of sexual difference—he began to pose to his colleagues the questions he had come to ask himself, namely, whether the standard was genuinely in the best interests of their young patients. The uniform responses to his questions, he told his audience in 2000, yielded two arguments in defense of the standard. First, "intersexed individuals," his colleagues told him, "could not possibly live normal lives as intersexed individuals and . . . the only chance they had for happiness and psychological well being was the establishment of a secure male or female gender identity. Second, there simply was no precedent for [such individuals] living as normal people in our society" (Daaboul 2000).

Just at the time that he was engaged in these conversations, Daaboul went on to say, he read *Hermaphrodites and the Medical Invention of Sex* (Dreger, 1998b), Alice Dreger's account of the Victorian "discovery" of hermaphroditism. From Dreger's history he learned that until the late nineteenth century, individuals with intersex were not automatically objects of medicine as he had been trained to see them; until the start of what Dreger calls the "Age of Gonads" (1870–1915) (29), people with atypical sex anatomies in England and France lived unremarkable lives. It couldn't be, Daaboul realized, that it was necessary to correct the bodies of individuals with atypical sex in order to secure their happiness. The category of "the normal," which he had been trained to see as natural and necessary, was all at once a historical artifact. "For me," he concludes,

> the study of history proved invaluable in my formulating an approach to intersex. The moment I realized that there was a historical precedent for individuals with intersex leading happy, normal productive lives I revised my approach . . . and have become a strong advocate of minimal intervention. The study of the history of intersex gave me the knowledge to improve and refine

my approach to this condition. Consequently, I am a better doctor to my patients. (Daaboul 2000)

Daaboul's account is compelling. It is a remarkable personal story of transformative insight ignited by the study of history and an understanding that truths one has taken for granted may be contingent—that is, neither necessary nor inevitable, but the result of human practices, actions, and ideas. In the case of atypical sex, these include truths about sex and gender, about normality and abnormality, about sickness and health. That is not to say that these categories, and what we take to be our natural responses to them, do not matter; they obviously do, for these categories are the ground from which we make sense of ourselves and each other. It is to say that what we may take to be "the way things are" could be different. Daaboul's reading of Dreger's historical account belied the training that had inculcated in him a certain vision of the way things are, of how they always would be. He now understood that many of the ways he had been taught to see the world and his patients ought to be challenged. It was this understanding, he says, that enabled him to be a "better doctor to [his] patients."

Daaboul's lesson in history invites a closer look at the meaning of the changes that prevailing beliefs, attitudes, and treatment concerning those with atypical sex have undergone. What may not be clear from Daaboul's account is the historical tension between competing views of atypical sex anatomies as a threat to the social body literally embodied by those with what was called "doubtful sex" (Dreger 1998b, 41), on the one hand, and the view that intersex is a danger to the health and well-being of those individuals with atypical sex anatomy, on the other. If this tension is not fully evident in his account, I would suggest that it is because the history turns out to be more complicated than Daaboul could have known at the time of his presentation. Daaboul's identification of his own training in the traditions of Wilkins and Money is right, I suggest in the first part of this chapter, but unraveling the threads that identify Wilkins and Money so closely lays bare important tensions in the ways that atypical sex anatomies are constituted as a "threat," first to the social order, and then to the individual who bears the alleged affliction. These competing views—the first marking the late nineteenth and early twentieth centuries, and the second the emergence from that period—intertwine in the mid-twentieth century, precisely at the point when the training Daaboul himself underwent as a physician was shaped. Existing historical accounts suggest that it was this dual constitution of the threat posed by atypical sex that prevailed at least through the end of the twentieth century. Using Daaboul's presentation as a guide, I want to clarify the historical developments that can help to make sense of how the commitments to care for "individual well-being" and what we might call "social adjustment/accommodation" may be at once in concord and conflict.

It is not often that ordinary people recognize that they are at a crossroads of historical change, and it is not entirely clear that when Daaboul made his presentation he was aware of the position he occupied in this regard. The explicit aim of his presentation was to argue for the importance of an historical sensibility, but more than a decade later we know that it is also evidence of his own place in the recent history of the medical management of atypical sex that begins with the founding of the Intersex Society of North America (ISNA) in 1993. In the second part of the chapter, I discuss another important element of this history: normalization. Michel Foucault's understanding of the power of "normalization" can help us make sense of the history of medicalization and its repressive influence; it can also guide our understanding of the significant changes that occur at the beginning of the twenty-first century, when the work of activists, academics, and a growing number of physicians critical of the standard of care resulted in the meetings of the U.S. and European endocrinological societies in 2005 and the publication of a groundbreaking Consensus Statement in 2006 (Hughes et al., 2006). These meetings heralded significant change, including the replacement of the nineteenth-century diagnostic nomenclature. Foucault's account of normalization is perhaps particularly helpful in examining and reckoning with what are evidently "repressive" effects of the history of medicalization, which in his view begin in the Victorian period, as well as what I argue we should regard as the positive possibilities marked by the changes announced in the 2006 statement.

Focused on removing sexual ambiguity, medical management of atypical sex anatomies since the mid-1950s has emphasized medical (and especially surgical) fixes for what might otherwise be understood in contemporary terms as social, political, or psychological matters of sexual identity. One might reasonably ask why it wouldn't be simpler to take intersex conditions out of medicine altogether, to "demedicalize" conditions that might otherwise count as ordinary human variations. The case for understanding differences in genital appearance as matters of variation is undeniably convincing, and yet there is an equally compelling case that some of the conditions with which genital variation are associated bring genuine health challenges that require not less, but substantially more, medical attention than has been afforded them. The best example, and the one on which this chapter focuses, is the case of congenital adrenal hyperplasia (CAH), a condition that in some forms poses grave dangers to an individual's health. Understanding the history of the medical management of atypical sex anatomies in general requires careful study of the treatment developed by Lawson Wilkins at Johns Hopkins University for treatment of CAH in particular. Wilkins's work is significant not only for the consequential advancements in the care of children with CAH for which he is rightly celebrated, but also because the surgical normalization of affected females with CAH became a generalizable model for managing atypical sex anatomies figured as a problem to "fix" in early childhood. While pediatric research on the pathophysiology of CAH begun by Wilkins still thrives today and continues to advance in major medical centers nationwide, including at the National Institutes of Health, it is striking that, given that CAH is a disease that may require lifelong management, there is no comparable work that investigates the effects and management of CAH into adulthood.[1] To understand how care for those with atypical sex continued to emphasize matters of appearance over those of health through the end of the twentieth century, we must look more closely at the history of medicalization of atypical sex. As different historians have provided detailed accounts of key eras that make up this history, we may trace a development in the treatment of atypical sex anatomies, but this history does not move in linear fashion. Rather, there is a kind of cyclic movement constituting atypical sex as a threat, first to society, then to individual well-being and back again.

From the Victorian Age to the Clinical Age: Circling Forward and Back into the Past

Dreger's *Hermaphrodites and the Medical Invention of Sex* recounts the moment at which the threat of doubtful sex becomes, for medicine, something that must be carefully measured, classified, and mastered. Interest in hermaphroditic bodies was at once entirely characteristic of the modernization of medicine that took place in Western Europe in the late nineteenth and early twentieth centuries, interested as it was in measuring, classifying, and mastering knowledge of the human body and its functions, normal and aberrant. It was also distinctive: hermaphroditism would prove an inordinately rich object of scientific and medical interest that combined medical and scientific curiosity and concern with managing a social menace.[2] The publication of the cases of hermaphroditism that fascinated and preoccupied late nineteenth and early twentieth-century physicians occurs just at the time that transcontinental dissemination of one's observations and findings became a mark of one's professional distinction (Dreger 1998b, 61). It is no coincidence that this period coincides with what Foucault identifies as the shift in medicine from a reliance on the judgment of individual patients with respect to their health to the expertise of the physician authorized to make judgments and to treat them. As Daaboul notes, it does not appear that immediately preceding the period that Dreger studies, atypical sex was the problem he and his cohort understood it to be. Furthermore, the cases that span the developments Dreger traces—of Marie-Madeline Lefort or Herculine Barbin in France, and Louise-Julia-Anna or "S. B." in England, for example—were cases of "mistaken sex" that posed significant challenges to a social order that depended on the clear and verifiable distinction between the sexes. Cases that did not present such challenges, one expects—because they were not written up and disseminated, or because people did not consult doctors or surgeons to the extent that they eventually would come to—were not extraordinary. In an era without sophisticated surgical practices, and in the absence of any genuine uncertainty of sex assignment by an individual or a physician, one would expect that the majority of cases of "genital ambiguity" that Daaboul would encounter in his practice at the end of the twentieth century would not have caused particular consternation in a social climate where anatomical variation would be unremarkable and not regarded as the problem it would become in the middle of the next century.

Attending to the gap that Daaboul identifies between practices at the end of the twentieth century and those preceding the "Age of Gonads"—before "hermaphroditism" became an object for modern European medicine to diagnose and to manage—requires that we look at the interval between the Victorian era and the period Daaboul locates in the mid-1950s, when John Money began work at Johns Hopkins University's pediatric endocrinology clinic. Daaboul's recounting of history falters here—not because he traces the origins of his own discipline to the work of Wilkins, the "father" of pediatric endocrinology, but because he so closely identifies the critical part of Wilkins's work at mid-century, when, we learn from historian Sandra Eder, it belongs to an earlier period, preceding the Second World War. The error turns out to be consequential for the understanding of the history, as we will see, because the objects of medical practice in the mid-1930s differ significantly from those twenty years later. Understanding that difference, I argue, is critical for identifying the ethical problems we must confront today. But there is a further wrinkle in the history of pediatric endocrinology (and psychoendocrinology) that we find in the corollary history of normalizing genital surgery with which pediatric endocrinology is also bound. Wilkins shared a number of pediatric patients with his senior colleague at Johns Hopkins, renowned surgeon Hugh Hampton Young, "the Father of American Urology," as described in his 1947 obituary (Wesson 1947, cited in Kenen 1998, 37). Young earned this title with his treatment of men with enlarged prostates, but he was also a founder of the *Journal of Urology,* still the leading journal in the field today. Young's extensive practice of surgical sex reassignment—what usually entailed the reshaping of sex anatomy of a child with typically male (46,XY) chromosomes so that the child could appear, and function, as a girl—locates him fundamentally as a late nineteenth-century figure who brings urological surgical practice into the modern era, even as his concerns and interests appear to have remained in the preceding era. In contrast to what appears to be Wilkins's interruption of the prevailing concern with doubtful sex as a threat to the social body, we might understand Young's to be a dogged insistence on this view, one that may have been motivated and reinforced by the surgical advances he pioneered.

In his account, Daaboul traces his once-secure faith in the standard of care to the specialized training he received, a training established by Lawson Wilkins. It was Wilkins's founding of a fellowship in pediatric endocrinology in the 1950s at Johns Hopkins Hospital that produced the leaders in the field whose influence continues still. According to Daaboul, Wilkins had trained nearly every physician who in the 1960s would go on to become program directors of pediatric endocrinology; for this reason, most pediatric endocrinologists practicing today, he says, are "descended" from Wilkins. That the Pediatric Endocrine Society was, from its founding in 1972 until 2010, called the "Lawson Wilkins Pediatric Society" is a testament to the abiding strength of Wilkins's legacy and its continued influence.

Wilkins's opening of a fellowship program occurred precisely at the point when the newly minted psychologist John Money began work at Johns Hopkins to assist Wilkins in the psychological counseling of, and research concerning, Wilkins's patients. Most anyone who knows anything about the medical management of intersex today will readily identify the prevailing standard of care with the work Money carried out from that time until his death in 2006. But those outside of the field will likely not recognize the importance of Wilkins's work, which occurred in the interval between the end of the European era that Dreger's history details (in the 1910s) and the beginning of the mid-1950s, the point to which Daaboul traces the origins of his training.[3] Indeed, the history in which Daaboul locates himself should more precisely be understood to have begun two decades before Wilkins's establishment of the fellowship in pediatric endocrinology, in Wilkins's 1936 opening of the endocrinology clinic in the nation's first pediatric medical center, Johns Hopkins University's Harriet Lane Home.

Sandra Eder's history of Wilkins's work fills in a picture that validates Daaboul's and his colleagues' loyal faith in their founding father and, by extension, their high regard for Wilkins's treatment of children with CAH, still the most frequent cause of atypical sex in girls throughout the world. CAH is a genetic disorder that involves malfunction of the adrenal glands. It affects males and females in equal numbers, and both may suffer from metabolic problems soon after birth (when it is usually detected) and throughout one's life. In the "classic," salt-losing form, it results in vomiting and dehydration and, if left untreated, can lead to death. Increased vulnerabilities—caused by ordinary illness or injury that can exacerbate various sorts of imbalances associated with CAH—are among the problems that require careful attention in early childhood and beyond. CAH also prompts premature development of bone growth, which ultimately results in adult short stature—a particular concern for affected boys—and of secondary sex characteristics. In addition to metabolic problems, what Wilkins called the "androgen push" may result in virilization of sex anatomy, which can make a male look, as Wilkins put it, like an "infant Hercules" (Eder 2012, 71) and can make a genetic female appear more like a male.

Wilkins's treatment was groundbreaking in a number of ways, but first and foremost for the detailed clinical understanding he developed of the disease and its effects. Wilkins's years of study of the disease led, in 1949, to his first attempt to determine whether CAH would be responsive to cortisone, reported by a Mayo

Clinic physician to bring dramatic relief of rheumatoid arthritis (Eder 2012, 73). Wilkins refined the administration of cortisone over several years. It did not lead to the promised cure of the condition, but when administered in the dose appropriate to each individual patient, cortisone could control the effects of CAH, which encompassed a range of what most would regard without controversy as ailments.

Examination of the history of CAH is a complicated matter. Though today it is clear that there is a close identification of genuine medical problems caused by CAH with the social problem atypical sex is taken to present, this was not always the case. Indeed, there is little evidence that "hermaphroditism" during the period Dreger studies was associated with any condition we would regard as a disease or malady, as most forms of CAH obviously are now recognized to be.[4] In other words, it was not the fact that atypical sex posed a medical danger that brought these bodies under special scrutiny in the Victorian period; instead it is their deviation from a standard of "the norm" that comes to be identified at this time and that is identified as a threat to the social body (Dreger 1998b, 166).[5] Rather than a concern with health, Dreger notes that the fascination with hermaphroditism was likely connected to challenges to sexual boundaries coming from new directions, particularly from first-wave feminists and homosexuals (26).[6]

The threat posed by the bodies of those with "doubtful sex" exemplifies what bioethicist Erik Parens calls "bad medicalization." Where medicalization takes nonmedical problems—"life or human" problems—and casts these in medical terms, bad medicalization constitutes the commission of a category mistake—that is, taking something to be a medical issue or problem that is really a social problem, for example. In other words, where medicalization is a matter of express, if problematic, translation, bad medicalization represents a more subtle and sinister phenomenon; mistaking one problem for another at the outset, a subconscious sleight of hand may result—and, indeed, has resulted—in the sorts of objectification that constrain people's lives (Parens 2011, 2–3). By stark contrast, the focus of treatment and investigation in Wilkins's clinic, from its founding through the end of the 1940s, was, according to Eder, not so much on genital anomaly as on the health and flourishing of his patients. Thus much of the treatment of CAH exemplifies what Parens calls "good medicalization"—that is, the identification of a malady or disorder that had not been previously identified, or had been misidentified, for example, as an individual moral failing. Indeed, the identification of CAH in the case of those with the salt-losing form of the disease would, in Wilkins's hands, become literally life-saving.

The historical trajectory that Daaboul briefly sketches in his account turns out to be a far messier business than was understood when he gave his presentation in 2000. Dreger documents the simultaneous fascination, disgust, and resentment regarding what appeared to be a sudden and dramatic increase in cases of hermaphroditism in France and England in the late nineteenth and early twentieth centuries (1998b, 27). Physicians' voluminous studies during this period made hermaphroditic bodies a spectacle, both titillating and threatening, and one that would be controlled by medical authority. This is perhaps best illustrated by Dreger's discussion of the photographic display of genitals literally presented by the hand of the unseen physician, a common motif in both photographs and drawings of atypical sex anatomies (47; see, e.g., H. Young 1937, 170). But the properly medical—and not only medicalized—treatment of CAH in Wilkins's clinic stands in contrast, which is not to say opposition, to the treatment of those with the identical condition only a few decades earlier. No longer did physicians theorize about the "psychic influence on the part of the mother," whose thoughts were believed capable of malforming the developing fetus in her womb (Dreger 1998b, 70); the new specialists at Johns Hopkins Hospital saw conditions that could alter the expected course of sex(ual) development as natural defects. Such conditions might be understood in terms of heredity but would no longer be taken to be a function of the "social" heredity of maternal influence, race, class, or education.

I do not mean to suggest that social mores did not have a critical role in Wilkins's understanding of what constituted the health and flourishing of his patients. Before Wilkins demonstrated the effectiveness of cortisone to manage the symptoms of CAH, which included progressive virilization in genetic females, it was his concern with the well-being of his patients that led him to support the assignment of these patients as boys, since they would "look too male to be able to live as women" (Eder 2012, 72). As Eder writes, even "before psychologist Dr. John Money formulated his theory of gender at Wilkins's clinic in 1955—namely that a person's gender role was learned after birth and could be in contradiction to one or more biological sexual characteristics—the idea of a 'better' sex that made sense socially but contradicted various biological sex determinants of a person was already put into practice in this clinic" (69). In other words, the "optimal gender theory" developed by Money, together with John and Joan Hampson, was not the "departure" from prevailing practice that most have taken it to be (e.g., Karkazis 2008, 55); rather, in important ways this theory extended Wilkins's practice of permitting virilized females to be raised as boys, to accept the anomaly of their atypical sex, and to adapt to the prevailing social standards in ways that created new possibilities for understanding the distinction between boys and girls, men and women.

One might argue that the assignment of virilized females as male was not a recognition of variation, but was instead an accommodation to a gender system that requires conformity to a structure that does not allow for the expression of "doubtful" sex. One could also argue that Wilkins's approach was not ethical, that it subordinated an individual's authentic expression of self to social norms that could not promote his or her flourishing. And yet Eder's account makes a compelling case that Wilkins's concern was indeed for the well-being of the individual patient, whose care must not be based wholesale on some "normal standard," but in relationship to himself (cf. Canguilhem 1991 [1966], 138). In Eder's words, Wilkins appreciated that variation "was a natural part of development and it was pressuring a child into a stage of development that did not fit its own biological norms that caused psychological problems" (2012, 72). For Wilkins, attending to an individual child's well-being should not occur in spite of social norms, but according to one's own individuality understood in relation to others and within one's world. Wilkins's approach was a departure from that taken by his nineteenth-century predecessors who had become focused on the question of "true" sex, the question that put the needs of society against those whose health and flourishing challenged the order on which it insisted. For Wilkins, the issue of sex assignment was—for good reason in the case of CAH—thoroughly entwined with that of a patient's physical and emotional health.

To better appreciate the significance of the standard of care for atypical sex, we must keep in mind that the primary cases in Wilkins's clinic were genetic females with CAH. As important as sex assignment was—and there is no doubt of its importance, as Eder's work documents (2010; 2012)—the fact that the disorder seriously compromised an affected child's physical health cannot be understated. That one of the most conspicuous signs of the disorder was atypical sex in females, and precocity in both males and females, helps us to understand how atypical sex could be more firmly established as a medical problem rather than a social problem at this time. The children treated with the severe salt-losing form of CAH were almost uniformly females, since their adrenal crisis was far more frequently identified by physicians with the "adrenogenital syndrome" than was often possible in the cases of genetic males, who lacked the more conspicuous genital anomaly that pointed to the systemic defect.[7] The enhanced ability to identify the disorder in affected infants together with the discovery of the drug that would make possible lifelong management of the disorder are rightly regarded as major advancements in pediatric medical care, comparable in many ways to the discovery of insulin in managing type 1 diabetes (Eder 2012, 75).

Drawing too bright a line between the treatment of doubtful sex associated with the era on which Dreger focuses in her study and that of the children and young adults with CAH in Wilkins's clinic risks obscuring the ways that the earlier treatment of atypical sex as a fascinoma and threat appear to be present in Wilkins's clinic. Focusing on the endocrinological advances that occurred with respect to CAH at this time, and the careful and individualized care that characterized Wilkins's model of pediatric endocrinology, it may be easy to overlook the ways that the distinctive approach to atypical sex that dates to Wilkins's treatment was partner to the surgical work of another pioneer, Hugh Hampton Young. As an historical figure, Young has one foot firmly in the "Age of the Gonads" and the other in the period in which Wilkins so prominently appears. Beginning in

1897—one year after he came to Johns Hopkins Hospital as an intern to learn surgery—he was appointed head of "genitourinary surgery."[8] Johns Hopkins was quickly transforming medicine from the low-status profession it had been until the late nineteenth century to a prestigious research-oriented profession emphasizing publication of research modeled on the sciences (Kenen 1998, 38). Young's extraordinary advances—all the more extraordinary because he had had no surgical training before coming to Baltimore—soon made the Johns Hopkins Hospital the leader in urological disorders as well as "the primary center for cases of so-called indeterminate sex" (Karkazis 2008, 43). In 1916, twenty years before Wilkins's arrival, Young established the renowned Brady Urological Institute. He began publishing his work on cases of indeterminate sex soon after.

If Wilkins's work ushers in a new era with respect to the treatment of atypical sex, in many respects his senior colleague appears to emerge from the preceding one. Given the undeveloped state of surgery at this time, normalizing genital surgeries had been rare, particularly in the United States. It was Young who began in the twentieth century to develop and refine the techniques that would mark the standard of care over the coming century. A leading figure in the history of the treatment of CAH, Young had understood that CAH was a disease affecting primarily the adrenal glands and had aggressively promoted adrenalectomy in the affected patients he saw at Johns Hopkins.[9] From Eder's work it appears that Young had an active, if sometimes contentious, relationship with the younger Wilkins. (Wilkins was skeptical of the value of adrenalectomy in particular, and his discovery of the benefit of cortisone rendered Young's approach obsolete.) For the sake of his patients' well-being, however, it appears that Wilkins supported the normalizing genital surgeries in which Young specialized, particularly clitorectomies of "large" clitorises (Eder 2010, 700).

Of all surgical interventions, the matter of clitorectomy remains today the most controversial. The history of clitorectomy in the United States does not begin with normalization of atypical sex, but has much deeper origins in the Victorian era, when "female sexual excess, sexual pathology, hysteria, and other mental states became associated with the female genitals" (Karkazis 2008, 148). Such pathology or excess could be defined simply in terms of erotic pleasure (see, e.g., Webber 2005), but this pleasure also came to be linked to a host of genuine maladies, including epilepsy.[10] It is not entirely clear what relation prevailed between what Eder describes as the "existing tradition" of clitorectomy at Johns Hopkins Hospital generally and its employment in cases of children assigned female in Wilkins's clinic specifically. Clitorectomy was, according to Eder, "neither discussed nor questioned in the patient records" she studied; her account suggests that clitorectomy was by then routinized in the clinic and "persisted through the introduction of cortisone and Money's gender concept" (2010, 700). If Young's 1937 textbook is any indication, it does appear that clitoral "amputation" was performed regularly in the case of uncertain sex. But even if the unremarkable use of clitorectomy was a legacy of an earlier era, it appears that there is a period in the West—which may be located in the early part of the twentieth century—when clitorectomy was employed almost categorically to resolve the disturbance that "doubtful sex" obviously provoked.

Young's surgical textbook, *Genital Abnormalities, Hermaphroditism, and Related Adrenal Diseases* (1937), was not only the first to address normalization of sex, but it was also "the first American treatise on the types of human hermaphroditism" (Karkazis 2008, 44). It compiles what was in the United States an unprecedented number of detailed case histories and accompanying photographs of Young's subjects, as well as careful drawings and instructions for surgical techniques performed on or recommended for them. If this, the main part of Young's text, published the year after Wilkins's arrival at the Harriet Lane Home in 1936, locates Young's major work at the very start of a new era of the treatment of atypical sex, the book's extended first chapter, "Hermaphroditism in Literature and Art," seems inspired by the thinkers of the previous century. Young's is an almost rapturous treatment of what he represents as a comprehensive overview of hermaphroditism beginning with the birth of the "extraordinary child" of Aphrodite and Hermes recorded in ancient Greek mythology known as Hermaphroditos. But "this amazing anatomical combination of both male and female was encountered long before" this time, in the Hebrew biblical story of Adam, originally both male and female, and then divided—an interpretation found in Jewish scholarship and then among Catholics during the period when Innocent III was pope (i.e., at the turn of the fourteenth century) (H. Young 1937, 1). Young presents an interesting critical reading of Ovid's story of Hermaphroditus, to which he finds "obvious objections . . . especially from a medical standpoint" (5), suggesting on Young's part a literal reading of the ancient sources. He also consults various authoritative religious texts that attest to the "fairly considerably frequency" (6) of hermaphroditism across the West. Ancient Greek sculptural representations document the presence, for example, of hypospadias (15), the condition in which the urinary meatus is not at the tip of the penis, but on the underside or base of the penis; statues such as these, he elaborates, inspired seventeenth-century German engravings and nineteenth-century French poetry.[11] Young ends this first chapter with selections from the long poem "The Hermaphrodite," composed by Samuel Loveman the same year Young's book went to press:

Out of the deep, immortal night
Came to me the Hermaphrodite,
Moonlight-breasted, pale, antique,
He spoke to me in deathless Greek:
. . . .

Long have I tarried, yet to me cries
The flame that follows the flame that dies;
I pass—but worship me, hold me still,
Body and soul inseparable.[12]

It does not seem precisely ironic that Young would end the first, presumably introductory, chapter of his monumental text with the poetic call to "worship" the body ("and soul inseparable") of one with atypical sex anatomy before devoting the remainder of the book to a careful study of the means of correcting the defects that constitute it. In this respect Young is a bridge between the two eras in which he lived and worked and to which he importantly contributed.

Whereas the late nineteenth century saw an explosion of scientific discourse and interest in both the body generally and the hermaphroditic body especially (an explosion that, if Young's introduction is any indication, also implicated cultural production in broader ways), the period that follows is focused not on generating discussion but on correcting the signs of difference, of working to ensure silence on the matter of doubtful sex. It is not that there would be less interest in, or research on, the intersexed body during this time. Indeed, research would proliferate, particularly in the United States, not only at Johns Hopkins University, where the new field of psychoendocrinology would be established in the 1950s, but also by the first of Wilkins's students at other centers. The production of knowledge aimed now to settle the matter of doubtful sex by normalizing the bodies of those with atypical sex before they became the problem they had been taken to be in the previous period.

Historian Alison Redick has argued that Wilkins's work in the 1950s ushered in a new era in which a team of specialists under his direction would shape the standard of care for the next fifty years. Wilkins's team was the first of its kind and included Howard Jones and William Scott, Young's junior colleagues in surgery, as well as the psychiatrists John and Joan Hampson.[13] Money had come to Johns Hopkins on Wilkins's invitation. He had been working with Frederick Bartter, an endocrinologist who was a sort of rival of Wilkins's in Boston, who had published work on cortisone and CAH at the same time that Wilkins did (Redick 2005, 293). With the Hampsons, Money made Johns Hopkins the center of research on sex variation, publishing in 1955 the five essays published in the *Bulletin of the Johns Hopkins Hospital* that comprised the new protocols for gender assignment in cases of atypical sex. They set out multiple variables of sex, including that which is assigned or announced at birth, the appearance of external genitalia, reproductive organs, hormone levels, chromosomes, and "gender role," that is, the sex with which someone identifies. Together these articles challenged what was at the time the commonsense notion that "biological markers of sex" told the entire story of one's sense of self. The theory elaborated there shifted the "truth" of sex understood as determined by biology to an understanding of sex as a production of society. This understanding provided the theoretical ground for "a treatment regime designed to ensure that future generations of intersexed infants developed unambiguously masculine or feminine identities" (Germon 2009, 24). The dominance of endocrinology and psychology that emerged at this time is also evident in the ascension of Young's junior surgeons, Jones and Scott, culminating in their 1958 publication of *Hermaphroditism, Genital Anomalies, and Related Endocrine Disorders*, the title only slightly modifying their mentor's masterwork. In place of the history of hermaphroditism in literature and art that opened Young's treatise, Jones and Scott's treatment of cases and surgical technique is supplemented by significant portions of text authored by Money, including "his freshly minted and rapidly circulating theory of gender role" (Redick 2005, 294).

Given the prominence Money assumes in the clinic at this time, it is no wonder that in his own historical overview, Daaboul presents the work of Wilkins and Money as of a piece. And yet the generalized model for the medical management of children with atypical sex that was developed in Wilkins's clinic in the 1950s appears to constitute a significant departure from the ethos that seems to have guided Wilkins's work during the earlier period, between the late 1930s and the mid-1950s. Wilkins's practice was focused above all on the individual health and well-being of his patients. But centering as he did on the case of CAH, the issues of health and of genital appearance became entwined to the extent they were no longer distinguishable. As a result, the standard of care formulated from the mid-1950s, which becomes entrenched through the better part of the century, seems in some ways to hark back to that earlier time, when hermaphroditism figured as curiosity and threat.

Normalizing Medicine

From Eder's account we know that before his success with the administration of cortisone, Wilkins often supported the assignment of virilized females as male. In other words, the work of Money and the Hampsons was not so much an innovation with respect to the notion of "optimal gender," but in important ways extended the practice of Wilkins's clinic that had encouraged virilized females to be raised as boys—that is, to accept the anomaly of their atypical sex—thus adapting to the prevailing social standards in ways that created new possibilities for understanding the distinction between boys and girls, men and women.

In the mid-1950s we find a moment when atypical sex was considered alternately and simultaneously—as twentieth-century philosopher and physician Georges Canguilhem puts it—an "anomaly," something that was merely unusual, "removed, in terms of one's organization, from the vast majority to which one must be compared" (1991 [1966], 133), and a "pathology," something that "interrupts a life course" (138). In supporting the male assignment of those virilized females, Wilkins effectively treated them in the terms that Canguilhem advanced in his study. Wilkins's response to his patients' difference took what we might today call the aspect of CAH that resulted in their gender variance (see, e.g., Menvielle 1998) as anomalous rather than pathological. As Canguilhem writes, "Pathological implies *pathos*, the direct and concrete feeling of suffering and impotence, the feeling of life gone wrong" (1991 [1966], 137). However unusual it might be to be female and live as a boy or man, the lives of Wilkins's patients—much as the lives of those individuals before the Age of Gonads for whom atypical sex had not posed a problem—had not entirely "gone wrong." They—and presumably their families, who may well have been aware of their child's or partner's difference—had adapted, which is, for Canguilhem, the condition of an organism's "normativity," the creative capacity to generate new norms of living.

One may also understand Wilkins himself to have adapted in response to his patients' needs, to have changed, to some degree, his own views of sex and its meaning. But when Wilkins understood that female genital ambiguity as a symptom of the generalized disorder of CAH was diminished by successful pharmaceutical management, his recommendations in favor of assignment of virilized females as boys changes. They are not, however, entirely reversed, as Eder finds in the case of the toddler "Charles" who enters the clinic in 1958. After diagnosis of CAH and confirmation of typical female chromosomal pattern are made, physicians recommended reassignment and cortisone treatment. Because the child was already two and a half, and the parents are recorded as feeling "strongly about raising [their] child as a boy," Charles underwent a hysterectomy and was prescribed hormone doses that would manage CAH *and* maintain his male assignment (Eder 2010, 698). But if Charles's story exemplifies the sort of adaption of which Canguilhem speaks, we must recognize that it also validated formalization of the treatment rationale that Money was at this time providing Wilkins's clinic, one that did not seek to recognize the distinction between anomaly and pathology, but rather imposed a "normalization" that would effect the close identification, if not conflation, of the two.

According to the theory developed by Money and the Hampsons, the formation of gender identity in early childhood is "malleable," that is, susceptible to social shaping that would provide the clear gender identity the researchers took to be necessary for psychosocial health. "Gender ambiguity later in life," however, "was pathological," as Anne Fausto-Sterling observes (2000, 63). The insistence by Charles's parents on his male assignment is consistent with the critical role that parents play in gender identity development according to this theory, taking one's identity to be a matter of social shaping rather than an expression of an individual's essential sense of self. Surgical normalization would ensure that a child would have no confusion about his or her assigned sex. As Fausto-Sterling explains,

> [While] such anatomical clarity was important for the young child, Money, the Hampsons, and those who followed their lead argued, it was even more important for the child's parents. As Peter Pan might have said, "they had to believe" in their child's gender identity for that identity to become real. Hampson and Hampson write: "In working with hermaphroditic children and their parents, it has become clear that the establishment of a child's psychosexual orientation begins not so much with the child as with his parents." (Hampson and Hampson 1961, 1,415, in Fausto-Sterling 2000, 63–64)

Even as Charles's case demonstrates a continuity between the kind of care delivered in Wilkins's clinic in the 1930s and '40s and the standard of care that dates to the mid-1950s, there are subtle yet important differences indicating that the recommendations in Charles's case mark a kind of crossroads in the trajectory of care in Wilkins's clinic. Preceding the period when the role of Money and the Hampsons gained prominence, we may see how the standard that Wilkins devised was concerned with his patient's well-being in the "normative" sense that Canguilhem describes. But the reassignment that Charles's parents were evidently pressed to consent to appears far more consistent with contemporary accounts of affected individuals and parents treated both at Johns Hopkins and at other centers whose model of care was shaped at Johns Hopkins during this period. The medical care in line with this model is better described in the terms of what Canguilhem's student Michel Foucault calls "normalization."

"Normalization" is not only a term employed by physicians to describe cosmetic genital surgery for those with atypical sex anatomies, but, following Foucault, it also has become a critical theoretical shorthand to signify the pervasive standards that structure and define social meaning. Medicine has played a central role in the modern development of the norm, and "medical power," Foucault claims, "is at the heart of a society of normalization" (1996, 197). In the ancient period health was conceived in terms of the harmonious functioning of the individual; medicine was regarded as "a set of techniques for curing ills and of the knowledge they require" (Foucault 1994 [1963], 34). This view of medicine would persist into the eighteenth century, but medicine would also come to "embrace a knowledge of the *healthy man,* that is, a study of the *non-sick man,* and a definition of the *model man*" (34; original emphasis).[14] Medicine assumes, as Foucault puts it, a "normative posture which authorizes it not only to distribute advice as to a healthy life, but also to dictate the standards for physical and moral relations of the individual and the society in which he lives" (34). The formulation of the understanding of the model man sets the stage for a further development in the nineteenth century that would see a subtle but important change from a focus on "health" to "normality."

For Foucault, the eighteenth-century standard of health was concerned with qualities that could be understood as specific to a particular being, namely, "vigour, suppleness, and fluidity, which were lost in illness and which it was the task of medicine to restore" (35). Such qualities were understood to a certain extent to be judged and regulated by the individual, through diet and exercise, for example, which entailed "the possibility of being one's own physician" (35)—the possibility, that is, that the evaluation of an individual's health could be determined and regulated only with respect to, and by, oneself, rather than a measure or command imposed from without. Nineteenth-century health, by contrast, "was regulated more in accordance with normality than with health; it formed its concepts and prescribed its interventions in relation to a standard of functioning and organic structure." Consequently, Foucault writes, the medicine that previously took as its object "the structure of the *organized being*" was transformed into "the *medical bipolarity of the normal and the pathological*" (35; original emphasis). It was no longer the judgment of the individual that mattered most, but that of "experts" who would be authorized to evaluate and treat the individual as prevailing standards dictated.

The late nineteenth-century development of the taxonomic system used to classify hermaphroditic "types" (Dreger 1998b) is exemplary of the periodization Foucault describes. This taxonomy was in use for more than a century. It dictated that females and males were defined as presenting only standard female or male anatomy, respectively, while so-called male and female pseudohermaphrodites and "true" hermaphrodites presented different mixtures of male and female anatomy (Dreger 1998b, 35–40).[15] Such divisions, together with the medical practices aimed to correct the abnormalities they denoted, may be understood to exemplify what Foucault calls "the art of punishing," an essential component of the society of normalization.

> The art of punishing . . . is aimed neither at expiation, nor even precisely at repression. It brings five distinct operations into play: it refers individual actions [or bodies, in the field of medicine] to a whole that is at once a field of comparison, a space of differentiation and the principle of a rule to be followed. It differentiates individuals from one another, in terms of following the overall rule: that the rule be made to function as a minimal threshold, as an average to be respected or as an optimum towards which one must move. It measures in quantitative terms . . . the "nature" of individuals. It introduces, through this "value-giving" measure, the constraint of a conformity to be achieved. Lastly, it traces the limit that will define difference in relation to all other differences, the external frontier of the abnormal. (Foucault 1979 [1975], 182–183)

The language of punishment may seem out of place with respect to treatment of intersex conditions. It would be far-fetched to claim that the physicians in Wilkins's clinic in the 1950s sought to punish children for their physical difference. And yet accounts of adults treated at that time and into the three decades that followed suggest a subjection to a "punitive operation" consistent with the exercise of power Foucault vividly describes in *Discipline and Punish*. Consider sociologist Sharon Preves's interview with "Tiger," who reports having had sixteen surgeries to correct hypospadias, spending most of his summer vacations in the hospital while friends went to camp and on family vacations (2003, 31).[16] Others recount chilling experiences of having their bodies repeatedly displayed in hospitals and public clinics. "Carol," Preves reports, was humiliated by what she called the "parades" of physicians, residents, and interns—in one visit she counted more than one hundred—who "touched, poked, looked, mumbled, and left" (67). Anthropologist Katrina Karkazis's interviews with adults recount the stern proscriptions they received against questions or comments about their surgically corrected bodies; others who had surgery as young adults report the performance of surgeries without their consent, making one twelve-year-old feel, in her words, "freakish" (2008, 221).

Following Foucault, we shouldn't see the punitive experience of these individuals as one that physicians or parents meant for them to have; what Foucault understands by punishment is better captured in the passive voice, referring not to an action intended by a particular agent or agents, but to an action occurring *through* them. The "offense" that provokes the punishment in the first place is itself similarly construed. Rather than conceived as a wrongdoing committed by an individual, normalization acts on "the whole indefinite domain of non-conforming"—for example, failing to achieve a certain level of performance or, as in the case of atypical sex, being born with unusual anatomy (Foucault 1979 [1975], 179). By contrast with the more familiar conception of a "judicial penalty" (183), this "penalty of the norm" is more helpfully understood as a new "rationality," a way to make sense of the practices and bodies that insists on homogeneity and so both fixates on—and aims to correct—individual differences figured as abnormal (199). The operation of normalization here exemplifies Foucault's provocative characterization of power as "both intentional and nonsubjective." "There is no power," he claims, "that is exercised without a series of aims and objectives. But this does not mean that it results from the choice or decision of an individual subject" (1990 [1976], 95).

The work of John Money may be an especially apt illustration of the operation of power that establishes, as Foucault writes, "the Normal . . . as a principle of coercion" (1979 [1975], 184). Karkazis's account of Money's work is among the most sympathetic and resists caricature of the psychological paradigm he and the

Hampsons crafted and that held sway for more than four decades. Their theory should not simply be described as promoting the malleability of gender, she argues. Money and his colleagues saw gender identity and gender-role formation as "complex processes involving both biological and social factors" (Karkazis 2008, 63). At this point, normalizing surgical intervention became widely accepted, she says, "because it seemed obvious to both clinicians and parents that a child would experience problems personally and socially with atypical genitals" (64).

Money's role in shaping the standard of care for treatment of atypical sex has been addressed in detail by many (e.g., S. J. Kessler 1998; Fausto-Sterling 2000; Karkazis 2008; Germon 2009). Most people who know something about the history of the medical management of atypical sex know some version of what has come to be known as "the true story of John/Joan." This was the revelation in the mid-1990s that the "success story" of a boy who had been reassigned female after a circumcision accident turned out to have been a sham. Rather than the successfully reared girl Money described in his published reports, Joan had rejected her role and was living as a man named David Reimer. He had married a woman with whom he was raising three children. Reimer was not born with atypical sex; a pediatrician's accidentally burning off his penis during a circumcision opened the way to the grim experiment with which the standard of care for those born with atypical sex has become entwined, both within and outside medicine. The truth of what had occurred was revealed for the first time in a 1997 article published in the *Archives of Pediatric and Adolescent Medicine,* by biologist Milton Diamond, an ardent and longtime critic of Money's, in collaboration with Keith Sigmundson, the Canadian psychiatrist responsible for ongoing management of the case near Reimer's home. The story was widely disseminated that same year with journalist John Colapinto's "The True Story of John/Joan" in *Rolling Stone* and received further coverage when in 2000 Colapinto published the extended story, together with Reimer's identity, in *As Nature Made Him.*

To Reimer's story have been attached many morals, among them (as Oprah would tell it) that "boys *will* be boys," that no amount of good intentions, surgical intervention, or social conditioning will change what is "biological fact." Despite the efforts made by Joan's parents, his teachers, the doctors at home in Canada who were treating him, or the team at Johns Hopkins to whom he and his family made annual visits, he would not be a girl. But the story has also been cast as one of the cruelty and singularity of Money's work. The story of John/Joan—"the true story"—is a sad and important moment in the history of the normalizing treatment, both medical and social, of atypical sex, but its significance now appears both lesser and greater than these two versions of the story would have it.

After the revelation of the outcome of Reimer's failed reassignment, the standard of care for those born with atypical sex anatomies largely remained—and in important ways, arguably remains—unchanged. There are at least two reasons for this. First, while many have treated Money's work as entirely original—he is responsible for coining the term "gender role," which would become influential far beyond the bounds of the clinic—Eder's documentation of Wilkins's influence on Money's understanding of the supposed flexibility of gender role, particularly of virilized females with CAH, attests to the ways that Money's theories were designed to conform with the practices Wilkins had established long before. Money's theory (and that of the Hampsons) that the gender identity of a person born with atypical sex might not be as settled as that of a typical fetus was not new. The crucial fact that David Reimer was born a typical male meant that his failed reassignment might not be at all meaningful in the treatment of those whose sex anatomies were not typical: the putative failure of the experiment of John/Joan could not carry the weight it might have where care for children with atypical sex was concerned. Indeed, that experiment alone, which featured Money in "The Sexes" column of *Time* magazine in 1973—by which point "Joan" was as a ten-year-old still ignorant of her reassignment and resisting her parents and doctors' attempts to "feminize" her—could be seen as an individual manifestation of hubris rather than cause for wholesale condemnation of the standard of care that was developed, after all, by Wilkins. And there are many who do not take the failure of this experiment as an invalidation of Money's theory of gender development, pointing, for example, to another case of *ablatio penis* (penile ablation) to demonstrate that a chromosomally typical male can be reared as a girl (see Angier 1997; Bradley et al. 1998; Glassberg 1999; Meyer-Bahlburg 2005b). However prominent he may have been, Money's role was not definitive of the standard of care for the management of atypical sex. The same year that the story of John/Joan broke, independent evidence challenging the routine reassignment in males without androgen insensitivity was also published (see Reiner 1997). It is perhaps for these reasons that once Money as a figure became nearly invisible, the importance of theories that had been so closely associated with him was nevertheless undiminished. In place of a robust theory about psychosexual development in children came a vague yet unrelenting concern with "normal appearance" and the "normal life" this appearance promised.

But the revelation of the story of what happened to David Reimer did have the effect of multiplying questions that practitioners like Jorge Daaboul were already asking at this moment. First and foremost were questions about the outcomes of gender reassignment and normalizing surgery. What happened to girls who had had clitorectomies? What of the chromosomally typical boys who had been castrated and raised as girls? These questions gave rise to still more questions: What had the children been told? What did their parents know; what did they understand? And would it be possible—and ethically permissible—to try now to find out the answers to these questions? Absent information about what had happened to the children and their families after medical interventions had been concluded, could the standard of care stand? When Daaboul explains in 2000 that "all of us trained in the tradition of Money/Wilkins followed their recommendations. We lied to the parents of intersexed children and we lied to the children and we subjected intersexed individuals to 'corrective' surgery," he makes plain the depth of the challenge that the standard of care faced at this time. And Daaboul was not alone: other pediatric specialists had developed similar criticisms by this point, including Bruce Wilson, William Reiner, and Justine Schober, all of whom published articles in the special issue of the *Journal of Clinical Ethics* edited by Alice Dreger (1998c). In the lead article of that issue, Edmund Howe, the journal's editor in chief, reported that Dreger had invited proponents of normalizing pediatric surgeries—John Money among them—to contribute to the special issue, but all declined (Howe 1998, 338, 342n3). That same year, Suzanne Kessler's important *Lessons from the Intersexed* appeared, as well as Dreger's own *Hermaphrodites and the Medical Invention of Sex*. The groundbreaking scholarly work produced at this time supported, and was in turn supported by, increasingly sophisticated advocacy on behalf of those with atypical sex, activism spearheaded by Cheryl Chase, the founder of the Intersex Society of North America, and by Dreger, who eventually joined Chase in leading ISNA. Broadening awareness of the harms wrought by what these advocates identified as the "shame and secrecy" promoted by the standard of care was evident. Intersex was entering public conversation with reports in the mainstream and alternative press, televised documentaries produced in the United States and Canada, and new novels such as Jeffrey Eugenides's *Middlesex* (2002). Physicians in the United States and Europe were also increasingly concerned about a standard of care that, physicians had finally to acknowledge, was based on little evidence of success. Despite what most have regarded as the indisputably good intentions of physicians, the routine ethical violations of accepted principles of bioethics promoted by the standard of care raised additional questions. What Karkazis describes as the "deep and divisive crisis" into which care for those with atypical sex had been driven, prompted specialists in the United States and Europe to convene in Chicago in 2005—a year after Reimer would commit suicide—to review and to revise the standard of care in which they had been trained.[17]

From Intersex to "Disorders of Sex Development"

The Consensus Statement that resulted from the 2005 Chicago meetings, published in 2006, recorded a number of significant changes to the standard of care, among them a rejection of the older claim of intersex as a "social emergency." Atypical sex is not a source of shame, these new standards insisted, and honesty on the part of caregivers would be imperative going forward not only for parents but also for children, who were to receive developmentally appropriate explanations about their conditions. Just as in 2000, when the American Academy of Pediatrics opened its statement with an acknowledgment of the importance of language in guiding care and influencing parents' understandings of, and relationship to, their children, the Chicago group recognized that the nineteenth-century nomenclature still in use shaped their own practices.

If variations on the term "hermaphrodite" "place[d] these patients outside the mainstream of society, relegating them to the realm of mythology," and if "intersex, with its connotation that such patients are somehow in an 'in between' state" (Aaronson and Aaronson 2010, 443), was likewise inappropriate, a new nomenclature was needed. This need was first identified before the Chicago meetings by the group comprised of Alice Dreger, Cheryl Chase, Aron Sousa, Philip Gruppuso, and Joel Frader.[18] New nomenclature would correct the misleading taxonomy that was "scientifically questionable" and "provide[d] little clinical help" (Dreger et al. 2005, 730). Based on outdated understandings that had been long proved flawed, the old taxonomy was intended not to guide the care of affected individuals, but instead "to sort confusing and sometimes disturbing anatomies into clear types." In the era in which the taxonomy was introduced and took root, gonadal histology was "a fashionable (though vague) explanation for gender and sexual behavior" (730). Classifying, and thus managing this confusion, was a nineteenth-century priority that all could agree was out of line with the aims of modern medicine, so there was good reason to revisit the issue of nomenclature. The group's proposal of the term "disorders of sexual differentiation" aimed to correct these problems, noting particularly the importance of nomenclature in guiding physicians' practice.[19]

The changes announced in the resulting consensus statement, published the following year, demonstrate another kind of circling forward and back into history, refocusing physicians on those aspects of conditions associated with atypical sex that have consequences for individuals' health rather than on the achievement of "normal appearance" that had previously constituted the principal aim of care. However, rather than "disorders of sexual differentiation," the term tentatively proposed by Dreger and her colleagues, the representatives of the U.S. and European groups settled on "disorders of sex development," which, because of the ambiguity in the term "sex development," had the unfortunate effect of re-invoking the nineteenth-century taxonomy from which the group apparently sought to distance itself.[20] Disorders of sex development (DSD) would now describe "congenital conditions in which development of chromosomal, gonadal, or anatomical sex is atypical" (Hughes et al. 2006, 554). Understanding something of the history of treatment, we can appreciate how this change would be genuinely progressive, an important break from the Victorian medicalization of bodies with atypical sex that saw in their anomalies not a risk to the health of those individuals but a threat to the social body. The change was also a response to the history so closely associated with the work of the case of David Reimer, for which the standard of care had so obviously and tragically gone wrong. What Chase, at ISNA, called "the concealment-centered model" of care had begun to appear more like a Victorian throwback than the enlightened medical care with which specialists in the tradition of Lawson Wilkins had prided themselves. The "patient-centered model" of care Chase outlined bore a far closer resemblance to the kind of care that Wilkins modeled before 1955, as well as the sort of care that physicians today would see as "good care." [21] For these reasons it is not surprising that the new nomenclature was embraced by physicians and replaced older terms in the medical literature (see, e.g., Pasteriski et al. 2010).

There was nevertheless strong opposition to the term "disorders of sex development" as evidenced first by the letters sent to the *Archives of Disease in Childhood* in the months following the statement's publication. Those objecting to the new nomenclature focused on the description of intersex conditions as "disorders," which they described as "stigmatizing" to the individual, who should be spared identification "as" a disorder (e.g., Baechler 2006; Cameron 2006).[22] For those who saw DSD to apply—largely as it had applied, both in the late nineteenth and early twentieth centuries, and then for those who had been labeled "intersex" as children—not to a condition, but to their person (e.g., Chase 2006), the appeal of taking atypical sex outside the domain of medicine altogether, to demedicalize conditions that might otherwise count as ordinary human variation, is apparent. And yet the proposed alternatives, such as "variations in sex development" (Diamond and Beh 2006) or "divergence of sex development" (Reis 2007; 2009), would not permit appreciation of the medical challenges faced by many individuals with intersex conditions during infancy or over the span of their lives.[23] Genuine health concerns have been a particular problem precisely because the focus of DSD has been on gender and genitalia that could be "fixed," supposedly resolved by pediatric specialists who did not follow their patients into adulthood and for whom specialized adult care has not been—and largely continues not to be—available, most strikingly for the chronic condition for which Wilkins's legacy is so strong, namely, CAH.

Foremost among the questions raised by objections to the use of "disorders of sex development" is the relationship of atypical sex anatomy to the constitution of personal identity: has intersex taken on in the late twentieth century the status of an identity, or is it a condition that is merely incidental to one's person? The objections to the change in nomenclature seem to take for granted, first, that there is a category of "intersex people" (e.g., Hester 2006, 47; Roen 2009, 35), or "intersexuals" (e.g., H. Young 1940, 201; S. J. Kessler 1998, 85; Fausto-Sterling 2000, 31; Preves 2003, 97) that would render the characterization of the condition as a disorder offensive. A second concern is related to the first, namely, that the pathologizing label would limit people's subjective possibilities by containing them within its terms. Underlying these two claims, I propose, is an implicit understanding of intersex(uality) as analogous to homosexuality.

There is every reason to consider the treatment of homosexuality, both historical and contemporary, alongside the medical management of atypical sex. At nearly every moment in medical investigation and the popular imagination alike, each has been implicated in the other. In the nineteenth century, "sexual inversion" was understood as "the tendency to embody physical characteristics associated with the opposite sex," mirroring an idea that "homosexuals were in some sense constitutional hermaphrodites" (Terry 1995, 135). This close tie between hermaphroditism and homosexuality has a longer history, however. According to Foucault, it was not the mixing of sexes in individuals that was threatening in seventeenth- and eighteenth-century France but the crime of making "use of their additional sex" through homosexual behavior (2003 [1999], 67–68). While the close connection between physical sex and object desire was, as Jennifer Terry notes, "eventually undermined as Freud's theories of sexuality gained greater notoriety and influence in the scientific community," fears about homosexuality have shaped popular discourse and certainly played an important role in the standard of care developed at Johns Hopkins even before Money's arrival (Eder 2010, 702). As Fausto-Sterling recounts in *Sexing the Body*, it would make sense for laypeople, particularly parents of children with intersex conditions at mid-century, to conflate homosexuality—still understood as a "disorder of psychologic sex"—with intersex.[24] "If," as she writes, "intersexuality blurred the distinction between male and female, then it followed that it blurred the line dividing heterosexual from homosexual." But even if parents made category errors that "pioneers" of medical management such as Money and John and Joan Hampson did not, Fausto-Sterling clarifies that heterosexual orientation nevertheless counted as a significant indicator of the success of medical management (2000, 72).[25]

This historical and psychic connection between homosexuality and intersex accounts for why resistance to the new nomenclature made sense on its face. It is, after all, the successful battle against the pathologization of homosexuality—its critical removal from the *Diagnostic and Statistical Manual of Mental Disorders* (*DSM*)—that has provided the foundation for the ongoing effort to secure social and political acceptance since the era of the "invert" (Bayer 1987). And certainly the intersex movement, from its inception in 1993, when Chase announced the formation of a support group for those with intersex conditions, has made use of the language and practices employed throughout the history of gay liberation and queer activism.[26] The very formation of the Intersex Society of North America was a reclamation of the term "intersex." Its publication of the newsletter "Hermaphrodites with Attitude" and the recording of the very first gathering of individuals with intersex conditions in the video *Hermaphrodites Speak!* (Chase 1996) evoke the rallying call for gay men and lesbians to "come out of the closets and into the streets," and bring to mind the contemporaneous activism of the 1990s practiced by groups like ACT UP and Queer Nation.[27]

It is not a mistake to see important differences in the ways that sex and gender are enforced. Ignoring the points where the experience and interests of those who are in some way "queer" diverge from those with DSD (a divergence that may occur as distinctive dimensions of experience even in a single body) risks obscuring the unique needs of those with DSD. These are the kinds of needs that medicine has ignored or marginalized to some degree in favor of a disproportionate, or in some cases even hysterical, concern with gender and genitalia. These include the "ordinary" kinds of health problems associated with diverse DSD, the sorts of challenges for which individuals with just about any other medical diagnosis would expect care as a matter of course.[28] CAH is not the only condition like this; hypopituitarism, a condition in which the pituitary gland does not produce typical amounts of different hormones it normally produces, is another example. Other conditions might require hormone replacement therapies as a result of the removal of gonads at risk for malignancy, or because gonads do not function at all (as is the case with some conditions), or their function is insufficient to prompt the pubertal changes that many individuals want.[29]

Where homosexuality was, as historian Jonathan Ned Katz (1995) put it, "an invention" of the nineteenth century, and the homosexual was, in Ian Hacking's (1986) terms, "a made-up person," disorders of sex development resist comparable characterization as productions of history.[30] That is not to say that there should not be histories of hermaphroditism. Daaboul's moving account of how an understanding of history dramatically changed his view of the standard of care and transformed the care he gave his patients is testimony enough of the value of such history. Even as there are what might be described as cultural constructions of hermaphroditism, many DSD are conditions that benefit from, or positively require, medical intervention. In this respect the history of intersex management may be more aptly compared with the storied past of a disease such as tuberculosis, as a medical condition whose "truth," as Hacking has put it, was slowly transformed by the late nineteenth-century discovery of the "brute fact . . . that [tuberculosis] is a disease transmitted by microbes." This discovery—of an underlying cause of a condition that had previously been attributed to a different sort of individual or societal "ill"—changed, but did not immediately displace, the earlier belief that "consumption was not only a sickness, but a moral failing, caused by defects of character" (Hacking 1986, 227). So while tuberculosis, unlike consumption, was recognized at last to be a disease caused by real and external pathogens, it was nevertheless considered in the United States "a disease of only some, not all people, essentially the immigrant and the poor, not the middle or upper classes" (S. Rothman 1994, 181).

The comparison between DSD and tuberculosis is a limited one: while some conditions (such as CAH and 5-alpha reductase deficiency, or ARD) can be heritable, DSD are not contagious.[31] Tuberculosis was associated with particular populations and activated government campaigns of public health; DSD are generally considered individual matters, and secrecy—intended to protect the privacy of individuals and families—is maintained.[32] The comparison may nevertheless serve to underscore the importance of attending to the underlying physiological condition of a disease or disorder, even as we take account of the abundance of social meanings at work—a dimension that the comparison to homosexuality, as I have suggested, risks minimizing. Invoking the historical case of tuberculosis suggests that there is room both for robust criticism of the stigma attached to the bodies of those who contract the disease (or those understood to be "at risk") and for appreciating the importance of treating the condition. If, at least for some period, social stigma and medical "truth" coexisted in the case of tuberculosis, we may similarly regard treatment of DSD to be in a state of transition.

The ongoing tension between treating intersex as a social problem (that has fallen to medicine to "cure") versus a medical problem (in the ordinary sense) is most starkly evinced by the fact that cosmetic genital surgeries for infants and children remain a significant component of care, so they understandably continue to occupy a central position in the controversy over treating affected children. The section on "Surgical Management" in the Consensus Statement reflects the equivocal position taken by medicine toward those with DSD. While surgery may be necessary to address specific problems caused by some conditions that carry a genuine risk of malignancy, such as "mixed" gonads, the statement's discussion of surgery foregrounds instead cosmetic procedures aimed at "normalizing" the appearance of the genitals. That the statement does not explicitly advocate surgery is a tremendous advance, but the acknowledgment that cosmetic surgery "relieves parental distress and improves attachment between the child and parents" should give pause. While, as the Consensus Statement admits, "the systematic evidence for this belief is lacking" (Hughes et al. 2006, 557) (and there's little sign that such evidence will be forthcoming), surgery is neither ruled out nor cautioned against. The statement raises questions about the real object of normalizing surgery, that is, for whose relief it is performed. Without substantial evidence or any apparent interest in an investigation that could produce such evidence, important aspects of the treatment rationale established in the United States at mid-century, while seemingly disavowed, were in fact reaffirmed.

2 "In Their Best Interests"
Parents' Experience of Atypical Sex Anatomy in Children

For Ruby, in memoriam

IN A STUDY conducted by psychologist Suzanne Kessler, college students were broken into two groups by gender. The women were asked to imagine that they had been born with "clitoromegaly," a condition defined as having a clitoris larger than one centimeter at birth. In response to a question regarding whether they would have wanted their parents to sanction clitoral surgery if the condition were not life-threatening, an overwhelming 93 percent of the students reported that they would not have wanted their parents to agree to surgery. Kessler reports, "Women predicted that having a large clitoris would not have had much of an impact on their peer relations and almost no impact on their relations with their parents . . . they were more likely to want surgery to reduce a large nose, large ears, or large breasts than surgery to reduce a large clitoris" (1998, 101).[1] These findings, Kessler reflects, are not surprising given that the respondents characterized genital sensation and the capacity for orgasm as "very important to the average woman, and the size of the clitoris as being not even 'somewhat important'" (101–102). Men in the study were faced with a different dilemma, the one facing parents of boys with "micropenis," a penis smaller than the putative standard of 2.5 centimeters stretched length at birth. Their question was whether to stay as male with a small penis or to be reassigned as female. More than half rejected the prospect of gender reassignment. But according to Kessler, "That percentage increases to almost all men if the surgery was described as reducing pleasurable sensitivity or orgasmic capability. Contrary to beliefs about male sexuality, the college men in this study did not think that having a micropenis would have had a major impact on their sexual relations, peer or parental relations, or self-esteem" (103).

In a separate study, Kessler and her team asked a different group of students to imagine that their child was born with ambiguous genitalia. Students in this study indicated they would make what Kessler describes as "more traditional choices" to consent to "corrective" or cosmetic surgery. Their rationales mirrored those of parents of children with atypical sex: students reported that they did not want their child to feel "different" and believed that early surgery would be less traumatizing than later surgery (103). Like parents over the last sixty years who have been faced with these difficult decisions, students did not reflect on the somatic experience of the child and with it the possibility of lost sensation that so concerned the students in the first study.

Kessler's paired studies confirm a kind of common sense that individuals, as individuals, are disinclined to compromise their erotic response for the sake of cosmetic enhancement. At the same time, parents, as parents, want what is best for their child, and the promise of a normal life figures prominently in that conception. The juxtaposition of the two studies raises the obvious, if nonetheless vexing, question: why would parents consent to procedures on behalf of their children that they would refuse for themselves?

The work of social theorist Pierre Bourdieu provides a powerful descriptive framework to account for what might be characterized as the ambivalence that marks parents' experience and the heavy responsibility they must bear to conceal that ambivalence from others and from themselves. As I learned from speaking to parents of children born with atypical sex anatomies, this responsibility is continuous with the vulnerability that attends all parents' efforts to do what is best for their children. All parents are, as parents, "vulnerable": in ways large and small they must rely on others in order to do their work as parents. And yet this vulnerability can be masked by parents' roles as protectors of their children (Kittay 1999; Lindemann 2006b). Though the parents with whom I spoke live thousands of miles away from one another, and a thirty-year difference separated the births of their children, their experiences were remarkably similar. All talked of their isolation as they carried the burden of the secrets doctors encouraged them to keep from their children, their neighbors, and their extended families. Those with grown children recounted the anger and despair of sons and daughters who could not have satisfying sex lives and who held them responsible for the silence to which they were subject. The situation of being a parent of a child with atypical sex anatomy presents a conflict in the intention to ensure "the best interests" of the child. The experience of those with whom I spoke reveals how parents' caring identification with their children may be forsaken in the well-intentioned effort to tend to these best interests.

The Imperative of Normality

While obvious on its face, the question of why parents would consent to normalizing genital surgeries is one of the most difficult raised by the conventional management of infants with DSD. Its difficulty lies, I think, in the fact that seeking answers demands that we investigate areas of understanding that are resistant to critical examination—areas we call common sense, or "what goes without saying." This is the realm that anthropologist and philosopher Pierre Bourdieu has called the "*habitus.*" It is not so easy to objectify a structure that natively resists such objectification, but understanding something of the mechanics of habitus promises insight into parents' experience. Bourdieu provides a number of ways of getting at how habitus works. It functions, he says, as "durable . . . dispositions," or "principles which generate and organize practices and representations that can be objectively adapted to their outcomes without presupposing a conscious aiming at ends or an express mastery of the operations necessary in order to attain them." It is at once a stable framework—a "structured structure"—and a dynamic "structuring structure" (1990 [1980], 53), ordering action and understanding in the seamless ways that we take for granted in ordinary life. Thus, as Bourdieu describes it, the understanding that is sustained by habitus is generally not a reflected understanding. Playing by "the rules" of habitus, in other words, does not entail an intention to follow the rules and does not require understanding or conscious recognition of the rules. For example, we take for granted the "fact" of sexual difference. That the world is comprised of men and women, boys and girls, orders our world and regulates practices in countless unreflected ways. That is not to say there isn't disagreement where questions of sex and gender are concerned. Indeed, controversy concerning what it means to be a man or a woman, what social roles and political rights these entail, is a thriving concern. But for the most part, sexual difference *as* sexual difference is not in dispute. In fact, sexual difference could be said to be the primary "structure" that itself "structures" the social order in which we move and make sense of the world. As such, it is also a structure that can be understood to make sense of us, that is, to place us in the world in ways that render the positions we occupy, the roles we play—as girls and boys, daughters and sons, mothers and fathers—intelligible; sexual difference provides order for the world and for our place in it.

Parents' wishes to have "normal" children and their fears about the consequences—for themselves and for their children—of living outside the norm are also products of this structuring structure. *Of course,* we might say, one wishes to have normal children; one could not wish for one's children anything but the easy path that normality promises. The concept of habitus marks this realm of the taken for granted, establishing that which is not questioned, what we could describe in philosophical terms as a kind of implicit normative order—a normative order that nowhere spells out the rules, that nowhere commands obedience to rules, but works to regulate practices in conformity with the prevailing expectations of a given society. If the medical management of children with atypical sex suggests that there are rules of normality that must be followed, these rules are not the rules of mere social convention, but something more along the lines of what might be described as a "cultural unconscious," conventions that are not considered and weighed and then thoughtfully enacted *by* individuals, but, should be understood to be working *through* individuals.

One might object that medical professionals—perhaps particularly John Money—have historically prescribed rules concerning gender. However, it does not appear that Money prescribed new rules of gender; rather, he formalized medical protocols that would be consistent with the rules of gender that were already in place. It was not Money who made the rule that there were "only two" sexes, only two ways to express or experience gender identity. However, to say that Money did not invent the rules of sex and gender is not to excuse him for the unethical practices and the deception he perpetrated on the scientific community and the public at large; nor does it absolve the physicians who continue to be faithful to his protocol despite the revelations of the deceptions Money engineered and promoted and the substantial harm that resulted. Bourdieu's analysis goes far, however, to suggest why Money's theories were so eagerly taken up by the medical community and why doctors continue today—often without explicit justification—to embrace the protocols established at Johns Hopkins.

What Kessler's paired studies suggest is that even as social conventions—of gender and of "good parenting"—powerfully enforce a discernible "regularity" in individuals' responses to given situations, these regularities, forceful as they are, can also be in conflict—an instance of competing habituses. Following Bourdieu, the conflict presented by the very appearance of ambiguous genitalia must be concealed lest it disrupt the taken-for-granted conceptions of normality that ground social practices. Parents of children with ambiguous genitalia, then, must not only bear the burden of the secret of their children's difference but must also be responsible for masking the tension produced by the necessity of concealing this difference. They must do so not only for themselves and their children but also for the sake of the preservation of the prevailing habitus itself.

Some Parents' Stories

From 1950 through the end of the century, parents make the briefest of appearances in the clinical literature on surgical correction of ambiguous genitalia in children.[2] The leading roles go to doctors who recommend and perform surgeries, and to the children themselves, who appear not so much as children but as discrete body parts: a hypospadiac penis in a "before" picture displayed urinating from a new meatus in an "after" picture; a large clitoris that is then shown after recession or trimming; or even a whole child with eyes concealed by a black patch to preserve anonymity. Neither sons nor daughters, but isolated organs or "subjects," such representations resist association with living children, complete with parents and communities. Despite the distorted images represented in the pictures, despite the difficulty one might face in imagining lives in place of body parts, parents' absence nevertheless becomes conspicuous when we consider the emphasis placed on parental response as a determining factor in the reported success of corrective surgery (e.g., Money and Erhardt 1982, 16). Thus, the silence surrounding parents' experience mirrors the silence parents are asked to maintain regarding their children's conditions.

As I discussed in my introduction, when I tried to make contact with parents of DSD-affected individuals in the spring of 2000, I encountered significant resistance and suspicion. Many parents thought that my interest was not actually in their stories or in their experience, but was instead a ploy to gain access to their children, of whose welfare they were so rightly protective. It was difficult for many parents, particularly parents of younger children, to understand why there would be any interest in their own stories. One reason may be owing to the unusual degree of isolation they experience, isolation that is consistent with the treatment protocol first advocated by John Money and accepted without significant challenge for more than three decades. Although parents of children with other congenital problems are urged to seek help, to join or form support groups, and to bring their children into contact with others like themselves, through the end of the twentieth century parents of children with ambiguous genitalia had not been given the opportunity to meet with other parents; nor was the possibility of consultation with mental health professionals with expertise in intersex or even gender development presented to them. At the same time that they were urged to keep the "truth" about their children to themselves, they were led to believe that the intersex condition has been corrected and that their children would grow up to be normal girls or boys. It may be easier to see why in this context parents found it difficult to understand themselves as subjects of interest in their own right.

Personal contacts introduced me to many of the parents of older and adult children I interviewed between May 2000 and August 2001; I found others, particularly those with younger children, through what were then new internet bulletin boards devoted to parents of children with medical conditions associated with atypical sex anatomies. Starting in 1993, when Cheryl Chase founded the Intersex Society of America, adults with intersex began to speak publicly about the debilitating physical and emotional effects of cosmetic genital surgeries; the disturbing questions raised by their stories had begun to be taken up by parents who faced, or who had recently consented to, surgeries for their children. Parents posting to these boards did not speak with the same voice; some wrote with confidence and certainty that their children had been "fixed," while others expressed anguish and confusion over their decisions. The parents who agreed to speak with me demonstrated a similar diversity, with a majority of those with older children critical of decisions they had once embraced. The mother I call Ruby was the first who agreed to speak with me, breaking a silence she had maintained for more than two decades. Both of Ruby's daughters, born a few years apart, had congenital adrenal hyperplasia. Girls and boys with the "classic," or "salt-losing," type of CAH (such as Ruby's daughters) require regular doses of the steroid cortisol, which they cannot produce on their own, as well as prescribed amounts of a salt-retaining hormone. Without such treatment, children will experience crises like those that brought both of Ruby's daughters close to death shortly after their births. While most DSD are not associated with medical conditions as severe as those suffered by Ruby's children, I begin with this story because it also highlights the distinctive nature and consequences of the treatment of medical and the cosmetic issues associated with DSD. It is also telling because despite significant refinements in cosmetic surgical techniques, Ruby's story presages the experience of parents ten, twenty, and even thirty years later.

Ruby's Story

Paige was born in 1961.[3] Doctors thought she was a boy. Her clitoris was enlarged, her labia fused. She was given a male name. But she became sick almost immediately. She couldn't breastfeed, she lost weight, and on New Year's Eve we took her to the ER. The doctors thought she was going to die, but one doctor knew about pediatric endocrinology, and transferred her to the children's hospital in the city. They diagnosed her with CAH and explained that she was female. She had no testicles, but a uterus and ovaries.

At three months, she hemorrhaged; her urethra was connected to her vagina. She had surgery, and they performed a clitorectomy at the same time. She had another surgery when she was two.

The same thing happened with my second daughter, Maggie. Everyone thought, "This one's the boy," but I knew. I just knew it was a girl, but we gave her a boy's name. When we brought her home she became very sick. So I insisted that I be sent to the children's hospital again. She was kept in the hospital for a long time, because the doctors thought that any talk about a son would upset my older daughter. At three months she had the clitorectomy. This was a female, and she needed to look like a female. They did leave tissue, but she had a series of infections and she had more surgeries—five by the time she was five years old. She has almost no clitoris left and massive scarring.

My daughters received medical care throughout their childhood. Once a month, sometimes more, we drove a whole day to get to the hospital. Fifteen hours there and fifteen hours back, with two active children in the backseat. And at the hospital I would have to fight the doctors. They would conduct a study on the salt levels and make my children sick, and I had to yell at them to stop. The doctors almost gave up on Maggie, and I took over a lot of her care. I had to dilate her urethra, and it was so hard. I did cultures for the doctors, too. I grew the bacteria, and the doctors would tell me what antibiotics to give her. I was the one who had to coordinate her care, and I was determined that my daughter not die because her mom didn't fight for her.

We were lucky to be part of these studies, though. As my daughters got older, they started to complain about the examinations. But somebody before my first child was born allowed these doctors—many doctors—to examine their child, to figure out what all this was about. Maggie is angry with me as an adult. She felt that she was raped, medically raped. And she's right. And I know how she feels. When you have a baby, you lose your right to modesty, and everyone is looking everywhere. But it was necessary, in my mind, just like when I gave birth. I told my daughters I wish we didn't have to do this. How would you feel having seventeen doctors look at you all at once? But it wasn't just that I felt a responsibility. This was a teaching hospital, and their treatment was being subsidized.

No one wanted to talk about the gender issues, how my daughters wouldn't play with their dolls. Both girls are gay. No one wanted to talk about that. Their father didn't want to deal with the gender issues at all, and his family thought that we had turned two little boys into girls. We divorced in 1976.

I had pastors who told me that they didn't know how to pray for me. And I told them, "I know how you can pray for me. You imagine a God who is bigger than all of these problems and you ask Him to help me."

As infants and young children, humans are vulnerable. Others, most often parents, must provide what these dependent beings cannot provide for themselves. Children who are ill or medically fragile are not exceptions in this respect; their needs magnify the needs that are common to all children—the needs for preservative love, fostering growth, and training for social acceptance (Ruddick 1989, cited in Kittay 1999, 33). As the needs of these children are magnified, so too are the corresponding demands upon parents with ill or medically fragile children. Those engaged in the practices of mothering will recognize the love that motivates Ruby's determination that her "daughter not die because her mom didn't fight for her." [4] Ruby's explanation to Paige and Maggie of the need to consent to invasive examinations reveals both an attempt to foster moral growth and to teach a difficult lesson in training for social acceptance. Other parents sacrificed their children's comfort so that doctors could help you, she tells them, and now we are obliged to do the same. And in life there are times that you must "go along to get along." Sometimes there's no choice.

Such lessons are ones with which Ruby herself had to grapple in the day-to-day care of her children. Having experienced the withdrawal of the support of her family—first by her in-laws, who believed she had robbed them of a grandson two times over, and then by her husband, who failed in so many ways to stand by his wife—Ruby found herself not only alone but also profoundly dependent upon the individual physicians managing the medical studies that subsidized her children's care. Refusal to consent to experimental treatments or yet another examination of her children's genitals would have put Ruby and her family at considerable financial, and thereby medical, risk. Caught in a bind of financial and medical exigency, Ruby could not really be understood to have had a choice in the matter. To refuse a medical intervention or examination would have effectively constituted a risk to her children's lives. This was a risk she would assume only at those times when she clearly perceived that an intervention itself posed a worse threat. That a mother would be faced with such a dilemma starkly underscores the special vulnerability to which Ruby was subject.

In *Love's Labor* Eva Kittay calls attention to the situation of those she calls "dependency workers," those who care for the "inevitably dependent." Parents of young children are dependency workers, as are those whose professional lives are dedicated to the care of the elderly or those with profound disabilities. As Kittay explains, dependency workers who care for the vulnerable are themselves vulnerable by virtue of a "secondary," or "derivative[,] dependency" (1999, x, 42; also see Fineman 1995, 162). The secondary dependency of parents is not always apparent in a culture in which parents' sovereignty over themselves and their children is presumed and valued. Although Ruby's situation is not different from that of any parent in this respect, it might be understood as an extreme variant of the vulnerability all parents face. Her vulnerability was most apparent with respect to physicians treating her children, but as Kittay's analysis makes clear, her vulnerability as mother to her daughters extended beyond the walls of the clinic.

The "Gender Issues"

What Ruby calls the "gender issues" form a part of any parent's child rearing. Training for social acceptance may require a mother to direct her daughter to behave at times "more like a girl" or teach her son to behave "more like a boy." In some cases a parent may come to believe that a social script dictating a particular gender behavior is not appropriate for her child. Parents with convictions concerning the problematic nature of gender scripts may resist the imperative that encourages them to direct their children to behave according to norms linked with a particular gender. For the most part, however, mothers generally harbor no doubts or anxieties about the "true sex" of their children. Absent such doubts or questions, a mother might shrug off a daughter's aversion to dolls. She needn't question whether her lack of interest is a sign that her daughter isn't "really a girl" or wonder whether she "did the right thing in treating her as a girl." Anxiety that parents may feel if a daughter prefers trucks or a son prefers dolls may be concerned not so much with their children's sex assignment but with the possibility that their child might experience homosexual desire, or identify as transgender. The difference between the kind of gender panic manifested by parents afraid that their "otherwise normal" girl or boy might be gay or trans and that experienced by parents of children with atypical sex anatomy is the fact that there's an apparently tangible "biological abnormality" to which the diagnosis of intersex points.[5]

As Ruby tells it, in her family's case questions about gender began with the criticism from her husband's family after they discovered that the children first announced as boys were, in fact, girls. In Ruby's memory there was no question that the surgeries would occur. She and her husband were informed of the necessity for genital surgery just as a parent would be informed that a child's congenital heart defect would have to be corrected. The consent to corrective surgery was not a question, but a printed form that she and her husband signed, like all the others concerned with procedures or administration of drugs their children required.

These issues came up again when the children were just about school age; Ruby remembers the support group that had been formed after doctors finally permitted parents involved in the long-term study of children with CAH to do so. While parents spoke about the challenges involved in staving off adrenal crises and communicating their children's medical needs to teachers and school nurses, the children played outdoors. Seeing their sons and daughters interact, parents began to take note of the fact that their girls and boys rarely split up along gender lines to play, and the parents of girls became interested in how similar their little "tomboys" were to the other girls in the group. Emboldened by her observations of the other children and understanding, for the first time, that she was not alone, Ruby started to raise questions. "*Why*," Ruby remembers insistently asking the doctors, "do my girls behave this way? And what can I do to help them be more like girls?" Most of the doctors at the hospital had no answers to her questions. One impatiently cut her short: "They're girls. What's the problem?" It is tempting to speculate that the repeated failures to respond meaningfully to Ruby's questions might be symptomatic of doctors' own anxiety over whether they had made the right decisions in the management of her daughters. Ruby herself suspected that it was the questions parents were beginning to raise that prompted doctors to withdraw their authorization of the support group and to take measures to ensure that it no longer met.[6]

Ruby understood that her job as a mother was to help her girls grow up to get along in this world. Being a female and acting like a man wasn't going to get them far. When Paige or Maggie had health problems associated with CAH, she insisted that her questions be answered; she could *do something* about these problems, whether that meant monitoring their cortisol levels or making sure they stayed hydrated. But when it came to the fact that her girls wouldn't "act like girls," she was on her own. It was here, where matters of gender were concerned, that support was conspicuously withheld by those charged with supporting her and where her own ability to provide support was undermined.

It would be many years before Ruby's daughters would be able to articulate the effects of the surgeries, and thus many years before she could understand the meaning of the consent she had provided. Ruby credits the close relationship she now enjoys with her older daughter, Paige, to hard work exploring these issues and to the help of a therapist Ruby sought out after her divorce. Ruby's involvement in Paige's life has also meant that she could be a resource to her close friend, another woman with CAH, whose mother never spoke to her about her condition. For many years, however, things were rougher with Ruby's younger daughter, Maggie, whose anger affected her intimate relationships as well as her relationships with her mother and sister. Ruby was—and remains—sympathetic to her daughter. She understands that Maggie's physical and emotional pain are constant reminders of the violation she experienced throughout her childhood. But her daughter's anger is difficult for Ruby, too, for it is a constant reminder of her role in inflicting the injury that caused it.

Vulnerability and Trust

As a parent, Ruby made decisions on behalf of her young children. Such is the responsibility of those responsible for meeting the needs of one who cannot meet them for herself. Kittay proposes the conception of a "transparent self" to describe the distinctive connection a dependency worker must try to maintain in order to make decisions for the dependent other in a responsible fashion. A transparent self is a "self through whom the needs of another are discerned, a self that, when it looks to gauge its own needs, sees first the needs of another" (1999, 51). While the achievement of a perfect transparency is not possible, Kittay advances the concept as a regulatory ideal to describe the attunement to the needs of another that is necessary to the successful performance of dependency work.[7]

In thinking about the standard cases of mothering, attunement to the needs of a child appears to take two primary forms. In the first form a mother can attend to the dependent child in ways that are sensitive to expressions of need that a child can express only imperfectly. For example, a mother can use attentive interpretive skills to discern whether an infant is crying because she is wet, hungry, or wants to be held. In the second form she can use what could be termed the "everyday social knowledge" she has as an adult to anticipate the needs that a child cannot. Such needs would include toilet training or skills required in social interaction with peers and adults. In addition, however, there is an array of needs to which a child may be subject and which the mother herself will require extensive assistance in order to satisfy. While a mother might be able to discern a child's discomfort in the common case of an earache, for example, she may not be able to discern the specific cause of the pain. Though the child may be able to express pain or discomfort, she cannot communicate what she needs to treat her medical condition; everyday social knowledge does not usually provide such professional/technical information. Where the two primary forms of attunement are not finally effective in meeting the needs of her charge, as in the case of an earache or other medical problem, the mother must depend on doctors' "expert knowledge" to both understand and respond to the needs of her child. Cases such as Ruby's are complicated by the fact that the expert knowledge she is offered as definitive of what her children need may not itself be attuned or sensitive to the genuine needs of her children.

In the paradigm case of a dependency relationship as Kittay sees it, three aspects define the labor of the dependency worker:

It is the work of tending to others in their state of vulnerability—*care*. The labor either sustains ties among intimates or itself creates intimacy and trust—*connection*. And affectional ties—*concern*—generally sustain the connection, even when the work involves an economic exchange. For the dependency worker, the well-being and thriving of the charge is the primary focus of the work. In short, the well-being of the charge is the responsibility of the dependency worker. (1999, 31; original emphasis)

To all appearances Ruby both understands and assumes her responsibilities in just the way Kittay describes. There can be no question that Ruby cares deeply about her daughters or that her concern for their well-being could be described as anything less than fierce. In the paradigm case of a dependency relationship, connection cannot but be understood as a necessary corollary of care and concern.

Where Ruby's own experience fell short of her ability to discern her daughters' needs, she learned what was necessary to identify them. More than thirty years later she remains an expert on her daughters' CAH symptoms, identifying imminent crises before her daughters themselves recognize them. And yet her connection to her daughters, particularly her younger daughter, Maggie, was strained for many years—the result, all agree, of the treatment of their atypical sex anatomies. It was not Ruby who performed the surgery or conducted the exams, but it was Ruby who—willing or not, witting or not—sanctioned these actions. The tragic paradox of Ruby's situation is precisely this: her caring and concerned attempts to fulfill her responsibility to her daughters' well-being led her to consent to actions that resulted in harm to her daughters and to an erosion of her connection with them that required sustained work to rebuild. Ruby's situation exemplifies how the imperative of care, itself shaped by habitus, works through parents and can direct us to ask how harm can result from "good" care.

If Ruby fulfilled her responsibility to Paige and Maggie the best way she knew how, her "knowing how" was tainted by the flawed expert knowledge on which she had to depend. The possibility of effecting harm in an effort to do right by one's charge is certainly a risk for any dependency worker. In this sense Ruby's situation exemplifies the sometimes perilous nature of dependency work generally. Ruby's marked dependence on, and vulnerability to, her children's doctors magnifies an important relationship not immediately apparent in examinations of dependency relationships, namely, the relationship of the dependency worker to the third party Kittay calls a "provider" (1999, 44). A provider is a person responsible for the supply or regulation of some significant external resources. A provider may be the head of a household, who supplies financial support necessary to the maintenance of a child or other dependent. In Ruby's case the provider who figures most prominently in her life and that of her children is the hospital medical team managing her daughters' care. Even as a provider enables a dependency worker to do her work by supplying necessary resources, a provider may also limit the autonomy of that worker by exploiting her dependency to carry out some other agenda, an agenda the provider himself might not even be aware of. The relationship between a provider and a dependency worker, like that between a dependency worker and her charge, then, is characterized fundamentally by inequality (45). Ruby's daughters received lifesaving care as a result of the beneficent intervention of their doctors. But at the same time, the doctors' management of what Ruby calls the "gender issues"—that is, their insistence on cosmetic genital surgeries and their failure to address issues related to the nonconforming behavior of her children—wreaked havoc in their lives.

Trust is crucial to the success of the relationship between a parent and child. The fraying of trust between Ruby and her daughters is not due to any questionable intentions on Ruby's part. Rather, it is Ruby's own vulnerability to her children's doctors that renders fragile her relationship with her daughters. Paige and Maggie experienced pain, momentary and enduring, physical and emotional, as a result of decisions in which Ruby participated. And yet, isolated by doctors and herself subject to forced collusion in the secrecy of her children's treatment, Ruby's own vulnerability was exploited and so exacerbated.

Precisely because inequality characterizes the relationship between parent and child, trust is essential to the success of that relationship (Kittay 1999, 35). If trust that an abuse of power will not occur is essential, the illegitimate exercise of power—domination—is anathema to the parent-child relationship (34). At several points Ruby's story illustrates the illegitimate exercise of power. Domination manifests itself in the physical scars on her daughters' bodies; it reveals itself in Maggie's difficulty in forming intimate relationships; and it is evident in the emotional rift that characterized Ruby's relationship with Maggie for so many years. At the same time, however, it is difficult to apply the term "domination" to a situation such as Ruby's. Domination, as most understand it, is associated with a willful agent of power, and while the illegitimate exercise of power has left its mark, it is nonetheless difficult to locate the agent who left those marks. Ruby, who went to such lengths to ensure her children's well-being, is an unlikely agent of domination. As Ruby tells it, the doctors, too, make for poor culprits: those recommending and performing genital surgeries do not intend harm; on the contrary, it was their firm belief that genital surgeries were essential to the healthy psychosexual development of a child born with atypical sex anatomy. Doctors who ask that patients make themselves available to colleagues and medical residents for repeated examination by medical personnel do not mean for patients to experience violation; rather, they understand themselves to be engaged in important educational work that advances medical progress. And yet the injury suffered by Ruby's daughters, by Ruby herself, and by the many others who have spoken out against normalizing genital surgeries, points to the exercise of power absent "moral legitimacy" (34).

Mary's Story

Twenty-five years after Ruby's first child was born, a young mother named Mary brought her twelve-year-old daughter, Jessica, to the pediatrician. The day before, Jessica had just come out of the shower after a ballet lesson when Mary noticed, out of the corner of her eye, a "growth" emerging from her daughter's labia. Mary had called the doctor, who agreed that Mary should bring Jessica in the following morning. Her daughter did not question why they would be going to the doctor. "Jessica was the type of child who never questioned me. She never spoke back. Never. Because she wanted to make me—us, her parents—happy, and not displease us."

That same day, Jessica's pediatrician sent her to a pediatric endocrinologist. A sonogram revealed that Jessica did not have a uterus, but undescended testes.

> The pediatric endocrinologist asked to speak with me alone. Jessica was in a different room. The doctor and I then sat and she explained to me that Jessica had XY chromosomes and Jessica would not be able to bear children. She also explained to me that this was something I should never, ever bring up with Jessica. I should never talk about it with Jessica. We should just take care of it as quickly as possible so that Jessica could live a normal life. I agreed to this because it was what [the doctor] asked me to do. I was very young at the time. I was just in my late twenties.
>
> Naturally I was shocked; I was stunned, I was saddened. I went home and told my husband, who had just come back from work. I told him all about it, what the pediatric endocrinologist said. I had never seen him cry before, but he just broke down and sobbed in my arms. That's when it impacted me the most . . . There were a lot of tears, a lot of feeling bad for Jessica, knowing that she couldn't have children naturally.

Androgen insensitivity syndrome (AIS) is a condition in which a fetus with a normal (46,XY) male karyotype is unable to absorb androgens in utero. In its "complete" form, AIS would result in a child with typical feminine external genitalia and undescended testes. Jessica, Mary would learn, had "partial" AIS. Her body could absorb some androgens, and at puberty an enlargement of the clitoris could result. Mary was instructed to tell Jessica that "her ovaries hadn't developed properly and they would have to come out." Jessica was not told that her testes would be removed because doctors feared they would become cancerous. Nor was she informed of the "clitoroplasty" that would be performed at the same time.[8]

Just a month later, Jessica was in the recovery room of the children's hospital. Mary remembers finding her daughter moaning in bed as she recovered from the anesthesia. She thought it was only from the pain, but Jessica has since told her that, having reached down, she realized that "a piece of her was gone." In the week that Jessica spent in the hospital, she was told nothing directly about the procedure she had undergone. Doctors did inform her, however, that she would have to return to the hospital in a week to evaluate the effects of what they called "the plastic surgery."

Mary remembers that before the surgery, immediately after, and in the follow-up evaluation, "scores of male residents would come in to examine" her daughter. Mary had consented to the examinations because she knew that her daughter was being treated in a teaching hospital. It was not until years later, when Jessica had obtained her medical records and confronted her parents with what she had learned, that Mary would hear from her daughter's mouth the terrible effects not only of the surgery and the deception but of the repeated examinations as well.

Looking back, it seems obvious to Mary that her daughter, who regarded her enlarged clitoris as perfectly normal, would have experienced the surgery and the examinations as painful violations. But if at the time Mary entertained such thoughts, she put them out of her mind. She remembers asking whether she should seek counseling for Jessica and, in response, was told the story of another girl with AIS who, as a teenager, had stolen a look at her records when the doctor was called out of the office. That girl, the doctors informed Mary, had had to be placed in a psychiatric institution as a result of learning "the truth." The surgery had taken care of the problem, Mary was told, and further discussion would only raise potentially damaging questions for Jessica. What was important was that Jessica look normal. If she looked normal, she would "be able to live her life as a normal girl."

A Failure of Identification

When Mary speaks of the importance of the "normal appearance" of her daughter's genitals, it is difficult to discern whether her remarks reflect her own concerns or those of the doctors. As Kessler reported in her 1990 article, appearance, as opposed to sensation, was the governing criterion determining whether genital surgery (and in some cases a change in gender assignment) was indicated (1990, 18–21).[9] Perhaps it should not be surprising that parents of children with atypical sex anatomies follow the lead of doctors when it comes to making sense of a condition they have most likely encountered for the first time and that was—and may continue to be—presented in ways that exacerbate the disorientation that it has provoked. Mary's response, as well as Ruby's, reflects the experiences of many other parents.[10] But in focusing on genital appearance rather than the experience of the child, a parent puts both her child and her relationship to her child at risk.

Mary's story underscores one of the recurrent themes implicit in Ruby's narrative, namely, what might be described as a *failure of identification* with her child. Parents, particularly mothers, are widely taken to have a kind of privileged knowledge of their children. Psychologists and other specialists in child development speak of the special attentiveness or attunement that a mother must cultivate in order to meet the needs that an infant and young child can express only imperfectly. Cultivation of this special connection is necessary in the child's development, and as a normal part of development it is also expected to diminish as the child grows and is capable of increasing self-sufficiency.[11] In the case of children with genital ambiguity, it appears that a parent may be forced to forsake this attunement to a child's needs or desires and put aside what her own common sense would tell her about her own desires and her own bodily experience in exchange for the promise of a child who will "look normal."[12]

It may be discomfiting for parents—or even, in the case of the students queried in Kessler's study, those simply imagining themselves in the position of parents—to focus on the feeling in a child's genitals; many parents may understandably resist what might be regarded as a kind of sexualization of their child. However, the case of children with atypical sex anatomy demands that parents take account of just those feelings in order to make an informed decision and fulfill their obligations as parents. To do that, parents require the assistance of the experts on whom they must rely when their own knowledge proves insufficient. It would have been interesting if the researchers in Kessler's team had asked the students participating in the first study—the study asking whether they would have wanted their own parents to have consented to surgery—what they would have done if faced with the decision of whether to consent to surgery for their children. If such questions had been included, it is possible that students in the first group would have been more disposed to identify with the children and to be more cautious about making cosmetic surgical decisions than those in the group asked only what they would do if they had a child born with atypical sex anatomy.

The juxtaposition of Kessler's studies suggests a conflict between the needs of an individual child and the norms and expectations that govern society. A parent's obligation to her child is complicated by the fact that socialization is also constitutive of her child's needs. But socialization, or the necessity to adjust one's behavior or person to the culture to which one belongs, is not generally taken to be a parent's primary obligation. As Kittay writes, "A mother, acting in a manner compatible with the norms of maternal practice, does not force her child to sacrifice the child's own well-being for another's benefit. Such coercion is not commensurate with a maternal practice that remains true to the well-being of the child" (1999, 71). When parents are presented with medical situations for which they can provide no context—and so are unable to make judgments concerning what is right for their children—they must rely on doctors to provide direction and advice. In place of the parent who has shared such a close relationship to her child, the parent becomes an agent of her daughter's violation. But parents who act as agents of violation are at the same time objects of domination. Their relationship with their child is compromised, and the parent, as a parent, is compromised by virtue of her inability to identify with her child.

Normality by Other Means: Sarah's Story

From my first interview with Ruby to one of the last I conducted in 2001—with the mother of four-month-old identical twin girls who were still recovering from surgery—there was a notable consistency in the experience they shared. All of their children had undergone surgery, and all, including those who had recently consented to surgery and believed they had done the right thing, expressed some degree of ambivalence.[13] Among the parents I interviewed, however, there was one story that was exceptional. Sarah's is a story that begins in the early 1990s, after an uneventful pregnancy, a natural childbirth, and a child pronounced a "girl." But, Sarah recounts,

> it was funny because I had an immediate intuition that told me they had gotten it wrong as they announced, "it's a girl." And I remember after he was born that there was a little bit of hesitancy with the nurses as they weighed and checked him. That morning [my son] returned from the nursery . . . and I could see from the pediatrician's face that something was wrong. But I kept thinking, I was prepared for everything! I had a birth plan with everything that I wanted to happen, accounting for every possibility . . . but this. Because I'd never heard of this.
>
> Gender is supposed to be a given. You have either a boy or a girl. But they said, "We have a problem: We're not sure your baby is a girl."
>
> "What do you mean? How can you not tell if a baby is a boy or girl? What's the problem?"
>
> "Well," the doctor said, he "couldn't find a vaginal opening." And I immediately began to think about all these terrible talk shows, because that's the thing you have a reference to . . . They said, "We have to do more tests."

The prospect of a newborn fit for the likes of daytime talk shows was a chilling one. The small hospital in which delivery had taken place was ill-equipped to deal with anomalies such as atypical sex, but having had a case several years earlier the doctors knew to summon experts and to maintain the privacy of the mother and child, "to protect us from other parents, who might be inquisitive about what was happening in the nursery." The secrecy and heavy mood of the hospital staff, together with Sarah's ignorance in the face of an unexpected—even unfathomable—event, cast a pall over the birth of her child. Her outlook quickly improved, Sarah remembers, with the thoughtful intervention of a labor nurse who "knew someone who knew someone with a daughter with CAH." It was that mother who came to the hospital the very next day and helped ease the anxiety and worry that a first-time, single mother faced at the frightening news of a child born with genital ambiguity. Another important source of support came from her own mother, a retired La Leche League leader who had helped raised Sarah to understand that although her child's doctors possessed an unmistakable expertise, history shows us that there were a number of things they had gotten wrong, particularly where a paternalistic approach to medical care of infants was concerned.[14] Sarah's own attendance of La Leche League meetings during pregnancy had equipped her for the birth and early raising of her child in a way that, she now reflects, gave her the resources to advocate for and raise questions about the care of her child.

Sarah hadn't wanted to name her child until she saw the baby. She had prepared on a single sheet of paper a list of possible girls' names on one side and a list of possible boys' names on the other. On both sides of the sheet appeared the name "Robin," which was, as Sarah saw it, the obvious choice for her new son.

Seeing that Robin was thriving, and tremendously relieved after having spoken with the mother raising a daughter with CAH, Sarah was able to dispel the frightening images that accompanied the announcement that her child might not be a girl. When they shopped for diapers that week, she and her mother wondered together whether it would make sense to buy those marked "boys" or whether the "girls" diapers were more practical, laughing when they caught the confused stare of an eavesdropping shopper.[15] Sarah and her mother went to the doctor for a first consultation with light hearts. They were singing, finally celebrating the arrival of the baby. They had brought a recording of a favorite song by the children's folksinger and educational psychologist Peter Alsop titled "It's Only a Wee Wee" (1997) and played it for the doctors and nurses during the visit, wanting to communicate that what had been presented (and initially received) as devastating news might not warrant such gravity. Although the song is intended to make light of gender difference, Sarah reheard the song in more literal terms after Robin's birth:

> As soon as you're born, grownups check where you pee
> And then they decide just how you're s'posed to be
> Girls pink and quiet, boys noisy and blue
> seems like a dumb way to choose what you'll do
> [chorus]
> Well it's only a wee wee, so what's the big deal?
> It's only a wee wee, so what's all the fuss?
> It's only a wee wee and everyone's got one
> There's better things to discuss!
> Now girls must use makeup, girl's names and girl's clothes
> And boys must use sneakers, but not pantyhose
> The grownups will teach you the rules to their dance
> And if you get confused, they'll say "Look in your pants"
> . . . .
> Now grownups watch closely each move that we make

Boys must not cry, and girls must make cake
It's all very formal and I think it smells
Let's all be abnormal and act like ourselves

For all her open-mindedness concerning gender roles, however, Sarah also understood that her initial distress on hearing the news of Robin's difference was not aberrant: this was how the world would see her child and, she believed, there was little hope for change. After a series of tests to determine whether Robin's body would respond to testosterone, she agreed, on her doctors' strong recommendation, to an initial series of surgeries, including primary hypospadias repair, cosmetic surgery of his scrotum, and relocation of his testes, which had not descended in utero.[16]

> At the time it seemed like the right thing to do, but I should have done more research then; by now I've talked to people who've had hypospadias repair, and they've gone through hell. It's all about peeing standing up, but the body has ways of undoing these surgeries. He's developed a leak . . . If I knew then what I know now . . .

Sarah's understanding underwent a transformation after the birth of Robin. She sought out adults with conditions like her son's and has heard the tragic stories of men and women who have undergone any number of surgeries (see, e.g., Devore 1999). When first presented with "the problem" of her son's difference, Sarah could imagine only the alternatives proposed by the doctors. From the adults with intersex conditions with whom she became acquainted she learned that the poor surgical outcomes were only a small part of the pain they experienced. They were robbed, she believes, of the signature experiences—the "normal kid stuff"— that she regards as crucial in a child's life: they didn't take baths with other kids, didn't run around naked in sprinklers in hot summers. Children with conditions like Robin's often made repeated visits to the hospital, spending school breaks at home recovering from surgeries rather than going to summer camp. While at first daunted by the prospect of preparing her child for a world hostile to his physical difference, Sarah came to believe that she didn't have to take on the world to care for her child, that is, to make him feel safe and to feel normal. Rather than focusing her energies on promoting a sense of normalcy through concealing Robin's difference and making it a secret, Sarah aimed through his childhood to facilitate the life experience that would normalize this difference:

> I developed friendships where [people] were supportive and knew about Robin, and then he did have kids to run around naked in sprinklers with, and he did have kids to take baths with, and he did all that normal stuff . . . Kids knew he was different, but that was okay, and he learned that everyone, really, looks different from everyone else no matter what mold they come from.

If Sarah's story is remarkable, it is not because her commitment to her child's well-being rivals that of other parents. But even as it stands apart from others' experiences—flying in the face of prevailing management of atypical sex anatomies—it is an approach to raising a child that exemplifies the same principles of common sense that informed the acceptance of the recommendations made to other parents. This fact may explain the intensity of the anger that adults who have undergone surgery demonstrate: the betrayal they experience is a measure of the distance they feel from their parents.

Perhaps the hardest lesson the experience of parents with atypical genitalia teaches is that there can be a conflict between caring for your child, in the sense of being attuned to a child's needs, and wanting "what's best" for your child. The conventional wisdom of what's best tells parents that their child should be spared the "mark of difference." While normalizing genital surgery promises the erasure of that mark, parents and their children are faced with a lifetime of concealment of that difference and with the shame and guilt that that concealment entails.

For Whose Sake?

Neither the doctors nor the parents with children with atypical sex anatomies can take for granted the fact of sexual difference, and yet they can, and generally do, continue to abide by its rules. The parents with whom I spoke shared an interest in maintaining the secret of intersex because others' ignorance or cruelty could harm their children. But did they do so for the children's sake? The silence that parents have maintained to protect their children protects parents, too, from a kind of guilt by association. As one parent of a girl with mixed sex chromosomes remembers asking before her birth, "What sort of people would give birth to a hermaphrodite?" While such a message cannot be attributed to doctors, their counseling of the parents with whom I spoke nevertheless suggests that their view could be characterized in similar terms: "what sort of *parents* would subject their child to life as a hermaphrodite?" The challenge for Ruby, Mary, and Sarah—the job of any parent—is not only to protect one's child but also to accommodate her to the world in which she lives. If, in the case of children with atypical sex anatomies, cosmetic genital surgery is presented to parents as a necessary adjustment, it is only too easy to understand why parents would consent to its performance.

Although parents are expected to be "attuned" to their children, such identification is discouraged in parents of children with atypical sex anatomies. Parents are not given the chance to imagine their children's lives in any way except as in need of immediate correction. Despite the fact that doctors know, for instance, that later surgeries are often less dangerous and more likely to produce desirable results—both with respect to appearance and the preservation of sensation—they nevertheless promote early surgery. They claim that children will experience less trauma if they are spared memories of removal of gonads or the excision of phallic tissue. For decades, doctors understated the eventual necessity of painful vaginal dilation in the case of the (majority of) children assigned female. The likely prospect of additional surgeries or other traumatic procedures in subsequent years has also gone unmentioned, as has the option of delaying surgery until the child is older. If, as the experiences of the parents I interviewed suggest, decisions were not made *for* parents, they could be understood to have been made *through* them: parents are not simple instruments of doctors' agendas. At the same time, however, their decisions cannot be regarded as products of an uncompromised agency. Similarly, doctors' failure to present a complete picture to parents may be seen not as a conscious and deliberate effort to mislead parents for the sake of maintaining a clear division between male and female, but as a function of habitus, which works, as Bourdieu understands it, to reproduce itself.

The very fact of atypical sex anatomy—that is, the material evidence that sex is not an either/or proposition, but rather exists on a continuum—poses a threat to the current construction of habitus—a threat that is managed by the prevention of the very possibility of posing questions about it.

> The *habitus* is a principle of the selective perception of indices tending to confirm and reinforce it rather than transform it, a matrix generating responses adapted in advance to all objective conditions identical to or homologous with the (past) conditions of its production; it adjusts itself to a probable future which it anticipates and helps to bring about because it reads it directly in the present of the presumed world, the only one it can ever know. (Bourdieu 1990 [1980], 64)

The dispositions that motivate the practices associated with normalizing genital surgery must be very narrowly concerned with the reinforcement of "the present of the presumed world." Consider doctors' resistance to reconsidering standard practices despite the publication of critical narratives by adults with intersex through the late 1990s, stories that resonated alarmingly with the "true story" of John/Joan.[17] Consider the insistence with which doctors promote surgical interventions similar to practices known in developing countries as "female circumcision," prohibited by U.S. federal legislation in 1996.[18] When the American Academy of Pediatrics declared the birth of a child with ambiguous genitalia a "social emergency" (2000, 138) without explaining the nature of this emergency, it was perhaps because there was little question of the threat that the revelation of intersex posed to the existing social order.

The clouding of the transparent self in the case of parents of children with atypical sex is a function of habitus. At the same time, Kittay's analysis indicates the presence of an imperative—itself the product of habitus—acting on the dependency worker to develop a transparent self that is capable of being attuned to what one's charge may experience and to act on behalf of that charge in a way that respects and aims to ensure the future agency of the child. While, as Kittay acknowledges, many forms of dependency can be taken to be natural or inevitable, the ways that dependency may be regarded and understood, and the ways that dependency work may be conceived, are neither natural nor inevitable. The normative force of the conception of the transparent self demonstrates the extent to which the very concept is embedded in habitus. But here the habitus functions at the same time to cloud the transparent self. In the abstract ethical terms of care we return finally to the apparently irreconcilable tension reflected in the questions raised by Kessler's research.

Kessler's paired studies point to a contradiction between what individuals would wish for themselves and what they would feel was "right" for their children. In the space of this contradiction, we may, or perhaps we must, ask: *What if* parents identified with their children as Sarah has done? *What if* parents opted to understand the decision to perform cosmetic genital surgery as the child's, that is, to forgo immediate corrective surgery until the child was capable of making the choice him or herself? Understanding the current management of intersex as a function of habitus suggests the radical potential of a dependency critique. If parents of children with atypical sex anatomies were to work to identify with their children, if doctors were to use their considerable authority to promote acceptance of genital variation instead of erasure, the prevailing habitus would shift. Not only would such a positive identification lead to improved relationships between parents and children, but it would also work against the conservative principles of habitus to effect social change.

3 Tilting the Ethical Lens
Shame, Disgust, and the Body in Question

Whom do you call bad? —One who always wants to put to shame.
What do you consider most humane? —to spare someone shame.
What is the seal of liberation? —No longer being ashamed in front of oneself.
—Friedrich Nietzsche, *The Gay Science*

OVER THE LAST fifty years, people with atypical sex anatomies have been objects of intense medical scrutiny. The term "intersex" encompasses a wide variety of conditions, the common feature of which involves some expression of sexual ambiguity: an intersex body's appearance doesn't match its karyotype or its sex of assignment; external genitalia or gonads are not distinctively male or female; or sex chromosomes are atypical in some fashion—there's an "extra" or missing X or Y, or even, though more rarely, a mosaic of chromosomes that includes a whole variety of combinations.[1]

The treatment protocols for infants and children with intersex conditions —which have frequently involved cosmetic genital surgery and sometimes sex reassignment—were originally formalized by psychologist John Money in the 1950s. For Money and his collaborators, "the problem" of intersex was the incongruence between the "biological sex" (which could be a confusing matter in cases of hermaphroditism) and what they called "gender role," the combination of one's social presentation and individual identity as masculine or feminine. Surgical intervention and hormone therapy, they argued, could facilitate this congruence. In their view, early intervention was necessary to ensure the consistent socialization—particularly with regard to parents' certainty about their child's sex of assignment—that would avert the "psychological disturbance" for which children would otherwise purportedly be at risk (Money 1955; quoted in Karkazis 2008, 55).

Perhaps even better known than the details of these pioneering protocols and the theories that ground them was the revelation in the mid-1990s that Money's career-making case of John/Joan was not the touted breakthrough featured in *Time* and in college classrooms, but a wrenching and wretched failure. In chapter 1 I recounted the story of the boy who suffered a circumcision accident and was then raised a girl, the story that stood for years as the evidence supporting Money's theory of the malleability of gender development and the soundness of what almost immediately became the standard of care in the treatment of children with atypical sex anatomies. Rather than being the successfully reared girl reported in national news, "Joan" rejected the role assigned him and lived most of his tragically short life as a man. But the story of the creation and acceptance of the treatment protocols gets stranger and more confounding still: Money's own research, presented in his doctoral dissertation—a study that involved a remarkable sample of 248 cases of individuals with intersex, did not support the direction his work took immediately after its completion.[2] His investigation of "the relationship of psychosexual conflict to the processes of psychopathology" in children with intersex conditions yielded what Money described as "disconcerting" conclusions: "One would not have been surprised had the paradox of hermaphroditism been a fertile source of psychosis and neurosis. The evidence, however, shows that the incidence of the so-called functional psychoses in the most ambisexual of the hermaphrodites—those who could not help but be aware that they were sexually equivocal—was extraordinarily low" (1952, 6). If individuals with intersex conditions do not, as Money himself reports, "break down under the strain" produced by their "manifest sexual problems," but instead "make an adequate adjustment to the demands of life" (10), we must ask what could have motivated his later recommendations to perform what are widely recognized to be disfiguring surgeries. And why would physicians have been so quick to adopt these standards (Karkazis 2008, 60) in the face of what would seem to be the likely concern that such surgeries would be damaging both physically and emotionally? As I also noted in chapter 1, Sandra Eder presents a compelling historical answer to the first question, namely, that Money's role at Johns Hopkins entailed not innovation of a new model so much as a formalization of the optimal gender approach developed by Lawson Wilkins. But understanding more about the influence that Wilkins, and then Money, maintained in the field does not go so far to answer the second question, regarding the eagerness of physicians to adopt these standards.

Cheryl Chase has argued that "the problem" of intersex is one of "stigma and trauma, not gender" (2003, 240). The trauma to which Chase refers is constituted in large part by the shame that appears so consistently to characterize the experience of children diagnosed with intersex, the wide variety of conditions now clinically termed "disorders of sex development." References to shame abound in the critical and narrative literature concerning intersex. And yet shame has not been a sustained focus of analysis in this work. This gap may be due to the fact that not only is it painful to think about shame, but it is also the case that reflecting on shame in this context requires that we consider the disgust that provokes it. The aim of this chapter is to ask what it would mean if disgust turns out to have had a dominant influence on the medical management of DSD. What would be the function of disgust, and what would be the consequences—material and moral—with respect to the shame it provokes?

Conventional ethical approaches may not provide quite the right tools to consider this affective dimension of the medical management of DSD, but Friedrich Nietzsche's *On the Genealogy of Morality* provides a framework that allows us a profound appreciation of its moral significance. Understanding doctors' disgust—and the disgust they promote in parents of those born with atypical anatomies—as a contemporary expression of what Nietzsche called "*ressentiment*" would direct us to focus not on the bodies of those born with intersex conditions, which have been the privileged objects of attention both in medical practice *and* in criticisms of it, but rather on the bodies of those whose *responses* constitute the initial force for normalizing practices.[3]

Though for Money "the problem" of intersex is gender and genitalia and for Cheryl Chase it is shame and stigma, both locate the problem in intersexed bodies. For both, the treatment of intersex is finally a matter of normalization. Money presents "normalization" as a positive, healthy intervention, a repairing of a malfunction, whether in nature (as in the case of chromosomal abnormalities) or wrought by human error (in the case of a hideously botched circumcision or administration of progestin in pregnant women). For Chase, normalization takes on a Foucaultian cast and marks the making of monstrosity (Foucault 2003 [1999], 71): the treatment of atypical sex anatomies makes of those with these anatomies horrible problems that medicine seeks to "fix," both in the sense of defining a new (and fixed) kind of pathological type and in the imperative to "repair" the abnormal anatomies marking this type. What George Annas described as a "'monster' approach" to ethics (1987, 28), developed with respect to emergency separation surgeries for conjoined twins, inspired an early argument against normalizing surgeries by Alice Dreger. Following Annas, Dreger (1998a) refers to the reasoning shaping normalizing approaches as "monster ethics," which can be summed up in this way: you (conjoined twins, or babies with atypical sex anatomies) are monsters, and we're going to make you human; after we make you human, the rules of human ethics will apply.[4] Seeing this moment of the production of monstrosity as an ethical problem calls us to consider more carefully Nietzsche's contribution to moral reasoning. Following Nietzsche's lead entails a redirection of the ethical gaze that casts "the problem" of intersex as a problem of ressentiment. Certainly I do not mean to suggest any equivalence in the positions of Money and Chase; rather, my aim is to locate the problem not in the bodies of those with atypical sex anatomies but in the ressentiment of "everyone else."[5] This is not to deny that intersex is also a problem of gender, as Money would have it, or a problem of stigma and shame. But casting the problem in Nietzschean terms, turning our attention to the agents of moral reasoning and not the objects, changes the way we understand these other problems and yields different responses to them. A Nietzschean approach provides clarity about the ethical questions we must recognize here, and also illuminates the metaethical construction of the questions that we pose.

I identify doctors' disgust—and with it, the corrective surgeries they recommend and perform—as contemporary expressions of the ressentiment Nietzsche sees as the source of our moral intuitions. Through understanding disgust in Nietzschean terms, we may better appreciate the shame that so often characterizes the experience of those who have been subject to the standard of care in the management of intersex. The inculcation of shame could be understood as a tool employed by what Nietzsche calls "slave morality." A thoroughgoing application of Nietzsche's concept of ressentiment also requires that we reckon with what at first might seem to be an unlikely dimension of the response that results in normalizing practices enacted upon the bodies of infants and young children: envy.

Interlude: With the Best of Intentions

Over the course of the year I interviewed parents of children with atypical genitalia, I was fortunate to have the opportunity to speak with some among the small group of physicians who had once recommended and performed cosmetic genital surgeries but later had changes of heart. Rather than continue this work, they had become allies in the emerging movement of resistance to these surgeries.

There was one physician I was especially interested in meeting, as his revelation of the moral wrong he had been committing was brought about by a sabbatical study in bioethics. By his own account, it was studying philosophy, particularly the work of the canonical thinkers in ethics whose work forms the foundation for contemporary bioethical guidelines, that made him ask, for the first time, whether the prevailing standard of care for those with atypical sex anatomies was in fact a violation of ethical principles.

For those of us who are repeatedly confronted by skepticism about the value of our discipline, the experience of this physician offers an extraordinary narrative with which to respond to questions concerning the "use" of philosophy that, as John McCumber reminds us, dates back to the origins of the discipline (2001, 29–30). Reading philosophy was not only personally transformative for this doctor, but it made a material difference in people's lives. Who knows how many infants and young children were spared unnecessary genital "correction" and with it the shame and isolation that have been so frequently experienced by entire families with children born with intersex conditions? Other physicians might be inspired by his example, and the effects of this doctor's encounter with philosophy would reverberate far beyond his own person and those of the patients he directly serves.

So perhaps it is understandable that I put out of my mind the exchange that almost immediately followed the tape-recorded portion of our interview. Before leaving him to resume his busy schedule, I was probably thanking this physician for his time, telling him again how admirable and important I found his story; in fact, it's likely that I was making a point much like the one I just made about the effects of his new understanding. But if the details so far in the conversation remain fuzzy, I do recall clearly what happened next. We had walked to another part of his office, and he stopped at a desk we were passing. "Just a minute," he said as he opened a file on the computer. A close-up digital photograph of an enlarged clitoris appeared on the monitor. Gesturing toward the image, he said, "But then you have cases like that. What are you gonna do with *that*? I mean, you can't leave it like that."

I only recalled this unsettling conclusion of my meeting when I heard a presentation by anthropologist Katrina Karkazis, who had been conducting interviews around the same time as I. She reports that an interview with a different doctor, "a very well-regarded surgeon," elicited the following response:

> Have you seen a baby with CAH? It's grotesque! You're the mother of a new-born with clitoromegaly [enlarged clitoris] and fused labia. Are you going to change the diaper every time? Are you going to hire somebody? Who's going be the caretaker? Are you going to let any neighbor change that child? Absolutely, positively not. You are tied to that child every minute of every day of every week of every month! You're not going to go on vacation. ("Dr. K" quoted in Karkazis 2005; 2008, 146)[6]

Hearing the frank expression of disgust by the surgeon here challenged me not only to remember the surprising exchange following my own interview with the physician I had understood to have renounced cosmetic genital surgeries for children; it also forced me to question what to me had seemed unthinkable to question, namely, the "good intentions" of doctors recommending and performing cosmetic genital surgeries.

Throughout the critical literature on the medical management of intersex, many researchers—myself included—have made a point of remarking on the good intentions of physicians recommending and performing corrective genital surgeries, the aim of which has been cast as an effort to "improve psychosocial functioning" (Parens 2006, xiv; Preves 2003, 62–63).[7] The basis for this understanding of "psychosocial functioning" has changed over the last decade or so. Though it was first explicitly based on Money's theories, particularly his claim that the development of a healthy gender identity depended on the congruence between the gender of (social) assignment and the appearance of the genitalia (see, e.g., Money and Erhardt 1982, 16), the current conception appears to be more loosely based on a tacit recognition of the imperative to "look normal" and the rewards that normality promises. Challenges to the standard of care have focused on the high price of these good intentions and the unfulfilled promise of normality. Many adults, including parents of children who have had normalizing surgeries, have spoken out about the grave harms that have resulted from well-intentioned interventions; some long-term studies have now documented, if only partially, the physical and psychosocial damage that has resulted from them.[8] By contrast, there remains little evidence of the vaunted success of "corrective" (or what some even call "reconstructive") genital surgeries. Physicians' frequent displays of photos of postsurgical genitalia reveal little of the psychosexual satisfaction of those who have undergone these procedures.[9] Erik Parens reports that in preparing for a Hastings Center project on "Surgically Shaping Children," which considered the medical treatment of intersex, "I asked surgeons who try to normalize the appearance of children with atypical genitalia to put me in touch with persons who were glad to have had the surgeries. I was told that such people had moved on with their lives and had no desire to draw attention to an anatomical difference that no longer existed" (2006, xvi). But if it is understandable that individuals who have had this surgery have no interest in sharing their experience, surely physicians who are morally obligated to provide informed consent (which requires, among other things, a report of long-term outcomes of treatment) would be eager to secure such information.

Critics of normalizing corrective surgery have mounted a campaign of resistance from two directions. First, they claim that the standard management of intersex is a violation of well-established bioethical principles, most saliently those concerning the requirement of providing informed consent, the avoidance of paternalism, and the requirement of truth telling; second, they highlight the failure of these practices to fulfill the promises—of preserved erotic sensation and, above all, of a normal life—made by the doctors recommending and performing them (see, e.g., Chase 1999).[10] I do not mean to suggest that the strategy adopted by critics of normalizing surgeries is not, or indeed has not been, an effective or appropriate one. My concern is whether there are important questions and ways of understanding the significance of the medical management of intersex that these strategies cannot accommodate.

Returning to my recovered memory of the "enlightened" doctor's response to a picture of masculinized female genitalia, I need to ask what can account for my own failure to reflect meaningfully on his response. It was more than my reluctance to recognize the expression of disgust by this particular doctor in response to the bodies of children with atypical sex anatomies. His disgust would also disrupt my willingness to attribute good intentions not only to him but to those physicians who continue to recommend and perform cosmetic genital surgeries. Once disgust enters the field of motivating factors, it becomes much more difficult to understand the intention to perform these procedures as "good," that is, "for the benefit of another." But if this realization came as a surprise, I also understood that it was only because I had not, in my own thinking about ethics, taken Nietzsche seriously enough.

A Nietzschean Turn

Nietzsche is infrequently taught in introductory courses in ethics, but even when he is, his project is often (mis)taken to be instituting a full-blown system of morality—albeit an untenable or repugnant morality.[11] Nietzsche's work in these cases is unflatteringly "compared and contrasted" with the two frameworks most frequently taught in ethics: the utilitarian approach, which takes results or consequences as central (and concepts of "good" and "bad" as primary), and the deontological approach, which takes intentions, principles, and the kind of act as most important (and the concepts of "right," "wrong," and "obligation" as primary). Utilitarianism is most closely associated with the work of nineteenth-century philosopher John Stuart Mill; the deontological approach originated a century earlier with Immanuel Kant. Rather than a theory comparable to those of Mill or Kant, Nietzsche's should be regarded as a critical intervention into those theories. Making the claim that the principles of ethics are not derived from "reason," but rather are products of history, Nietzsche unsettles the foundation of conventional understandings of morality, including our very conception of goodness. The work of maintaining these foundations, Nietzsche suggests, requires a "forgetting" (1998 [1887], I:1) of this history.

In considering how Nietzsche can help illuminate the case of the medical management of atypical sex, we cannot simply apply Nietzschean "principles" to the ethical problems raised by the standard of care, as we might in the case of deontology or utilitarianism. What his work provides instead are powerful tools to appreciate what motivates both the accepted management *and* the failure to apply conventional ethical standards to it. Nietzsche's genealogy of morality, for example, directs us to look at the recent historical development of the bioethical standards that are understood to guide medical practice.[12] We could follow that line of thought in investigating the ways in which bioethics as a field has been effectively neutralized as a philosophical practice by its limitation to providing answers to questions posed by doctors, rather than identifying questions ethicists may deem most salient. Here I pursue another direction to which Nietzsche's analysis directs us, following the trail of ressentiment, which he identifies as the origin of our understanding of "goodness" and "morality."

The first part of the *Genealogy of Morality* recounts the history of what Nietzsche calls the "slave revolt in morality," which, he writes, "gives birth to [moral] values." Nietzsche's characterization of his work as "historical" can be confusing for those unfamiliar with it. His recounting of the genealogy of morality is what it sounds like, namely, a tracing of the development of how morality has come to have the shape it has—in short, how moral values have come to have value. But the sociohistorical development he takes to have decisively shaped those values is, as Nietzsche scholar David Allison sees it, not "meant to be an accurate historical portrait." The slave revolt of morality is, a "'symbol' of the 'struggle' between different moral evaluations that occur, [according to Nietzsche] 'all across history'" (see Nietzsche 1998 [1887], I:16; Allison 2001, 220).

When Nietzsche locates the birth of morality with this "slave revolt," however, he does not mean that before the slave revolt there were no values or "moral designations" (1973 [1886], 260). But those values associated with the people Nietzsche describes as the "noble" are mostly foreign to our thinking of morality today; they belong to another time and place that we herald as the birthplace of philosophy but whose moral order was made all but unrecognizable by a tradition that Nietzsche traces to the Jews and culminating in the triumph of Christianity. This moral system, Nietzsche charges, was born of hatred, of powerlessness, and, above all, of an envy of the powerful "nobles," what Nietzsche calls ressentiment (1998 [1887], I:10).

What was once understood as "good," Nietzsche writes in *On the Genealogy of Morality,* was what was noble: "good=noble=powerful=beautiful=happy=beloved of God" (1998 [1887], I:8). The inversion of the values that made nobility and power "evil" was effected by those lesser mortals—"'the slaves,' or 'the mob,' or 'the herd'" (I:9), who, in a state of what Nietzsche describes as "unfathomable hate (the hate of powerlessness)," declared instead that

> "the miserable alone are the good; the poor, powerless, lowly alone are the good; the suffering, deprived, sick, ugly are also the only pious, the only blessed in God, for them alone is there blessedness,—whereas you, you noble and powerful ones, you are in all eternity evil, the cruel, the lustful, the insatiable, the godless, you will eternally be the wretched, accursed, and damned!" (I:7)

The feelings that gave birth to contemporary understandings of "the moral," what Nietzsche terms the victorious "morality of the common man" (I:9), are profoundly negative. In opposition to the nobles' "triumphant yes-saying to oneself," slave morality emphatically "says 'no' to an 'outside,' to a 'different,' to a 'not-self'" (I:10). Rather than motivated by the life-affirming love of oneself, then, ressentiment is a life-negating "hate"; it is "the revenge of the powerless" on "the other" and the transformation of the other into a "monster" (I:10), who must be punished by being made to feel bad about himself, to feel, in a word, *shame* (II:7).

Shame as Harm; Disgust as Violation

In the movement to challenge conventional medical management of intersex, the shame that adults with intersex conditions experience as a consequence of that treatment is repeatedly cited as the primary harm. Indeed, these individuals report that rather than resulting from their atypical genitalia or from possessing a karyotype that is incongruent with their phenotype, it was the treatment aiming to correct or conceal these conditions—that is, to "normalize" their bodies—that resulted in their experience of "isolation, stigma, and shame—the very feelings," sociologist Sharon Preves observes, "that such procedures are [understood to be] attempting to alleviate" (2003, 63, 78, 81). As one young adult interviewed by Preves puts it:

> The primary challenge [of being born intersexed] is [in] childhood; parents and doctors thinking they should fix you. That can be devastating not just from a perspective of having involuntary surgery, but it's even more devastating to people's ability to develop a sense of self. I have heard from people that are really shattered selves . . . The core of their being is shame in their very existence. And that's what's been done to them by people thinking that intersexuality is a shameful secret that needs to be fixed. So I think for most people the biggest challenge is not the genital mutilation, but the psychic mutilation. (65)

The almost forty adults with intersex conditions that Preves interviewed locate different sources of the shame they experienced, but all of the sources are related to their medical "treatment." Perhaps most prominent among these sources were the repeated genital examinations to which they were subject, both pre- and post-surgery, conducted without their consent (Preves 2003, 66–68; see also, e.g., Hawbecker 1999, 112; Moreno 1999, 138; Walcutt 1999, 200; Morris 2006, 7–8). Children with intersex conditions have found themselves subjects of medical schools' grand rounds, sometimes involving manual stimulation "to assess genital responsiveness and size" (Preves 2003, 73). Here shame is provoked through a kind of hyper-visibility, also exemplified in the photographs appearing in scholarly research and textbooks (Dreger 2000, 162); many of those Preves interviewed report painful memories of photo sessions (2003, 69). Another source of shame may be identified in the imperative to make intersex invisible, manifested in the secrecy that parents and children are forced to maintain and which early surgery is intended to ensure (Chase 1999, 147).

As noted earlier, although shame, together with the secrecy and isolation that generally accompany it, is frequently specified as a harm in the conventional management of intersex, there is surprisingly little in the critical literature concerning the nature of this harm and its consequences, both for the individuals who have been subjected to this treatment and for our understandings of the moral harm that this experience of shame marks.

Why is it that this experience of shame has not been more thoroughly investigated? It may be that it is simply understood that the suffering that shame entails is like no other. Psychologist Silvan Tomkins, whose work on affect has recently been so influential, describes how shame is "felt as an inner torment, a sickness of the soul" (Sedgwick and Frank 1995, 133). "There is no feeling more painful," Jennifer Biddle writes in a feminist analysis titled "Shame" (1997, 227). Perhaps it is for this reason that even those critics committed to uncovering—and so alleviating—the shame experienced by individuals with atypical sex anatomy who have been subject to unnecessary or nonconsensual medical intervention have remarked upon, but not investigated, this shame. "Shame is a painful thing to write about," Elspeth Probyn has observed. "It gets into your body. It gets to you" (2005, 130). While one might want to expose the shaming of a child and the ethical violation that produced it, a deeper treatment of this shame can draw one in to the pain it involves.

In highlighting this kind of derivative pain—pain caused by reflecting on a painful experience—however, I do not mean to suggest that the shame felt is shared equally by the critic and the person who has herself been subject to the violations that persons with atypical sex anatomies have endured. Indeed, one of the characterizing features of shame is the feeling of isolation with which it is associated—a function of the objectification that produces this feeling (see, e.g., Biddle 1997, 227–228). Here, we should consider a third reason that may account for why shame has gone largely uninterrogated in the critical literature: Thinking about the experience of shame necessitates that we consider its source, namely, those who provoke it. But even as objectification appears to be an obvious corollary of medical management of whatever kind, the contemporary bearers of the medical gaze themselves largely escape scrutiny in the critical literature.[13]

Of course there are good reasons for emphasizing the experience of those with intersex conditions. Precisely because so much of the pain associated with medical management finds its source in the secrecy and isolation that have been explicit components of treatment protocols since their origins in the 1950s, for critics the work of exposing these practices and bringing the voices of those with intersex to the fore has rightly been a priority. Although doctors are certainly represented in the narratives of those with DSD, they do not appear as full-fledged villains, intent on eradicating genital ambiguity wherever it may be found. Rather, they are more frequently portrayed as well-meaning, if insensitive, characters, concerned with doing "what's right" and doing it well, even as they appear to have no compunction about violating well-established bioethical principles that are apparently accepted in every area of practice save this one (Dreger 1999a, 16). If they consistently decline to ask the difficult questions concerning the consequences of their actions, we may sympathetically attribute this failure to the narrow focus of their specialties—for example, the fact that pediatric endocrinologists and urologists typically have little contact with their patients once they become adults.

But such a generous treatment of what nevertheless appears to be an obvious ethical failure within the terms of most conventional moral frameworks is not entirely at odds with a Nietzschean analysis that emphasizes neither good intentions nor bad, but rather ressentiment, a kind of affective response. Following his lead, we might understand the unapologetic flouting of their own codes of ethics to exemplify Nietzsche's contention that the morality that putatively protects us is actually destructive of much of the pleasure in life and in body that Nietzsche would value.

If it is "ethical" to perform surgeries in response to disgust—disgust that appears to be experienced by doctors, or that is projected onto or even promoted in, parents of children with atypical genitalia—one can certainly understand Nietzsche's contention that morality, as it has developed historically, is a "will to negate life" (1967 [1872], preface:5). This will develops out of, or in conjunction with, ressentiment. "While the noble human being lives with himself in confidence and openness," Nietzsche tells us, "the human being of *ressentiment* is neither sincere, nor naïve, nor honest and frank with himself. His soul looks obliquely at things, his spirit loves hiding places, secret passages and backdoors, everything hidden strikes him as his work, his security, his balm" (1998 [1887], I:10). This secretive insincerity suggests both fear (such as the fear of being found out) and shame (the constant need to keep hidden). We can see this ressentiment in the doctors' expressions of disgust and in their assumptions that of course parents will want to keep the knowledge of their children's atypical sex hidden from absolutely everyone else.

It will help to spell out more clearly the nature of the disgust I take to have been expressed by the physician whose interview I mentioned earlier, as well as by those physicians interviewed by Karkazis. In her critical ethical analysis of disgust, Martha Nussbaum highlights the distinction between what she calls "primary-object disgust" and "projective disgust."[14] Primary-object disgust is "standardly felt toward a group of primary objects: feces, blood, semen, urine, nasal discharges, menstrual discharges, corpses, decaying meat, and animals/insects that are oozy, slimy, or smelly" (2010, 15). This sort of disgust, following Darwin, is a human adaptation, thought to protect us from disease or infection.

"Projective disgust," by contrast, "is shaped by social norms, as societies teach their members to identify alleged contaminants in their midst" (16). Unlike primary-object disgust, projective disgust does not seem to have a direct connection to our shared animal being but takes advantage of the associations of primary-object disgust by means of what experimental psychologist Paul Rozin and his colleagues describe as an "opportunistic accretion of new domains of elicitors to a rejection system that is already in place" (2008, 764). Nussbaum offers the example of the way that people or groups can be marginalized, stigmatized, or made "other" by means of a fantasied association with primary-object disgust. "Jews are not really slimy, or similar to maggots," she writes, "although German anti-Semites, and Hitler himself, said that they were. African-Americans do not smell worse than other human beings, although racists said that they did" (2010, 16–17). Projective disgust exemplifies that emphatic no-saying "to an 'outside,' to a 'different' to a not-self'" (Nietzsche 1998 [1887] I:10) that Nietzsche casts as characteristic of ressentiment.[15]

Nussbaum's claim that disgust is a "powerful and central" means of marginalization resonates with Nietzsche's analysis of the pervasive character of ressentiment—more specifically, with the foundational quality it bears in shaping social attitudes and behavioral norms. But precisely because projective disgust is unlike primary-object disgust in its historical and cultural specificity, projective disgust proves surprisingle unstable. Nussbaum observes that when projective disgust "is removed (when, for example, aversion to physical contact with a racial minority is no longer present), other modes of hierarchy tend to depart with it" (2010, 17). Recognizing the vulnerability of projective disgust to dissolution also brings into relief the arduous nature the work that maintaining this state of disgust may entail. The strident efforts to prevent lesbians and gay men from marrying come increasingly to be seen as an ethically suspect, anxious attempt to maintain a social order that makes the superiority of some—in the form of the supposedly neutral status of legal personhood—dependent on the inferiority—or legal sub-personhood—of others (Nussbaum 2010).

Following Nussbaum's analysis, it is easy to see why disgust would be an effective means to shore up support for a social order organized to a significant extent around sexual orientation:

> Sex involves the exchange of bodily fluids, and it marks us as bodily beings rather than transcendent beings. So sex is a site of anxiety for anyone who is ambivalent about having an animal and mortal nature, and that includes many if not most people. Primary-object disgust therefore plays a significant role in sexual relations, as the bodily substances people encounter in sex (semen, sweat, feces, menstrual blood) are very often found disgusting and seen as contaminants. (17)

In the area of sexuality, the line between primary-object and projective disgust can be thin, in other words, and can manifest itself as readily in misogyny (17–18) as it does in the stigmatization of homosexuality.

In the medical management of atypical sex, it may be as important as it is difficult to distinguish between what Nussbaum regards as a kind of natural and ethically uncomplicated experience or expression of primary-object disgust and the ethically perilous projective disgust she criticizes. We might attribute this difficulty to the disgust (and revulsion and fear) that another scholar of law and humanities, William Ian Miller, claims are provoked by "the highly dangerous and vulnerable" genitals and their excretions, that is, "normal" genitals behaving "naturally" (1997, 101–105).[16] What distinguishes the general disgust provoked by "normal" genitals from the particular disgust atypical genitals are supposed to evoke is the distinctive urge to fix or correct these genitals; it is this urge, I propose, that marks the medical management atypical sex as an expression of ressentiment.

If we accept Miller's point that genitals generally are "disgusting," it would seem that if atypical genitals provoke disgust, it is not because these genitals in particular are so obviously abhorrent. Granted, close-up medical photographs can promote a sense that one is beholding something shocking or terrible (Wall 2010), but it does not seem that atypical genitalia would do so any more or less than would similar close-up medical photos of typical genitalia splayed or prepared for surgery. Another point that we may count against the claim that atypical genitalia provoke disgust where typical genitals do not is the fact that, as a number of anthropologists have documented, this response is not universal.[17] However, it is not necessary to look outside our own cultural context to substantiate the claim that it is *not* the case that "everyone" is disgusted by atypical sex anatomies. Since the beginning of intersex activism, it has been clear that there is some significant number of individuals with what would be considered atypical sex anatomies who have not been subjected to normalizing surgery. Some— probably a minority of such individuals—joined ISNA in the 1990s, but even limited anecdotal evidence suggests that there are many more who did not. Many times over the years people have confided in me that their sex anatomies, or the anatomies of present or former romantic partners, are atypical. Their anatomies had not been "medicalized" but were taken to be normal or, if not entirely ordinary, then certainly not pathological.[18] Dr. Alder, one of the physicians with whom I spoke years after the interview with the doctor I discussed at the beginning of this chapter, recounted an experience from his early general practice with adults that turned out to be influential when he later began to treat children with atypical anatomies. On two separate occasions he saw women who, he was surprised to find on examination, could have been diagnosed with a pathologically large clitoris. Both women were in long-term marriages to men, and when he asked each of them whether she had faced any challenges because of the size of her clitoris, both were puzzled by the question. Each reported having a satisfying sex life and had not been aware that there was anything unusual about her anatomy; nor had their husbands made any mention of their partners' anatomical difference.

These stories suggest that the disgust that doctors may experience, and appear to presume in parents and society at large, is not of the order of primary-object disgust, but is instead a projective disgust, a disgust that impedes an ethical wish to treat others with dignity and respect. In fairness, however, it is not only the doctors who demonstrate this presumption of disgust, as we have already seen in the study conducted by Suzanne Kessler discussed in chapter 2. Recall that a majority of college students who were asked to imagine that as parents they were faced with the decision to consent to cosmetic surgery for a child with an enlarged clitoris or to reassign a male with a micropenis, reported that they would make decisions consistent with the current standard of care (S. J. Kessler 1998, 103). Kessler's study itself supports the view that this disgust is projective, for individuals imagining *themselves* with atypical genitalia do not feel an immediate need for correction. Even if one is persuaded that the motivation for normalizing surgery may be found in projective disgust, however, there remains an important ethical question about how parents are to navigate what might be a hostile climate for their children.

Nietzsche's characterization of the effects of ressentiment is helpful in thinking about the contradiction posed by Kessler's paired studies. One response to the question of whether to perform normalizing surgery is to seek answers in our own bodies, which could provoke an unflinching challenge to the prevailing standard of care. More typically, as Nietzsche's account of the enduring legacy of slave morality predicts, the "norm" successfully keeps the "human being of *ressentiment*" (1998 [1887], I:10) "within limits *inter pares* by mores, worship, custom, gratitude, still more by mutual surveillance, by jealousy" (I:11). Rather than look to and with and in our own bodies in order to imaginatively consider the somatic experience of children, we are concerned instead with "appearances" of bodies. The question we must pose here remains why this consideration for our own erotic potential appears to fail, as Kessler's paired studies indicate it will fail. Returning to Nietzsche, we should recall the origin of the ressentiment, the noble's goodness inspired in those who effected the transvaluation of value: it was envy.

Enviable Ambiguity

On the face of it, envy would not seem to have any place in the medical management of intersex. Being born with atypical genitalia has proved "perilous" to those so diagnosed over the last century (Holmes 2008); medical management has taken as its object not simply a "condition," as is generally the case, but what medicine seems to regard as a kind of (pathological) personhood. That is to say, doctors have focused their attention not on treating disease (and, as should be clear from the story of Ruby's children, which I discussed in chapter 2, there are serious and even life-threatening disorders associated with some intersex conditions). Instead, doctors have focused on "fixing sex," that is, "repairing" bodies that are neither clearly male nor female and so reinforcing the normative ideal of "unambiguous" sex. There seems very little that is enviable in accounts of those subjected to corrective genital surgery; the documented physical harms and the emotional scars described are chilling; the insistent publication of these harms by affected individuals, their families, and allies has led finally to changes in medical thinking and practice that were unimaginable just a decade ago.[19]

But if thinking about envy in this context seems misplaced, asking whether envy is playing a role in what has functioned as standard medical practice yields some immediate possibilities: what comes readily to mind is the myth of Hermaphroditos, or what some have (mis)taken as the romantic view of a primordial "wholeness" that Aristophanes describes in his tale of the round people in the *Symposium*—an image that has become a kind of fixture in contemporary theorizing. Scholar and activist Morgan Holmes remarks with considerable disdain on the appropriation of intersex "as a mascot for sex radicals," who cast "intersexuality" as a "liberatory state that will free us from the bonds of compulsory heterosexuality" (2008, 44).[20] The pitfalls of the sorts of idealization to which Holmes points are many, and we must be particularly aware of the ways they can divert attention from the material harms experienced by individuals with DSD and by their families. Following Nietzsche, we must ask what happens when we understand these divergent responses—those associated with the medical and parental imperative to "normalize" intersex bodies, on the one hand, and those of the "sex radicals'" (which I take to be a shorthand for the sort of instrumental idealization of atypically sexed bodies), on the other—as two sides of the same coin. That is to say, what if this idealization marks an envy that is motivating harmful interventions in the first place?

We do not generally understand objects of envy as vulnerable; more typically we understand vulnerability as the experience of being somehow "less than" and consider *agents* of envy to be standing in admiration of those they see as more privileged, better endowed. In this we perhaps unconsciously hark back to the envy inspired by the noble "good ones" of whom Nietzsche speaks in the *Genealogy,* those who felt themselves to be "powerful . . . and high-minded" (1998 [1887], I:2) not through comparison to another but *prior to* any comparison (Scheler 2007 [1915], 32): "The 'well-born,'" Nietzsche writes, "simply felt themselves to be 'happy'; they did not first have to construct their happiness artificially by looking at their enemies, to talk themselves into it, *to lie themselves into it*" (1998 [1887], I:10; original emphasis). I think it may be challenging to grasp the sort of goodness that entails a "completely naïve and non-reflective awareness of [one's] own value and . . . fullness of being" (Scheler 2007 [1915], 31). But we need to attend carefully to the lessons of Nietzsche's genealogy of morality, for it was precisely the envy this noble sort of goodness aroused—the ressentiment of the powerless—that provoked the "slave revolt in morality" (Nietzsche 1998 [1887], I:7), displacing the whole ancient system of valuation. The concept of good that finally triumphed is not itself grounded in a noble goodness, but is the product of ressentiment, of "revenge, hatred, malice, envy, the impulse to detract, and spite" (Scheler 2007 [1915], 25). Understanding the prevailing conception of morality in terms of Nietzsche's analysis of ressentiment demands that we investigate the nature of an envy that resulted in, as Nietzsche writes, the "radical revaluation of . . . values" (1998 [1887], I:7). Coming to terms with the way the standard of care could be motivated by envy provides an important possibility for intervening in these practices.

I am prompted in this line of inquiry by Jane Flax's reading of Freud's *Three Essays on the Theory of Sexuality* in "The Scandal of Desire: Psychoanalysis and Disruptions of Gender" (2004) and by Judith Butler's treatment of that work and

The Ego and the Id (1997).[21] Both Flax and Butler describe Freud's characterization of gender as an arduous achievement made compulsory by culture and history. Cultural narratives, Flax writes, "naturalize . . . socially constructed gender norms" and thus "represent gender as an inevitable consequence of anatomical differences" (2004, 57); the achievement of a neat social division into male and female, man and woman, belies what Freud identified as the "bisexual"—what Flax calls the "polysexual"—character of individuals. Despite appearances, Freud maintains, we are not so very clearly male or female; that is to say, our apparent maleness or femaleness is a function of our continuous attempts to overcome what we could awkwardly describe as our fundamental "two-sexedness."[22] For Freud, these divisions between "biological" sex, gender expression, and sexual desire are not so easily parsed; each is—as the history of medical management of intersex has demonstrated—inextricably intertwined with the other in the cultural imagination. In this view the extraordinary measures that have been employed to "normalize" bodies with atypical sex are symptomatic of the effort to enforce the binary division of sex that is required by our society and enforced within families; it is the standard to which individuals are, as Foucault would say, "made subject."

If Freud's narrative of sexual development demonstrates how the assumption of "the positions of 'masculine' and 'feminine' . . . [are] the effects of laborious and uncertain accomplishment" (Butler 1997, 135), it also points to the *losses* suffered in the process of coming to occupy, and then maintain, these positions (135; Flax 2004, 55–56).For Freud, the polymorphous desire that marks the infant's embodied experience must be restricted. Children are made to understand that erotic possibilities for, on, and in our own bodies must be constrained and limited. "Freud's views," Flax writes, "suggest that such conditioning remains unstable and not without cost . . . The narrowing of desire robs many aspects of life of their eroticization and possibilities for pleasure. Proper object choice has to be policed by social prohibitions, self-discipline, shaming, and violence" (2004, 56). These are losses that are not forgotten, but repressed; they are the unmourned loss that constitutes what Freud called "melancholic identification" (Butler 1997, 134). To the extent that this melancholia marks foreclosed possibilities, embodied futures that cannot be lived (139), we can perhaps begin to make better sense of how the idealization of so-called ambiguously sexed bodies might be significantly connected to the medicalized imperative to "normalize" these bodies.

In what Freud understood to be normal development—that is, the development that results in the assumption of an unambiguously masculine or feminine identity—subjects must forsake an originary polymorphous sexuality. Taking up these new roles—living what is, in the psychoanalytic account, a kind of fiction of binary sex that is so successfully rendered as to be taken for granted—is an imperative of our society. But making as if "natural" gender norms that are in fact "arbitrary and changeable" requires considerable work: "individuals, families, and other social structures require pervasive and persistent effort to acquire and enforce them" (Flax 2004, 57). Butler's discussion of the melancholia entailed by the assumption of binary gender roles makes clear the high psychic price that must be paid for the achievement of unambiguous gender and the notions of sex and sexuality with which it is bound. Flax's account helpfully casts the price of this achievement as a kind of *sacrifice*.

As Flax discusses it, the concept of sacrifice is enormously rich; I will focus in particular on the layers of sacrifice manifest in the complex of responses provoked by the fact of atypical sex. According to Freud, there are losses we all suffer, psychic and material sacrifices everyone must make, in the assumption of sexed identities. But these sacrifices are not equal. Feminist arguments from Mary Wollstonecraft forward could be understood in these terms as criticisms of the ways that women have been made disproportionately to bear these sacrifices. Flax takes as an example the way in which, in resurgent "demands for a return to 'family values,'" women are made to unduly bear this sacrifice through their restriction "to traditional enactments of wife and mother" (2004, 62), adding, "Feminist attempts to alter gender relations stir up intense anxieties and threaten many apparently unrelated aspects of psychological and social organization. People may feel driven to protect existing gender arrangements by an unconscious fear of disrupting basic ways of organizing life" (63).[23]

Another way these sacrifices manifest themselves may be found in the example on which Nussbaum also focuses, namely, in what Flax several years earlier described as "the profound uneasiness many people experience at the demand for institutional recognition of same-sex partnerships."[24] Following Freud, Flax understands this uneasiness as "a fear that a too easy acceptance [of marriage equality] might undo those repressions [of polymorphous desire] so painfully acquired. Having invested in these sacrifices," she continues, "*we want to deny an excess of pleasure to others*" (2004, 56; emphasis added). In addition to the melancholia that Butler describes, Flax here points to a distinctive affective response: the repressed envy (of homosexuality) that awakens the fear of undoing its repression. This characterization exemplifies perfectly Nietzsche's concept of ressentiment: the solution to the envy of another's pleasure (or strength or beauty—their "good") is to deny another the pleasure that one cannot pursue oneself; making "good" one's own pleasures requires the denigration if not the active spoiling, undoing, or undermining of the other's. This envy is not conscious, as Freud argues in *Civilization and Its Discontents* (2005 [1930]), but built into our society's history.

The role of anxiety in this envy can be observed in the ways that demands for conventional sexual expression—whether with respect to one's role or one's desire—intensify during times of social instability; anxiety and envy work together to enforce particular social arrangements. Accounts of doctors' and parents' responses to the birth of children with atypical sex testify to the anxiety provoked by non-normative bodies. Understanding how this anxiety is already entwined with the envy of ambiguous sex, in which otherwise foreclosed possibilities seem to remain open, we may begin to reckon with how the ambiguity of intersexed bodies awakens these affects and come to terms with the ways these affective responses are then enacted upon infants and young children as well as the consequences of these actions. To understand the consequences of the envy I'm describing here—the envy inherent in ressentiment—I return once more to Nietzsche's *Genealogy* and examine his identification of envy with the destructive impulses it inspires in its contrary effort to create—or recreate—value.

The Envy of Ressentiment: Spoiling

For Nietzsche, as we have seen, the foundation of our moral system of value is the product of a resentful hatred of the nobles' goodness/beauty. He argues that it was the envy of the "priests" that drove the inversion of morality, making virtue out of weakness and those elevating values we have "inherited" (1998 [1887], I:7): the distinctively Christian values of humility, compassion, and submissiveness that displaced the noble "good" and rendered "evil" the strength and beauty with which that good had been identified.[25] But it is important to clarify what this envy entails and how this envy can be understood to be functioning indirectly, where there doesn't appear to be a specific object. Despite its considerable shortcomings, Max Scheler's phenomenological study puts envy at the center of the experience and expression of ressentiment in contemporary culture and can help us make sense of what may initially seem like a strange way of understanding the phenomenon.[26]

Scheler reminds us that because ressentiment is an inversion of noble morality, prominent elements of the prior morality will persist but will be expressed in ways that distort their antecedent expression and meaning. Take revenge, for example; seeking vengeance for wrongs committed against oneself or another may be understood to belong to a noble morality to the extent that these acts aim to discharge the damage done and so exorcise the feeling of powerlessness that "being done wrong" may instill. "There will be no *ressentiment*," Scheler writes, "if he who thirsts for revenge really acts and avenges himself, if he who is consumed by hatred harms his enemy, gives him 'a piece of his mind.'" So, too, in the case of envy. The envious person will

> not fall under the dominion of *ressentiment* if he seeks to acquire the envied possession by means of work, barter, crime, or violence. *Ressentiment* can only arise if these emotions are particularly powerful and *yet must be suppressed* because they are coupled with the feeling that one is *unable* to act them out—either because of weakness, physical or mental, or because of fear. (Scheler 2007 [1915], 26–27; emphasis added)

What distinguishes the envy borne of ressentiment, a repressed or "impotent" envy (29), is not a genuine desire to possess a given quality or thing; instead, that envy comes to be a "hatred against the owner, until the latter is falsely considered to be the *cause* of our privation" (30; original emphasis). Ressentiment is constituted by this confluence of envy and revenge—envy of the noble good and revenge against those who appear to withhold that good. According to Scheler, when revenge is repressed, the very "imagination of vengeance, too, is repressed—and with it the emotion of revenge" (27). The result is a state of mind that seeks to depreciate, to deny the positive value of a thing or person. Denigration of this sort is an effort, he tells us, to lessen the discomfort of powerlessness to take revenge or the inability to possess something desired. Continually frustrated, the person adopts what Scheler calls a "*ressentiment* attitude"; "envy, the impulse to detract, malice, and secret vindictiveness . . . [thus] become fixed attitudes, detached from all determinate objects" (46). That envy or revenge (or for Scheler, envy in tandem with revenge) comes to be disarticulated from particular objects is especially important in understanding the impact of ressentiment on the standard of care for intersex, because ressentiment is characterized as a whole attitude that cannot be understood to be directed at a single person or trait. What Scheler describes as the "repressed impulse" for revenge or envy "becomes more and more detached from any particular reason and at length even from any particular individual . . . [I]t turns into a negative attitude toward certain apparent traits and qualities, no matter where or in whom they are found" (43). Scheler's analysis provides considerable insight into how it can be that physicians caring for individual children promote, and parents seeking to act in their children's best interests may allow or even actively seek out, risky, often harmful, and almost always nonconsensual, normalizing interventions on the atypical sex anatomies of children.

Bringing Scheler's analysis of the envy associated with ressentiment into conversation with the Freudian account of the losses entailed by the assumption of binary gender roles can help us make sense of how the envy of ressentiment is operating in the medical management of intersex, how central a role it has played in the creation of the standard of care, and the authority it continues to command in the field—and this despite (or actually because of) the way that it is repressed and made unrecognizable as envy. Melanie Klein's treatment of envy in the landmark essay "Envy and Gratitude" resonates with Scheler's but helps us to shift our focus from the very constitution of moral value writ large to the individual development of value and, in particular, the value that is one's own worth.

Like Scheler, Klein defines envy as a sensation of anger provoked by another's enjoyment or possession of something one wants. What she calls "the envious impulse" is not only the experience of this anger but also an accompanying wish to "take [what is desirable] away or spoil it" (1975 [1957], 181). Klein's account of the infant's "primary envy" (of the giving mother's breast) (183) provides a means of understanding a deeply felt and yet inarticulate destructive impulse that strikes not only at the envied other but at the envious self as well.[27] Envy, Klein says, interferes with enjoyment (of the mother's giving breast—that is to say, of the other's generosity) and so "undermines the development of gratitude" that is, for Klein, central to the individual's development.

> There are very pertinent psychological reasons why envy ranks among the seven "deadly sins." I would even suggest that it is unconsciously felt to be the greatest sin of all, because it spoils and harms the good object which is the source of life . . . The feeling of having injured and destroyed the primal object impairs the individual's trust in the sincerity of his later relations and makes him doubt his capacity for love and goodness. (1975 [1957], 189)

Here Klein clarifies, as perhaps Scheler cannot, the high ethical stakes entailed in bringing to awareness the operation of envy and its "disturbance," as she puts it, of love. The envious impulse that strikes the infant in its primary relation to its mother extends throughout the lifespan. It lies also in the potential disturbance of parental love (or perhaps better, the projection of this disturbance by physicians onto parents) in an envy that may be awakened by the sexually ambiguous body of the child.[28]

I do not think that Klein's account requires us to understand individual parents of children with DSD as envious of their children. Rather, her account of envy and the impulse to spoil can help to make sense of the impulse to "fix"—that is, to normalize—the bodies of children with atypical sex anatomies despite evidence that the sorts of intervention entailed by surgeries or hormonal treatments are not necessary in pathophysiological terms. It makes sense perhaps especially of Money's odd insistence on the importance of congruence between sexual anatomy and gender identity. It isn't that those with intersexed bodies are exempt from the demands of assuming binary gender roles like "everyone else"; people with atypical genitalia are born into the same social world, the same habitus, as the rest of us. But if they are subject to the same rules and expectations, if the same cultural imperatives subject them, too, their anatomies belie that imperative; they do not allow the achievement of masculinity and femininity to look seamless, natural, inevitable. It is not simply that their bodies point to a truth about what gender "really" is, but also that those with such anatomies *cannot* do this thing that the rest of us must and for which we must sacrifice. That is why they are enviable. And that is why their "enjoyment" of ambiguity must be spoiled.

Unlike Nietzsche and Scheler, however, Klein's account of primary envy also provides the alternative affective response to the primary experience of infant feeding, namely, enjoyment and the gratitude that can accompany enjoyment. The feeling of gratitude, she informs us, can "mitigate destructive impulses, envy and greed" (1975 [1957], 187). For Klein, the capacity for enjoyment and for security in the sense of possessing a good object is critical for the development of a sense of one's self as good (187) and provides the wherewithal to tolerate the experiences of "envy, hatred, and grievance" that arise in one's life as a matter of course. Following the line of criticism regarding envy and its consequences from Nietzsche through Scheler and Klein, the problem of how to frame a robust ethical response remains. Roslyn Diprose's concept of "corporeal generosity" provides a rich possibility for shaping such a response.

Corporeal Generosity

The failure of conventional approaches to the ethical violations—violations that I understand to be committed both in the recommendations and performance of appearance-altering surgeries for infants and children and in the affective expressions that motivate these surgeries—speaks to the need to consider the limits of these frameworks and to identify new approaches. Diprose defines corporeal generosity as an openness to the other—an openness that is always already a part of our existence as embodied beings in interaction with others, but is at the same time impeded by that very existence. "Through habit and in accordance with the institutional setting in which my corporeal identity is constituted," she writes, "I develop a pattern of existence that leans toward certain practices and cannot tolerate others" (2002, 55).

Diprose develops her analysis of generosity particularly with respect to those we regard as "other," whether racial or sexual; she is concerned more generally, too, with relationships that seem to structurally entail objectification such as that experienced by the patient in the clinic. Although Diprose is not explicitly concerned with treatment of intersex conditions, the remarks she makes with respect to the salience of sex and sexuality in "the clinical encounter," in which the body of a patient is given "to a stranger whose body seems exempt from scrutiny . . . yet is an agent of normalization" (108), are illustrative of doctors' relationships to infants and children with these conditions. But if we expect a kind of affective "parsimony," as Diprose nicely puts it, from doctors who are trained to view their patients "from a distance" (see Diprose 2002, 35–40), what is striking in the medical management of intersex is how the position of *parents* of affected children can shift in the clinical encounter. Parents may become themselves distanced with respect to the doctor (for the stigma of difference their children bear in this setting may be attached also to them); but to the extent that they become identified with the doctors who are caring for (that is, seeking to normalize) their child, parents may seek to distance themselves from this stigma of difference borne by their child by making of their own child "the other."[29]

Perhaps because we typically understand parent-child relationships—with certain qualifications—to be characterized by a "corporeal generosity," we may hesitate to identify its diminution in or withdrawal by parents in the cases of children with intersex.[30] But I think we must consider this possibility as an effect of medical management; that is to say, it is the labeling of children with an intersex condition as "abnormal" by physicians that promotes the kind of distancing between parent and child that makes the child an "other" whose body must be altered as a condition of gaining entrance to the family and of being granted the love that entrance should guarantee. Not only in their own experience of disgust, then, but also in their projection of this disgust onto parents and every person a child might encounter, doctors foreclose the generosity that we might understand as the child's birthright.[31] Consider a response to the recommendation against routine cosmetic genital surgery on infants made by a Hastings Center working group appearing in the *Archives of Pediatrics* (Frader et al. 2004). In an invited critique, a pediatrician writes that while the recommendations of the working group may be ethically sound, the successful outcome for a child with intersex depends on parents' "ability to accept and unconditionally love their child" (Eugster 2004, 428). The physician writing here does not elaborate; it is as if a "deformity" such as a larger than average clitoris or a smaller than average penis would indubitably inhibit the love—the "unconditional" love?—a parent would feel for a child.[32] But I want to propose that if in attending to the atypical bodies of children our attention is focused on expressions of ressentiment, it will become our ethical obligation to attend instead to the bodies of doctors and of parents.

There are nevertheless significant barriers to fulfilling this obligation. Recognizing "that the clinician is a body" (Diprose 2002, 119) subject to the affective states entailed by ressentiment is the first step. At the same time, we must reckon with the ways that this body, cloaked in authority, is "shielded from the medical gaze" (114) and removed from view. For this reason, the more immediate obligation must be attending to the flourishing of the children whose difference has made them objects of envy and vulnerable to harm by physicians, as well as by their parents. But recognizing the presence of ressentiment requires that we attend not only to the intersubjective relations between parents (or physicians) and a child with atypical sex anatomy but also to the relationships parents and physicians have to themselves. This obligation might finally be better understood in the terms Nietzsche offers in *Gay Science*:

> *One must learn to love.*—This is what happens to us in music: First one has to *learn to hear* a figure and melody at all, to detect and distinguish it, to isolate it and delimit it as a separate life. Then it requires some exertion and good will to *tolerate* it in spite of its strangeness, to be patient with its appearance and expression, and kindhearted about its oddity. Finally there comes a moment when we are used to it, when we wait for it, when we sense that we should miss it if it were missing; and now it continues to compel and enchant us relentlessly until we have become its humble and enraptured lovers who desire nothing better from the world than it and only it.

But that is what happens to us not only in music. That is how we have *learned to love* all things that we now love. In the end we are always rewarded for our good will, our patience, fairmindedness, and gentleness with what is strange; gradually, it sheds its veil and turns out to be a new and indescribable beauty. That is its thanks for our hospitality. Even those who love themselves have learned it in this way; for there is no other way. Love, too, has to be learned. (1974 [1887], 334; original emphasis)

Learning to love, in Nietzsche's terms, is the enactment of a corporeal generosity; it entails changes in the one who "must learn" to love. Distinguishing what, following Gail Weiss, we might term an "embodied ethics" (1999, 158) from an ethics of ressentiment is the embodied transformation of the one who loves. Rather than seeking changes in the bodies of children with atypically sexed anatomies, the imperative for change is located in the bodies of parents, in physicians, in the rest of us.

4 Reassigning Ambiguity
Parental Decisions and the Matter of Harm

Some key elements of the medical management of atypical sex in children have changed since the late 1990s as adults with intersex conditions, and their parents, have spoken out about how the standard of care has affected their lives and as these stories have become an ever more powerful testament to the physical and emotional damage wrought by their treatment. Increasing numbers of pediatric specialists now reaffirm the good intentions that motivated earlier practices, but they also acknowledge the clinical ignorance, even clinical arrogance, that governed care—especially the failure to convey to parents what one group of practitioners describes as the potential side effects of surgery, including the likelihood of damage to erotic sensation (e.g., Dayner et al. 2004; see also Lee and Houk 2010, 1). More recently, researchers have also reported on the lack of certainty or confidence among physicians themselves with regard to the standard of care (Karkazis et al. 2010). Today, specialists in the treatment of DSD have embraced informed consent; a new model of "shared decision making" (Dreger et al. 2010; Karkazis and Rossi 2010) is coming to the fore.

These are indisputably important changes. And yet it does not appear that there has been a significant reduction in normalizing surgery. One reason may be a persistent sense that normalization remains an imperative. A prominent form of this understanding is expressed in physicians' claim that without surgery parents will be unable to bond with their child. The child's good depends on her parents loving and accepting her (e.g., Eugster 2004, 428). These physicians seem to agree that if the condition of that love is the normalization of the appearance of atypical sex, then surgery is indicated. But what if the performance of these surgeries has the opposite effect? What if it turns out that normalizing surgeries impede the love they are meant to facilitate?

In the previous chapter I proposed that normalizing surgeries may be motivated by an unconscious wish to spoil the enviable ambiguity the bodies of children with atypical sex are taken to exhibit. This suggestion may not be persuasive to some, particularly to those parents and physicians responsible for making decisions regarding the care of affected children. "Spoiling" entails some kind of harm. And there continue to be those who believe that many of the children treated twenty, thirty, or forty years ago experienced no harm, notwithstanding the fact that the chilling lessons from these years would seem to be succinctly captured in the recognition by the U.S. and European endocrinological societies in their 2006 Consensus Statement that what these children experienced at the hands of their doctors was "trauma." Indeed, the statement not only acknowledges the trauma experienced by children subjected to repeated genital exams, displays, and medical photography; it also recognizes the trauma experienced by affected individuals who have not been provided full information about their conditions or treatment they underwent as infants and young children (Hughes et al. 2006, 558).[1] And yet the nature of the harm effected by these medical encounters is not specified. Nor does there appear anywhere in the statement any acknowledgment of harm that might result from resisting the impulse to normalize children with atypical sex anatomies. That is to say, nowhere does the statement suggest that parents' decisions or doctors' recommendations *against* surgical intervention could adversely affect the child himself or herself. Instead, the physicians write, "It is generally felt that early surgery . . . relieves parental distress and improves attachment between the child and the parents," though, the authors note, "the systematic evidence for this belief is lacking" (557). For all the valuable developments the statement marks, the treatment of atypical sex in children remains exceptional. It is exceptional because the treatment is not directly for the benefit of the child, but for the parent, and only thereby for the benefit of the child.

Parents of children with atypical sex are described in the literature as confused or frustrated (Malmqvist and Zeiler 2010, 133), anxious or disoriented (Gough et al. 2008, 503–504). Of course, these are characterizations that may obtain with respect to any number of medical conditions that occur in the neonatal period. Confusion or frustration would be a likely result if a child is experiencing trouble breathing or has an irregular heartbeat that cannot easily be explained. If there has been no indication of a problem during pregnancy, and one's child is suddenly removed to a neonatal intensive care unit, there is every reason to expect that new parents will experience anxiety and disorientation. Yet I know of no other pediatric condition for which the standard of care is based on the relief of the parents rather than the care of the child. This is not to say that relief of parental distress has no place in medical management of intersex conditions; indeed, advocates and critics of the standard of care would agree that attending to parents' distress at the birth of a child with unusual anatomy is of critical importance for ensuring the care of the child in their charge and for the well-being of a parent whose own sense of self may be deeply unsettled. Parents of children born with unusual anatomies, Alice Dreger writes,

> [may] suddenly find themselves unsure about their *own* social and familial role. How are they supposed to act? What are they supposed to think, feel, do, say? They know only how normal parents are supposed to behave, but they can't be normal parents if they don't have a normal child. They seek surgical "reconstruction" of a normal child in part because they feel like they will know

> how to be a parent to that child, whereas they often feel uncertain how to be a
> parent to this one. (2004, 57; original emphasis)

This matter of parental responses to their children's anatomy merits more sustained consideration than is reflected in the current approach, focused as it is on "erasing" the problem. When physicians say that surgery is "what parents want," we should ask, specifically, what it is that parents ultimately want—that is, what they mean ultimately to achieve—and whether surgery will satisfy these aims. If what "normal parents" want is the best chance for their children to flourish, we should not take for granted that normalized appearance guarantees flourishing. In fact, what limited evidence exists suggests that surgery does not provide parents relief or reassurance in the long term.[2] We might seek such evidence in other cases of appearance-normalizing surgery where similar questions have been posed. Cassandra Aspinall, a social worker on a craniofacial team, who was born with a cleft lip and is herself the mother of a child with a cleft lip and palate, observes that parents may rush into normalizing interventions to relieve worry about differences in their children's appearance. "In their efforts to protect their children," she observes, such parents may "end up creating exactly what they so desperately want to avoid: fear, anxiety, and depression" (2006, 17). My aim in this chapter is to examine the nature of the harm that results from the prevailing model of medical management insofar as it focuses on relieving parental discomfort.

Evidence of the harm caused by the most prominent features of medical management since its beginnings in the 1950s has been substantial: physical and psychosocial injury caused by clitorectomy in girls with clitoromegaly, castration and sex reassignment in boys with micropenis (e.g., Reiner 2006), and performance of uncomfortable vaginal dilation in young children following vaginoplasty or the creation of a neovagina; psychosocial damage stemming from the emphasis on maintaining the secrecy of a child's sexual ambiguity from the child and extended family and from the trauma provoked by genital exams and medical photography. These are among the accepted practices that appear to have changed dramatically in the last ten years.[3] That change must be credited to those who have given voice to the suffering they have endured together with the recognition that the prior standard of care entailed violations of accepted principles of bioethics, most obviously those concerning informed consent (Tamar-Mattis 2006, 85–88) and the avoidance of paternalism.[4]

And yet the many harms that have been enumerated do not precisely capture what may be the greatest risk posed by the standard of care. This is a harm of another kind, the prevention of which is less easily conveyed—or even recognized—within the terms of accepted principles of bioethics. To describe the damage that occurs at the level of what French phenomenologist Maurice Merleau-Ponty calls the "body schema"—an injury to one's sense of self that is neither reducible to nor separable from our somatic being—provides a starting place for understanding the particular harm that normalizing genital surgery in infancy and early childhood may entail. For Merleau-Ponty, our embodiment is not a contingent aspect of our selves, as so much of philosophy has maintained.[5] It is not a mere object, though it *is* an object, for others and for ourselves. Rather, Merleau-Ponty indicates that the body, while the center of our being as subject, cannot be disentangled from its status as an object, defined and understood by other embodied subjects in the world. Merleau-Ponty's phenomenology, together with the psychoanalytic account of the early development of subjectivity with which he was so closely engaged, is an invaluable resource for understanding this harm, one that arises precisely because parents and physicians operate with what turns out to be a keen understanding of the importance—indeed, the primacy—of "the other's" view of the self in the constitution of subjectivity.

The first part of this chapter provides a sketch of this phenomenological analysis. In the second part of the chapter I turn to the narrative of a young man who underwent sex reassignment and normalizing surgery as an infant. When I got to know him more than ten years ago, I knew him as Kristi, a young, funny, and engaging lesbian and intersex activist. What I relay here is the result of a conversation we had in 2010, after I had become reacquainted with him as Jim. Still young, funny, and engaging, and now a straight man, Jim agreed to help me consider this problem of harm through reflecting on his own experience. His story captures what, following Suzanne Kessler (1990; 1998), we may take to be a characteristic episode in the history of medical management. It also offers insight into the lasting effects of early normalizing surgeries and into the consequences of living with the secrets and silence that have accompanied such interventions, thereby revealing the material and symbolic harms that prevalent forms of evidence in the field inadequately capture. While some may see in his story only the terrible consequences of a gross medical error in judgment, something that better informed physicians would never have committed, much of his treatment and the motivations for his treatment are continuous with the standard of care today that makes of atypical sex a condition "like no other."

Lessons learned in other fields—most strikingly, in this case, lessons concerning the harms effected by closed adoptions—were long ignored in DSD care, thus reinforcing the uniqueness of atypical sex.[6] The persistent ignorance of knowledge gleaned from analogous cases is evident in the account of Jim's sister, Mary Katherine. In Mary Katherine's story we may find more evidence of an unexpected harm—a collateral harm—that may be experienced by a child whose sibling's body has been subjected to normalizing surgery. It took many years before parents appeared in the clinical literature as objects of study and concern rather than as gateways (or obstacles) (Bing and Rudikoff 1970) to the normalization that physicians assumed was required by the social order. Work concerning parents re-

mains in its early stages. There is as yet no work in the field that addresses the effects of medical management of DSD on siblings. Mary Katherine's story suggests
that harms suffered by individuals treated for DSD may be visited upon the family
as a whole. Attending to these harms, I conclude, speaks to the need in medicine
for another kind of moral framework that may provide better guidance for parents and physicians in caring for children with unusual anatomies.

The Body Schema and Its "I Can"

Merleau-Ponty emphasizes that as embodied subjects, we are "ambiguous" (e.g.,
1962 [1945], 198), subject and object, perceiver and perceived (236–237). This ambiguity denotes the irreducibly "dynamic" (100) space that makes experience possible. Recognizing this dynamic, we must reckon with the fact that our bodies
themselves cannot be objectified in the form of an "I think." Merleau-Ponty explains that

> my awareness of [my body] is not a thought, that is to say, I cannot take it to
> pieces and reform it to make a clear idea. Its unity is always implicit and vague.
> It is always something other than what it is, always sexuality and at the same
> time freedom, rooted in nature at the very moment when it is transformed by
> cultural influences, never hermetically sealed and never left behind. Whether
> it is a question of another's body or my own, I have no means of knowing the
> human body other than that of living it, which means taking up on my own
> account the drama which is being played out in it, and losing myself in it. (153)

This is to say, "I *am* my body" (198; emphasis added). Taylor Carman summarizes this point nicely when he explains that for Merleau-Ponty, the body schema,
our implicit understanding of the body I inhabit, "is not a product but a condition of cognition, for only by being embodied am I a subject in the world at
all: 'I am conscious of my body via the world,' . . . just as 'I am conscious of the
world through the medium of my body'" (Carman 1999, 220, citing Merleau-Ponty
1962 [1945], 82). Consciousness understood in Merleau-Ponty's phenomenological
terms, then, cannot be understood as "a matter of 'I think that' but of 'I can'" (1962
[1945], 137). Consciousness is not simply a function of cognition, of thinking, as
we might conclude from Descartes's meditations on certainty, but must already
be a matter of embodied engagement in the world and with others. The sense of
the "I can" Merleau-Ponty describes cannot be understood in terms of conventional conceptions of the autonomous subject and the meaning of the intentions
that issue from this subject.

This notion of embodied consciousness has proved especially appealing to
feminist philosophers such as Iris Marion Young, who have found in Merleau-
Ponty's phenomenology a rich theoretical framework within which to identify the
ways that the objectification of women inhibits the "I canness" of the body. Ac-

knowledging how possibilities for engagement may be forestalled or spoiled by what Young describes as an inhibiting "self-consciousness of the feminine relation to her body" (2005 [1980], 44), the objectification she makes her own, is important for understanding the particular harm I want to identify in the medical management of atypical sex anatomies.

Even as feminists have found promising tools in Merleau-Ponty's analysis, however, they have commented on the ways that the gender neutrality of his account of subjectivity finally "reduces the specifically intersubjective experience of the body manifest in an encounter with another embodied person to the corporeal dynamic operative with the body proper (*le corps proper*)," and so neglects the ways that gender difference shapes the experience of this body (Stawarska 2006, 92; see also Weiss 1999, 2). The "body proper" refers to the image of the body that emerges after the point of an infant's development called the "mirror stage," a period marking individuation. Feminist phenomenologists see a conflict between Merleau-Ponty's concept of embodied subjectivity that is always already engaged in the world and with others, and the conventional conception of the autonomous subjectivity that lingers as a stubborn trace in his work, covering over the kinds of objectification that inhibit the "I canness" of the body. The tension that feminists have identified in Merleau-Ponty's work, I suggest, mirrors the tension at work in debates over ethical decision making in the care of children with atypical sex anatomies. Equivocations over the importance of familial love and acceptance in the literature supporting the standard of care may be owing to a concept of subjectivity that looks much like that concept feminist phenomenologists have both criticized and found so promising. As embodied subjects, in other words, our sense of ourselves is developed via our engagement with others and with the social and political institutions of which we are a part. For Merleau-Ponty, subjectivity cannot be reduced to objectification, and yet, as feminists have argued, objectification and the violent "setting apart" that it entails must also be a product of our intersubjective experience. Affirming, as Merleau-Ponty does, the rich fabric of intersubjective experience, however, it can nonetheless be difficult to account for the points in which violence can occur.[7] In feminist criticism of the covering over of the losses suffered as a result of objectification, we may find an analogous concealment of the losses that can occur as a consequence of normalizing genital surgeries in infancy and early childhood. Attending more closely to Merleau-Ponty's account of the development of human subjectivity may resolve the tension present in his earlier account and provide better tools with which to appreciate the nature of these losses.

Being Seen, Being Loved: Conditions of Human Emergence

In lectures Merleau-Ponty delivered on the work of seventeenth-century thinker Nicolas Malebranche in 1947–1948, lectures that closely followed the publication of Merleau-Ponty's *Phenomenology of Perception*, we may find a corrective to the limiting notion of the "body proper" on which his early published work focuses (Merleau-Ponty 2001 [1968]). Judith Butler provides a compelling reading of these lectures that considerably enrich Merleau-Ponty's account of subjectivity in her essay "Merleau-Ponty and the Touch of Malebranche" (2005). She offers there an unexpected and moving consideration of "the primary conditions for human emergence" (204). "On one hand," Butler writes,

> this is a theological investigation for Malebranche. It is not only that I cannot feel anything but what touches me, *but that I cannot love without first being loved, cannot see without being seen, and that in some fundamental way, the act of seeing and loving are made possible by—and are coextensive with—being seen and being loved* . . . But Malebranche in the hands of Merleau-Ponty—Malebranche, as it were, transformed by the touch of Merleau-Ponty—becomes something different and something more. For here, Merleau-Ponty asks after the conditions by which the subject is animated into being. (195; emphasis added)

Butler suggests that the "fundamental inquiry into the animating conditions of human ontology" that occurs here may supplement (and perhaps complete) the important work on "The Intertwining—The Chiasm" that remained unfinished at Merleau-Ponty's death. "This chiasm," she explains, "is the name for the obscure basis of our self-understanding, and the obscure basis of our understanding of everything that is not ourselves" (198). That obscurity is resolved for Malebranche in the mystery of a divinity that mediates the subject's "passage through alterity which makes any and all contact of the soul with itself necessarily obscure" (199). In Butler's reading, this connection between human and God as he manifests himself in this obscurity provides a way of understanding the complex underpinnings of what Merleau-Ponty called the "I can" in the *Phenomenology of Perception*, for it "is by virtue of this connection, which I cannot fully know, between sentience and God, that I understand myself to be a free being, one whose actions are not fully determined in advance, for whom action appears as a certain vacillating prospect" (199). Human freedom—that is to say, one's possibilities for becoming—remains mysterious; it is not located "in" the subject, and yet its animating conditions, beyond the subject, exceed its ability fully to objectify them.

At the end of her essay Butler suggests that we might understand these lectures to constitute Merleau-Ponty's recasting of "psychoanalysis as a seventeenth century theology" (203). While the "material needs of infancy are not quite the same as the scene that Malebranche outlines for us as the primary touch of the divine," she writes, "we can see that his theology gives us a way to consider not only the primary conditions for human emergence but the requirement for alterity, the satisfaction of which paves the way for the emergence of the human itself" (204). Individuals who have undergone normalizing surgeries provide a privileged opportunity to examine the conditions that "pave the way" for this emergence and the conditions that impede it.

Criticisms of the standard of care of intersex conditions that focus on the suffering caused by past treatment speak evocatively to "the requirement for alterity"— the need for the "seeing" and "loving" (m)other. While criticisms of harm committed in the past, as well as uncertainty of outcomes for interventions performed today, are recognized by most pediatric specialists who continue to recommend, or present, normalizing surgery as an "option" (Parisi et al. 2007, 355), they persist in seeing normalizing surgery as an important and perhaps even necessary means of securing parents' love. The problems of the past—which many physicians report they relay to parents faced with decisions about normalizing surgery today (355)—are understood to be the result of the inadequate surgical techniques of the past (e.g., Leslie et al. 2009). Reducing these problems to technical matters, however, precludes consideration of what may be more consequential questions concerning the effects of normalizing surgery, however improved.

The account of the mirror stage offered by Jacques Lacan provides an explicit psychoanalytic account of human emergence that Butler sees as implicit in Merleau-Ponty's reading of Malebranche. Lacan's discussion complements Merleau-Ponty's reflections by providing a ground for recognizing the particular harms that normalizing surgeries can effect, given that they are performed precisely during the period (between the ages of six and eighteen months) that Lacan identifies as the critical inauguration of this process of subject formation.[8] Bringing Lacan's account together with Merleau-Ponty's engagement with Malebranche provides an important insight into a kind of harm that is difficult for physicians, and perhaps even for those who experience it, to name, identify, or understand. Located at the junction of the corporeal and the psychic, it is neither precisely corporeal nor psychic, which may account for the challenge in recognizing what may be at stake for the child, her siblings, and the family as a whole, in parents' decision to normalize children's sex anatomy.

During the first few months of life, before the process of individuation begins, the infant relates to its body and the body of its mother in terms of their parts: the fist, the foot, or the nipple it finds in its mouth. The mirror stage marks the beginning of a process of identity formation in which the infant, starting at about six months of age, encounters what it takes to be its own unified image. This is, Lacan remarks, a joyful moment, arousing so much interest that the baby works to surmount the challenges of its inability to stand, devising the means to prolong its first recognition of itself as a whole body (1977 [1966], 2). But the "flutter of jubilant activity" evident at this moment is not only the delight the infant takes in the image of its own body but also his delight in recognizing the "persons and things" around him, including his own animated gaze and the mother the baby also sees reflected in the mirror.[9]

Many who write on the mirror stage emphasize the alienation that the recognition of one's body, distinct from other bodies, brings. As Merleau-Ponty writes, the "objectification of his own body discloses to the child his difference, his 'insularity,' and, correlatively, that of others" (1964 [1960], 119; cf. 129). At least at the beginning of his exposition of the mirror stage, however, Lacan does not emphasize alienation so much as the vulnerability of the baby, the observation that its joyful (mis)recognition of a unified image of itself comes at the moment when the baby is "still sunk in his . . . motor incapacity and nursling dependence" (1977 [1966], 2).[10]

In *The Imaginary Domain,* Drucilla Cornell argues that the "Lacanian account allows us to understand just how fragile the achievement of individuation is, and how easily it can be undermined, if not altogether destroyed, by either a physical or symbolic assault on the projection of bodily integrity" (1995, 38). The fragility of this achievement is owing to the dependency of the infant on the other, because the other enables the infant to repeat the experience of its mirror image, the experience that conveys its sense of bodily integrity as vital to the child's developing sense of self. Cornell explains:

> In this way, the sight of another human being, including the infant's actual image in the mirror, or in the eyes of the mother or primary caretaker, is crucial for shaping identity. This other, who, in turn, both appears as whole and confirms the infant in its projected and anticipated coherence by mirroring him or her as a self, becomes the matrix of a sense of continuity and coherence which the child's present state of bodily disorganization would belie. (39)[11]

Given the importance of the other's role in this founding moment of subject formation, we must ask what the implications of normalizing genital surgery during this process of mirroring could entail. What effect might the changing of the body's appearance have for the child? How might the pain of postsurgical recovery figure in what is, from a psychoanalytic perspective, a critical period in development? What changes might occur in the ways those significant "others"—those whose eyes serve as mirrors to the infant—relate to him?

If we are discouraged from asking such questions because of the paucity of good evidence we can gather from such an investigation, we should recall that it is precisely because of the fear that a parent will not relate well to a child with an atypical sex anatomy—that is, will not serve as a good mirror—that normalizing genital surgery remains the standard of care. But the fact that the sort of evidence most everyone wants is not forthcoming should not (as it largely has to this point) justify the unchecked performance of normalizing surgery in children too young to consent to these surgeries. It isn't that physicians do not see cautionary tales in the experiences of those whose surgeries occurred ten or twenty or forty years ago; they evidently see in these stories errors or inadequacies of technique. Thus, though they no longer justify these surgeries as a means of improving sexual or reproductive functioning, the questions they ask remain technical. Such questions demonstrate physicians' assumptions that these interventions promote affective, social functioning. In the experiences of those who are able to articulate their experience as adults, we find challenging responses to the recommendations of physicians to normalize a child's appearance and to parents' agreement—or sometimes urging—to do so.

Jim's Story

Jim did not know anything about his sex reassignment until he was twelve years old. Company had arrived one evening at the house, and Jim was with his mother in her bedroom while she finished getting ready. "I don't know why she chose then, but she told me that I was born a hermaphrodite and that I'd have to take pills to look like all the other girls." Jim—then called Kristi—recounts that this news, not that he would need to take hormone replacement, which he didn't really understand, but of his ambiguous sex, brought feelings of excitement, fear, and exhilaration. It was for him a kind of affirmation, a "recognition that there was something wrong with me, that there was a reason I was unhappy and riddled with anxiety." It wasn't that Jim always "knew" that he was born male; he describes instead a sense of distance from his body, an "ineffable" sense of being out of place that was beyond his grasp, finally brought nearer by his mother's revelation.[12] Perhaps it remained just out of his reach because his mother never told him about the two surgeries he had had—first at about thirteen months, and later, when he was three and a half—to remove a smaller than normal penis and undescended testes.

Jim's account of his childhood is a story of two different bodies. One was a model of athletic prowess. An accomplished soccer player despite the physical disadvantage entailed by not having hormone-producing gonads, he remembers how the soccer field was where he was "truly happy," where he felt "very much in [his] body." But as he got older, even that experience took on what he describes as the "grayness" that characterized his life off the field: "All the girls around me started to change, to look more like women, and more beautiful . . . I had to go to the doctor to have my change take place." The exhilaration Jim felt at twelve, when his sense of his difference from his peers was affirmed, flattened in later adolescence when he learned "I would need to take all these pills and put on weight, and develop these breasts." Even so, he remembers, "I experienced my body as a success on the field. It didn't come easily. The older I got, the more I was surrounded by girls who were better and better." On the field, Jim's body was fluent in what sociologist George Herbert Mead called the "conversation of gestures" (Mead cited in Weiss 2008, 64) that organized it. There, all the players "were encouraged to behave the way that I behaved naturally, which was aggressive, and focused . . . thinking about the game."

Despite, or maybe because of, the dull unhappiness he felt off the field, the resentment that he felt toward his teammates who were as conversant in the feminine gestures off the field as they were in those—athletic, unmarked, masculine—gestures on it, Jim didn't resist the vaginoplasty his mother presented him as "a matter of course" when he turned eighteen. From his narrative, it doesn't seem that he saw vaginoplasty as a means of joining the girls in being the women they seemed so effortlessly to become; rather, it seems that his assent was a measure of his indifference to his body, to what happened to his body, when it wasn't engaged athletically. Presented as "what happens next," it did happen.

Cornell remarks that the mirror stage "is not a stage in the traditional sense," because one never completes it" (1995, 39).[13] That is to say, the "coherence" that passing through the stage is supposed to secure is never finally achieved, and yet it is this sense of coherence, or imagined coherence, that grounds one's identity, one's sense of self. Put in other terms, the "self" the infant sees in the mirror is not "already 'there.' . . . Instead, the self is constituted in and through the mirroring process as other to its reality of bodily disorganization, and by having itself mirrored by others as a whole" (39).[14] Jim's description of a secure sense of self, of bodily integrity on the soccer field, reflects what he describes as the consistent approval he received, particularly from his father. But when he was not in training, when he was not playing, the disorganization, the "grayness," returned. In his account, the vaginoplasty he came to despise was a somatic insult that provoked a deeper discontent, an inability to forget his body as he had previously done. It was also an obstacle to intimate relationships and, as he would learn later when he consulted with a physician, potentially life-threatening: vaginoplasties of the type Jim underwent had proven to be vulnerable to cancer growth (see Schober 2006, 605–606). About a year after the surgery, Jim would look into his medical records and find out what had been taken from him.

It would take a few more years before Jim would seek medical help. By that point he had long stopped taking the female hormones he was prescribed as a teenager. His body consequently weakened with osteopenia (a condition where bone mineral density is lower than normal) and the onset of osteoporosis, his anger competing with his depression, Jim found a knowledgeable and compassionate physician and began a trial of testosterone therapy.[15] He did so with some trepidation, not because he feared transition, but because of his concern that it might not have any effect: "I was worried because when I was born, my genitals didn't fully develop, the [doctor's] concern was that my body didn't respond to testosterone." If hormone therapy wasn't effective, Jim was afraid that he would be truly, as he put it, "up a creek." But it did work. The wonder in Jim's voice is evident when he recalls that his "body really sucked it in, absorbed every bit, like it was hungry for it. It was magical." It was magical because everything changed—his body first and then the ways that others related to him. Recovered fully from the osteopenia, "demedicalized," as his doctor proclaimed him, he sought removal of the vaginoplasty.[16] Jim was a new man.

A New Man, the Same Kid

Jim's triumphant recreation of himself is a remarkable testament to Merleau-Ponty's observation of the way that a body's sense of being "geared onto the world" is marked by the ways that one's body and its intentions may be welcomed by the world. For the first time (at least off a soccer field), Jim describes the experience of what Merleau-Ponty characterizes as "a certain possession of the world by [his] body, a certain gearing of [his] body to the world"; his intentions "receive the response they expect from the world" (1962 [1945], 250). In stores, at work, his interactions with people demonstrated a marked difference; he experienced an unfamiliar ease as he related to and among others as a man.

But his experience also confirms Merleau-Ponty's claim that our existence "always carries forward its past, whether it be by accepting or disclaiming it" (393). This claim is perhaps best exemplified by the fact that those who knew Jim as Kristi see the same person. It is not that he has not changed or that his friends, family, and longtime acquaintances were really seeing Jim all along, nor is it that he is still Kristi. When people—those who knew him as a child or young adult, and his relieved mother—say that Jim is "the same kid" or remark that he "hasn't changed at all," they are speaking to a continuity in their sense of the person they know and love: his humor and gentle compassion, his resilience and edge. For those who knew Kristi and now encounter Jim, Merleau-Ponty's observations about our experience of the present and its relation to the past come to life.

> With the arrival of every moment, its predecessor undergoes a change: I still have it in hand and it is still there, but already it is sinking away below the level of presents; in order to retain it, I need to reach through a thin layer of time. It is still the preceding moment, and I have the power to rejoin it as it was just now; I am not cut off from it, but still it would not belong to the past unless something had altered, unless it were beginning to outline itself, or project itself upon, my present, whereas a moment ago it *was* my present. (1962 [1945], 416–417; original emphasis)

The way that the meaning of one's past can be changed by the present—a past that paradoxically retains its integrity notwithstanding that change—conditions the possibility for the "reinvention" Jim has effected. It may be helpful here to draw on Merleau-Ponty's use of the image of "sedimentation" to understand how this is possible. One might imagine one's experiences forming layers of sediment, constituting a foundation for the stream of understanding that is ongoing. Merleau-Ponty cautions us to see sediment not as "an inert mass in the depths of our consciousness" but as a ground that also conditions the possibility for the "spontaneity" that creates for Merleau-Ponty the "world-structure . . . at the core of consciousness." Newly acquired thoughts or ways of seeing "draw their sustenance from my present thought, they offer me a meaning, but I give it back to them" (1962 [1945], 130). Novel thoughts or understandings of our experience can provide surprising new directions for consciousness and create new layers of sediment. Following Merleau-Ponty's metaphor through to understand the effect of a change such as Jim's, one might consider the effect that a particularly heavy rain or other disturbance could have on its flow: its appearance and movement may be dramatically reshaped, and yet its new appearance and direction would remain continuous with its previous incarnation. This notion of sedimentation provides a way to understand how an individual experiences oneself and one's body as it becomes "habituated" to itself and its environment. It also speaks to the ways that intersubjective experience—the ways that we make sense of one another in gesture and speech—figures in the experiences we take to be "individual" but that must also be understood as formed and shared with others. The impression that Jim is the "same person" speaks phenomenologically to how Jim and those who knew him as Kristi coexists with—and not despite—the significant change he has undergone.

Jim's transition to living as a man is not the first time he experienced a significant shift in his view of his own past, however.[17] When his mother told him that he had been born different, "special," as she said, he saw his previous experience with new eyes, a perspective that changed his understanding of the past as he lived it in the present, laying down new possibilities for the future. When he finally learned years later that being born "special" prompted his castration and the removal of his penis, there was another shift, one that does not diminish his evident attachment to and love for his parents but that nevertheless complicates it. As he puts it, "I never had any doubt that my parents loved me; I also never had a doubt that they were riddled with multiple prejudices about me and I . . . wished they were smarter and filled with less fear than they were." Learning of the surgery brought a still different perspective on himself and his world. But understanding, as his parents and all those who care about him would come to understand, the consequences of his sex reassignment, they were also able to see, and so to mirror, this new man, "the same" lovable kid, before them.

Distorting the Mirror

Jim's story—a story still in progress—should direct us to consider with care the nature of the psychosocial injury resulting from the secrets and silence maintained by families about their child's condition, secrets kept from extended family and neighbors and from affected children themselves. Cheryl Chase observes that the "primary source of harm described by former patients is not surgery per se, but the underlying attitude that intersexuality is so shameful that it must be erased before the child can have any say in what will be done to his or her body" (1999, 147). In *Intersex and Identity*, sociologist Sharon Preves elaborates on the consequences of the erasure Chase describes, particularly with regard to identity formation. It is precisely because our relations with others are central to our sense of self that physicians and parents believe that atypical sex anatomy must be corrected—and thereby concealed—lest individuals suffer.[18] Drawing on Charles Horton Cooley's concept of the "looking-glass self" (1964 [1902]), Preves summarizes the sense of self that her interviews confirm in this way: "I am not what I think I am. I am not what you think I am. I am what I think you think I am" (2003, 21). Such a characterization captures something of one's everyday sense of self in the world and leads us to see the destabilizing effects of finding out that "what I think you think I am" turns out to be wrong, because the information that you (e.g., mother or father) have provided me does not reflect what you think I am at all.

To better appreciate what it means to see identity as an internalization of one's perceptions of what the other sees, we should examine the significance of the revelation that Jim experienced, most acutely at nineteen, that what he had understood to be his parents' and others' "thinking" of his own self was at odds with the view presented in his medical records. What was shocking to Jim was not the knowledge of his sexual difference—that he had understood, if incompletely, years earlier. What was shocking was learning of surgeries that had occurred when he was too young to remember and discovering that his parents and others had withheld information from him that would allow him to make sense of his experience.

Discussion of disclosure of a child's condition in the 2006 Consensus Statement is brief:

> The process of disclosure concerning facts about karyotype, gonadal status and prospects for future fertility is a collaborative ongoing action which requires a flexible individual-based approach. It should be planned with the parents from the time of diagnosis. Studies in other chronic medical disorders and of adoptees indicate that disclosure is associated with enhanced psychosocial adaptation. (Hughes et al. 2006, 557–558)

This acknowledgment of the importance of disclosure, like so many acknowledgments of the harm of past practices, is laudable. The brief analogous mention of what is known about the experience of those with chronic illness or who have been adopted is worth further investigation for understanding not only the benefits of disclosure but also the considerable risks that failures to disclose may entail.

There is now an abundance of evidence that a failure to disclose different aspects of a child's adoption is harmful. Whether concealing the fact of the child's adoption entirely (in periods in which adoption was maintained as much as possible as a secret) or obscuring certain aspects of it (as is the case in "closed" adoption), decades of research reveal a variety of resulting problems, most notably difficulties in identity formation.[19] Psychologist Janet L. Hoopes describes the conclusions drawn by any number of psychologists starting from the mid-twentieth century who have attributed such difficulties to adoptees' experience of "being cut off" from "an essential part of [themselves] . . . [that] remains unknown" (1990, 152). Since the 1940s, psychologists have worked to identify the emotional difficulties faced by many adoptees as a function of not sharing a "blood line" with their families, what the literature characterizes as "genealogical bewilderment" (152). Today, the importance of knowing oneself through knowing one's forebears—that is, the importance of knowing one's biological or genetic origins—is entrenched in the field and provides increasing traction for a claim to a "right to know" one's origins, including access to information about one's birth parents or gamete donors.[20]

That many of the problems associated with adoptees' sense of "shame, embarrassment, and lowered self-esteem" are mitigated by the process of open adoption, however, does not support the claim of a natural imperative to know one's origins; the changes prompted by open adoption suggest instead that the source of the harm lies in the "secrecy, anonymity, and mystique surrounding traditional adoption placement" (e.g., Baran and Pannor 1990, 317). Following this analysis, it isn't the "not knowing" that damages a person's sense of self, but the revelation that others have actively prevented one from knowing something important about oneself or something considered significant by others. Following Cooley's notion of the looking-glass self, we may see that what is damaging is the discovery that the sense you have of others' view of you has been shrouded, or, in psychoanalytic terms, that the mirroring on which you have relied for a coherent sense of self bears too attenuated a resemblance to yourself; the image one has relied on is no longer recognizable.

Whether owing to closed adoption or to secrecy surrounding normalizing genital surgery, the common experience of being shamed by having "the truth about oneself" withheld by others is striking. Examining this common thread of shame provides a direction for understanding the nature of the injury of withholding the "secret" of one's identity. Certainly the historical imperative of concealing the shameful conditions of adoption—from the "illegitimacy" of a child's birth to the infertility of an adoptive couple—has motivated the entire spectrum of closed adoption practices.[21] There is little question that the imperative of concealing a child's atypical sex, both surgically and socially, is similarly motivated. One should not wonder that the pernicious effects of this secrecy would likewise express themselves as narcissistic wounds, that is to say, injuries to one's sense of worth. Nor, following the more recent history of open adoption, should we be surprised that an individual's being adopted should be something, if not entirely unremarkable about oneself, that we might better see as an ordinary feature of a unique self.

A Sibling's Story

There may be another way that lessons from other instances of concealment, and other instances of extraordinary involvement of medicine in children's lives, can be instructive here. When I asked Jim about his sense of others' perceptions of him in his youth and now as an adult—as the girl, Kristi, and now as Jim—he said that the person I should really speak with was his younger sister, Mary Katherine. As soon as Mary Katherine and I began to talk, I understood that Jim's suggestion that I speak with her was not only a response to my question about others' perceptions of him growing up. His sister's experience was also a critical part of the more fundamental question he and I had been discussing about the consequences of the medical intervention for which his body was the explicit object, but the effects of which, he understood, had extended beyond his body and person. What he experienced as an infant, and then as a young adult, had had profound effects on his sense of self. Though he knew that his parents had each been affected in different ways by their own roles in his treatment and in raising him as Kristi, he was now learning that those effects had been visited upon his sister as well.

As adults Mary Katherine and Jim are close, but both agree they had little in common growing up in their parents' house. Their earlier memories of their childhood together look a lot like those of other siblings four years apart: Jim remembers Mary Katherine as the annoying little sister "constantly clamoring for attention"; Mary Katherine felt ignored by her older sister, who challenged and defied their parents in ways she did not dare to. Things got a little better, Mary Katherine remembers, when Kristi went off to college. The physical distance was consonant with the emotional disconnection Mary Katherine felt from her sibling. Plus she had her parents to herself.

Finding a bottle of the estrogen drug Premarin at home one day, Mary Katherine gathered her courage—both siblings keenly recall how unwelcome questions were in their house—and asked her mother why her older sister took these pills. "When you're older, we'll tell you," her mother responded. Unsatisfied with her mother's response, but unable or unwilling to press further, Mary Katherine took advantage of finding herself home alone one day to conduct an internet search. She was perplexed when she found that Kristi's pills were "female hormones for women who were going through menopause." Mary Katherine wondered, "How can my young sister be going through menopause?" She held on to her questions until her first year of college, when another session at her family's computer revealed her sister's browsing history and she found herself on the website of the Intersex Society of North America, with which Jim had made contact. Mary Katherine remembers she "read everything" on the site that explained about atypically sexed bodies and how they were medically treated. Finally seeing the pattern in the accumulating shards of information, she confronted her mother, who "admitted that '[Kristi] wanted to tell you while [s]he was here, but we asked [her] to wait.'"

Mary Katherine knows that in withholding the truth of her sibling's medical history her parents were trying to protect her. But it wasn't clear to her what hard truths they were trying to protect her from. Was it her brother's surgeries? Ambiguous sex? Her parents' decisions? Their own vulnerability? Whatever the fearsome something was, Mary Katherine felt instead "shut out," like she wasn't "part of this family." Mary Katherine now sees the early distance she felt from her family as a product of keeping her out of the secret that shaped all of their lives. She knows that Jim didn't find out the full story himself until he was almost through college and that he wanted to tell her. She resents her parents for keeping Jim from sharing what he had learned, from letting Mary Katherine *in*. He knew, as she doesn't think her parents knew, that she was "important enough to include me in." She recognizes how the sadness she feels for the child and teenager she was is also a result of the anger and grief she continues to feel on behalf of the brother she loves.

The therapist Mary Katherine began to see after her father's passing suggested to Mary Katherine that she was grieving the loss of the sister who is no longer. Certainly she is aware that her mother "misses Kristi, or grieves the loss of her daughter." Both her mother and father struggled mightily to use the right name, the apposite pronoun, when they talked to or about Jim, reverting frequently to the name they had given him after he was born, seeing him still as the girl the doctors had persuaded them was their child. Mary Katherine adapted far more easily to Jim's transition than did her parents, and she visibly bristles even now at any reference to Jim as Kristi, even when recounting memories of events that occurred before Jim's transition. Unlike her mother, Mary Katherine says, "I'm not grieving my sister . . . I don't—I don't miss that person . . . I never got to know that person, and that person couldn't get to know me. It was an impossible thing."

The therapist's proposal that Mary Katherine grieves the loss of her sister is obviously a point of frustration for Mary Katherine. It mistakes the source of the feelings that Mary Katherine is struggling to sort out. The anger the therapist's mistake provokes may also be explained by the implication that the decision to reassign her brother as a girl in infancy was somehow proper, or acceptable, that her sibling was once "really" her sister. Could it be that the therapist was not able to see that Mary Katherine's anger had another source because the therapist herself sees "Kristi" as the original sibling? If this is the case, the therapist unwittingly discounts Mary Katherine's own lived experience; she thus reenacts the stance of Mary Katherine's mother, whose insistence on seeing her oldest child as a girl had so many consequences, unintended as everyone must agree, on Mary Katherine's own sense of self.

Collateral Harm

Even if Mary Katherine didn't feel that she knew the sister with whom she shared a house growing up, it is clear that her sibling was a critical part of her life during those years. That fact might not have been so clear to her as when she learned that it was the secret, or multiple secrets—of Jim's birth, of the surgeries in infancy and young adulthood, of the hormone replacement—that had shaped her own experience in ways she has now begun to identify and understand. She remains sensitive to what she always took to be Jim's privileged position in the family, the respect and admiration he seemed to command from his parents despite—or maybe because of—his resistance to them as a teenager. Mary Katherine was not aware of Jim's uncomplaining acquiescence to what went mostly unspoken even to Jim himself and can now make more sense of the continuity between what she sees as her brother's preferential treatment in childhood and that special relationship between Jim and their mother that still leaves her feeling like a third wheel. As a child she could only understand the special attentions her sibling received at bedtime as evidence that her parents loved Mary Katherine less than Kristi.

There is no discussion of siblings in the clinical or critical literature concerning atypical sex, although study of siblings of children with serious illness, particularly of mental health outcomes for siblings of those with chronic disease, is now quite developed (e.g., Williams 1997). An emerging literature documents the experience of siblings of children with disabilities (e.g., Meyer 2009). Common themes are evident with respect to siblings of both those with illness and those with disability. Most striking is the salience of "feelings of isolation and anxiety . . . jealousy, conflicting feelings such as guilt and anger, and loneliness" (Houtzager et al. 2004, 591). Mary Katherine is keenly aware of the jealousy she feels even today: "My mother treats my brother differently from the way she treats me. I feel like my mother has more—positive feelings for him . . . like she dotes on him. It may be because she doesn't see him very often or maybe she feels guilt . . . I'm jealous of their relationship when we're together." A good deal of the experience psychologist Jeanne Safer describes in *The Normal One: Life with a Difficult or Damaged Sibling* (2002) captures the challenges Mary Katherine faces. Safer talks about the ways that those who have siblings with a disability, or other sorts of difficulties, can be made to feel invisible in their families. In discussing the consequences of feeling "shut out" by her parents in their efforts to shield her from the knowledge of her brother's condition and his treatment, Mary Katherine reflects on what she describes as her own feeling of "impairment." She is critical of her own insecurity, of the ways she finds herself "seeking acceptance, seeking attention." She also describes a kind of self-consciousness that gets in the way of her relating with others: "I worry about what I say, [I hold] back my feelings. I have a hard time communicating . . . and connecting with people on a deep emotional level." She guesses that these feelings are common to those who have had experiences like hers. Safer's account confirms Mary Katherine's suspicions. Even if they are not aware of a sibling's condition (Safer 2002, 57), "normal ones" can experience "chronic overlooking [that] happens when desperate, overwhelmed adults . . . try to cope with situations that no parent bargains for, and few have emotional resources to balance. As a result, many healthy siblings grow up with a hunger for attention that is never satisfied and that seems wrong to feel. Their needs, so consistently ignored, become invisible to themselves" (94). Mary Katherine's story is like many of those Safer tells. But it departs from nearly all of them because Mary Katherine and her brother, Jim, have opportunities for ongoing discussion, mutual understanding, and reconciliation that many siblings Safer interviewed do not, opportunities that Mary Katherine would not have had, one gathers, with Kristi.

Now looking back, Mary Katherine can start to make sense of what Jim describes as his envy of what he took to be his sister's ease in her body and in the world. Jim could not have known, just as Mary Katherine could not have known, how their parents' feelings and experiences affected their treatment as children. After their father's death, it was Jim who discovered the separate journals their parents kept during a marriage retreat years earlier. When asked "to describe their happiest moment as a married couple, they both separately said the birth of my sister." Their father added his regret that he didn't have the larger family he had envisioned for himself, Jim remembers, "but," his father wrote, "the risk of having another 'Kristi' was too great." In the end it is hard to identify who is, in Safer's terms, the "damaged" sibling. Because Jim's story is an extraordinary one, marked less by ongoing struggle than by reinvention, the challenges that Mary Katherine faces can now be more easily discerned, more readily acknowledged, including by Mary Katherine herself.

For all the differences between the relationship Mary Katherine describes between herself and Kristi, and that she now enjoys with Jim, there remains one point of continuity. Mary Katherine now recognizes that her feelings of inadequacy, the questions about her own lovableness as a child, result from her comparing her parents' treatment of Kristi with how she was treated. As a child, she could only imagine that the closeness she saw between her parents and Jim was a reflection of Jim's superiority or of her own inadequacy. Certainly Kristi's status as the firstborn child might also have been a factor and could explain what Mary Katherine sees as the privileged place that Jim occupies still. When Mary Katherine talks about the jealousy she continues to experience when she is with her brother and mother, she acknowledges having had "envious" feelings toward her brother, feelings that appear to have given way, as Melanie Klein (1975 [1957]) remarks, to the gratitude she now experiences in what she and Jim can share, namely, the sort of private history common to siblings who grow up under the same roof, and who can understand, as only siblings can understand, the ordinary outrages parental misdeeds provoke, even if the misdeeds include using the wrong pronoun to refer to one's sibling. With Jim, Mary Katherine says, "I can be myself; I can say anything," and her brother will understand. She is obviously grateful for his advice in her professional work and appreciates the pleasure, too, of being her brother's abiding ally.

Psychoanalysis, Safer observes, is "strangely silent" on the matter of siblings (2002, 29).[22] The emerging literature concerning those with siblings with a disability, disease, or disorder of whatever kind nevertheless suggests the importance of siblings in one's formation. Mary Katherine's narrative, and those increasingly available in print and online, point to the significant ways that siblings figure in the mirroring parents provide.[23] Mary Katherine's narrative shares common threads with these emerging narratives, but is unlike them to the extent that her narrative and Jim's converge in ways that each is beginning to recognize. Both Mary Katherine and Jim felt betrayed by their parents, and both felt that something important about them, something central to who they are, was withheld from them. The revelation of what Mary Katherine's parents had done—to Jim, to her, and in retrospect, to their relationship with one another—changed her vision of her parents. The images her parents now reflect back to her, in life (her mother) and in death (her father), are not finally reconcilable with those she had before. In Mary Katherine's story, as in Jim's, as in the innumerable stories of closed adoptions, we can see the damaging effects of the keeping of secrets and the effects of the revelation of secrets kept. We must recognize, too, that in seeing its own imagined wholeness reflected in her parents' gaze, the child sees also her parents' gaze directed at her sibling(s).

The Possibility of an Embodied Ethics

Jim's story provides an entrée into understanding the consequences of a treatment rationale grounded in satisfying the needs of parents or society, rather than those of children (as well as insight into how these can be sharply distinguished where we might not expect them to be). In making the aim of treatment the relief of parents' suffering, and seeking to resolve or diminish that suffering by altering the child's body, by making it tolerable, the child *is not seen*. Making the love of parents for a child conditioned on the child's appearance puts that love in question; however good the intention, "the effect may be otherwise" (Dreger 2006b, 261). Indeed, as Adrienne Asch puts it:

> By undertaking [cosmetic] surgery before children can voice feelings about their bodies and their lives, the most loving parent can unwittingly undermine the child's confidence that she is lovable and loved. It is confidence in that love and lovableness that provides the foundation for dealing with what life brings. (2006, 229)

The confidence in one's parents' love that Asch sees as vital to a child's flourishing also participates in the enigmatic becoming that Merleau-Ponty identifies in his reading of Malebranche. This confidence may be understood as a condition of the possibility of the embodied "I can," the place where the body's materiality and consciousness meet and engage in the world and with others.

From Jim and Mary Katherine we learn that damage to the "I can," to the corporeal schema, can result from, or perhaps is more likely to result from, the kind of affective assault constituted by secrets and silence, and not only from scalpels. In their stories we see how half-truths, what is spoken and what goes unsaid, are integrated into their senses of self. Jim's life is testament to the ways that the mirror stage is fragile and ongoing. In showing how one's sense of self can so easily be damaged, his story also demonstrates how this fragility enables the possibility of refashioning a self on the sedimented foundation of one's experience, of what has come before. Merleau-Ponty's concept of sedimentation can help us better understand how such change is possible and, indeed, how such change occurs in all of our lives, if not always with the triumph that Jim can claim. Mary Katherine struggles as she comes to terms with the vexed privilege of how her "normality" made her invisible, of how not being seen has impeded her ability to see, especially her ability to see that she has experienced harm. Mary Katherine did not suffer the surgeries performed on her brother's body, and yet the damage she is coming to recognize is damage, like her brother's, at the level of the corporeal schema.

The exploration of an "embodied ethics" I have begun here must concern not only the status of the child as subject—or perhaps the children as subjects—but the parents' subjectivity as well. As Gail Weiss describes it, an embodied ethics is "grounded in the dynamic, bodily imperatives that emerge out of our intercorporeal exchanges and which in turn transform our own body [schemas], investing and reinvesting them with moral significance" (1999, 158). Ethical reflection on parenting is often understood in terms of a parent's responsibility to support the development of a child's sense of self; bioethical discussions of such responsibility are framed largely in the familiar Kantian terms of autonomy and consider dilemmas of treating children in terms of the "rights" of parents to make decisions on behalf of beings who are not yet but will likely someday be bearers of these same rights. A phenomenological account of the enactment of the responsibility a parent has to a child emphasizes quite a different ethical dimension, revealing the ways that parents' "acting upon" their children must also, at the same time, entail *being acted upon.* This is the philosophical gloss on what Alice Dreger (2010b) writes in her *Psychology Today* blog:

> If you want to be a parent, start getting used to the fact that your children will change you as much as you change them. I now know far more than I ever thought I would about trains, airplanes, and Australian native species thanks to my son. I am also more patient, more organized, more disorganized, more sleep deprived, and more in love with him than I ever thought I'd be. If you would not have your child explicitly manipulate your identity as a condition of loving you, do not begin your relationship with your child by doing the same.

The ethical imperative articulated here—an embodied ethical imperative— should perhaps be understood as an essential supplement to, rather than replacement of, conventional approaches to bioethics. The imperative to which Dreger points is not one of "unconditional love"; it is instead an acknowledgment that parents' love, together with the caring work that constitutes parenting, should be understood to shape not only the child but also the parent herself. It is because specialists of DSD are focused on the child that parents' feelings and responses are given so central a role in the decisions made in the child's care. Were an embodied ethics to be taken seriously, however, it seems evident that the standard of care would change. Its objects of intervention would shift from what is now represented as an exclusive focus on the well-being of "the patient" to include those who care for him, that is, to make the adjustment of the parents to "the child they weren't expecting" (Dreger 2006b) a focus of care rather than a motivation for treatment decisions of the child that might not be in her best interests. Such an ethics may not easily be reduced to rules or immediately assessed via indicators of "quality care." The kind of phenomenological interrogation toward which Merleau-Ponty directs us offers resources for further investigation of the ethical challenges and requirements of caring for children with atypical sex anatomy. Before turning to these, I believe we need to better understand the obstacles to such an ethics as they present themselves today.

5 A Question of Ethics as/or a Question of Culture

The Problem of What Is and What Ought to Be

TRYING TO UNDERSTAND and to describe the nature of the ethical violation entailed by the standard of care for the treatment of atypical sex anatomies has been the focus of my analysis thus far. The aim of my project up to this point is much like those of others working in the humanities and social sciences who have criticized the practices associated with this standard. For all the power and cogency of that body of work, and for all the change that has occurred, the standard of care that makes normalization of the bodies of children with DSD the first and best option remains largely intact. The individual and collaborative work that has laid out ethical problems entailed by the standard of care—by Suzanne Kessler, Anne Fausto-Sterling, Cheryl Chase, and Alice Dreger, and then by those working in their wake—has not resulted in making cosmetic normalization a problem of another time. Trying to understand how it can be that the revelation of ethical violation has not resulted in change equal to that revelation is the focus of this chapter and the one that follows.

Already we have a good sense of some of the barriers to recognizing ethical problems that are salient in the standard of care: the apparently unassailable "fact" of sexual difference functions as a ground for social meaning and organization. It may be difficult now to appreciate that as late as the 1990s most physicians did not see themselves as "having a position" on atypical sex anatomies and the standard of care until activism made clear that there was even a possibility, or need, of doing so (S. J. Kessler 1998, 119). In *Lessons from the Intersexed*, Kessler writes that the 1996 American Academy of Pediatrics' "Position on Intersexuality," issued in response to the picketing of their annual meeting, was "intended to bolster the medical viewpoint that early genital surgery is necessary for the emotional and cognitive development of intersex/ed children." That is to say, the statement was an assertion of the noncontroversial status of the standard of care; it reaffirmed the claim made by one specialist in DSD care that medical practice takes place within "the context of what *is* rather than what *should be*" (120; original emphasis). But as Kessler sees it, the issuing of this statement marked a victory for activists who had, "for the first time, forced a medical group to publicly acknowledge that intersexuality was something about which a view could be taken" (159n62). Perhaps this is the moment at which the "conceptual, moral and practical messes" that hermaphroditism posed in the nineteenth century (Dreger 1996, cited in S. J. Kessler 1998, 120) took root in the twentieth. Twenty years after the founding of the Intersex Society of North America, it appears that one of the biggest messes remains the persistent refusal of physicians to see the ethical problems posed by the standard of care *as* ethical problems. Kessler diagnoses this problem as one owing to physicians' views that their practices are "constrained by real world demands," that is, that they have no choice but to normalize anatomies that disrupt taken-for-granted notions of how things are in the world. But in so doing, physicians refuse to recognize that they are themselves *"creators of that world"* to which they belong and that their practices serve to reinforce such notions (1998, 120; emphasis added).

Recognition by specialists who care for children with DSD that their professional work is not only shaped by culture but also functions itself to shape culture may not be easily achieved, because the standard of care for the management of atypical sex anatomies has been formulated not with respect to what we might characterize as the "natural function" of bodies so much as with appearances of bodies, the standards of which are, as physicians acknowledge, determined by one's location in a particular cultural context. But examination of questions such as these is typically not considered by physicians as part of their work. Most of what are considered to be ethical questions in medicine—by physicians themselves, as well as by bioethicists—do not challenge the goals of medical practice, namely, the "good health" of the individual or population. For the most part, the application of bioethical principles has focused on ensuring the soundness of the *means* of achieving that "good." Suspect or conspicuously bad means of achieving a "good outcome" may corrupt that goal—this would be one way of casting the history of eugenics, for example, but the goal of medicine itself has rarely been the object of criticism. Two decades after the beginning of intersex activism, physicians readily grant that the means by which children's bodies have been normalized has effected harm. And yet, because the care of those with atypical anatomies may call into question the good of the goal of medical treatment in this case—that is, "normal sex appearance" (conflated, as it is, with "normal gender expression")—the act of ethical reflection has been taken to be at odds, or somehow in tension, with medical practice.

Sorting out the ways that this tension manifests itself is no simple task. It is not only a matter of recognizing that sound arguments laying out the ethical violation that the standard of care entails have not resulted in the fundamental changes one might expect; it is also necessary to try to understand why the history of the medical management of atypical sex anatomies looks increasingly like a history of moral failure. The experience of the woman I call Andrea, diagnosed with congenital adrenal hyperplasia in the 1950s, provides an opening for examining this history in more detail. Her story is remarkable because it appears that a great deal of time and deliberation went into her treatment by doctors at a place and time when so many physicians, if not ignorant about the function of the clitoris, believed nevertheless that partial or complete removal of a larger than normal clitoris was the best decision for patients.[1] Unlike her peers with CAH, however, Andrea was spared the worst of the treatment to which they were subject. As she related her story in conversation with me, it struck me that we might find there an instance in which doctors demonstrated awareness of the ethical questions raised by what Kittay (2006) calls "the desire for normality." But if, as I discovered in later conversation with one of her physicians, we could find such an instance of ethical grappling with normalization in Andrea's story, it was not exactly as I had expected or, frankly, hoped.

Desiring Normality: Andrea's Story

I spoke with Andrea—Andie—in 2011 for the same reason that I spoke with Jim: I sought insight into the nature of the harm effected by the standard of care. Their experiences share some common features: both had childhoods marked by surgeries in late infancy and later years, about which, they were given to understand, they should ask no questions; both made frequent visits to the doctor intended to feminize their bodies, and both had troubling questions about their sexual desire for other girls. Unlike Jim, whose chromosomal sex was male and who was reassigned female in infancy, it appears that Andie was quickly identified as a girl with the "classic," salt-losing form of CAH. As a result, she would need far more regular visits to the doctor to regulate her hormones; her medical health could be so fragile that having an ordinary flu could result in hospitalization.

Born to an upper-middle-class Reform Jewish family in a large metropolitan city a few years after the end of the Second World War, Andie sees her story as characteristic of an historical moment. At mid-century Ashkenazic Jewish children in the United States were being increasingly identified with CAH, an autosomal recessive disorder that had not been well identified in previous decades.[2] Children who appeared perfectly healthy at birth would suddenly be in crisis—adrenal crisis, as it became clear—and could die within days of onset. Before the wider availability of newborn screening programs, misdiagnosis of CAH was common and mortality was high. More information was gleaned in the late 1940s, most importantly by Lawson Wilkins (Eder 2010; 2012), and research on optimal regulation of the condition is ongoing. Today children are typically identified prenatally (owing to family history) or soon after birth, a result of the newborn screening that became more common beginning in 2001 and is now universal in the United States and much of the developed world. But from the 1950s through to the end of the twentieth century, certain children with CAH benefited from being born in areas where there was greater prevalence of the disorder, which promoted broader familiarity in newborn nurseries and emergency rooms.[3] Andie was among those children who were fortunate to be identified at birth. As she tells it, this larger history of the increasing identification and understanding of CAH is critical for appreciating her treatment as a child and young adult. But just as critical to making sense of her experience, she believes, is the cultural legacy of assimilation she inherited along with the genetic mutation that results in her body's failure to produce cortisol. Born after the Second World War, Andie says, she received the strong message that it was important

> not only to be assimilated Jews but to be unnoticeable. At this time, not only Jews—but maybe particularly Jews—were warehousing kids with Down Syndrome . . . and there was this strong, maybe unspoken desire to fit in and to not have anybody speculate about you . . . I think there was this not only societal thing about having a child that was "right," but having a Jewish daughter who was "right."

Having a clitoris that looked more like a small penis would be one of those things that was not right—not for her family and not, she says, for herself as an older child.

Andie's thoughts about what motivated her care, and her willing cooperation in it, resonate with Kittay's reflections on normality at this time and place and her own experience as a Jewish immigrant to the United States at just the moment Andie discusses. In the years after the revelation of the horrors of the Holocaust, Kittay writes, "normality was deeply sought and deeply desired." The desire for normality was a kind of desperate and encompassing desire, where

> all that was regarded to be outside the normal—be it a revolutionary philosophy, an atypical sexuality, a deviant body, an unruly mind, a history of brutality, and surely grandparents, aunts, uncles, and cousins sent to the gas chambers—all these were banished from sight and from memory so that life could assume a predictability and stability that contrasted with war conditions. (2006, 91)

Internalizing this message despite or because of her differences as an immigrant, a Jew, and someone whose life was marked by her parents' horrible suffering, Kittay remembers, "I desired above all to be normal, to be like everyone else, to hide the pain of abnormality" (91).

When Andie decided in her thirties to finally confront the pain that had until that time been unspeakable, she began by asking her mother for details about her early diagnosis and treatment. Her mother remembered only that she was "circumcised," maybe before they left the hospital. She did not recall much about the surgery that Andie clearly remembers undergoing when she was eight. Andie would learn as an adult that this was among the very first clitoral recessions, a surgery that did not cut any sensitive clitoral tissue, but concealed it by moving most of the visible portion of her clitoris under her pubis.[4] "I remember a lot about the sutures," she begins. "I was present for that surgery, although I know I distanced myself from it in many ways . . . Dissolving sutures were new, and I remember pulling [them] out . . . and then, going back for the follow-up, they were 'miraculously dissolved!' And I remember thinking [I needed to take them out myself because] 'well, you hurt me the last time you were there!'"

Andie was not given much information about what kind of surgery she would have on that day, but she can recall vividly many of the details of the events that precipitated it.

> Something happened at summer camp the year that I was eight . . . I remember where I was standing; I was getting out of my bathing suit, and a counselor maybe, or another girl, saw that I was different and pointed out how different I was . . . I don't remember what was said, but I remember that in October after that summer (it was October because we were starting to wear sweaters), I finally approached my mother, and I remember thinking, "She'll know how to answer this."

When Andie gets to this point in the narrative, she pauses, and her voice catches, remembering the gumption and fear and hope she felt as she approached her mother with the question she had held since that day at camp.

> I asked her why—why I was different from other girls. And I can remember her saying something like, "Oh, sweetheart, what makes you say that?" and I must have told her what happened that summer, and . . . I was really hoping she would say, "You know, all girls are different, and some girls have bigger breasts and—*all girls are different*." And what I remember was getting to the doctor pretty quickly after that. And I remember the genital check, and I remember that my mother was kind of standing over my shoulder, to see, and I don't want to say that there was an audible gasp from her, but I remember that there was this body language-like withdrawal, and I remember that this [doctor] with another doctor in practice with him—both endocrinologists . . . and I remember his brother [another pediatrician] being called in to the room, and having a discussion over my body. And as I'm looking up at [the three of] them, they are not at all connecting with me. They are looking at "this body."

As traumatizing as these memories are for Andie—the cruel or merely curious counselor or fellow camper who called attention to her bodily difference; her mother's alarm, first when Andie asked why she was different, and then, in the doctor's office, when her mother saw what the doctors saw; the coldness of the doctors' objectifying gaze looking down at her body—she also remembers how strongly she wanted relief from these moments. She remembers how much she wanted to be normal.

Reflecting on her desire for normality growing up, Andie remembers another surgery that occurred several years later. When, at fifteen, she still had not gotten her period, her doctors recommended she undergo what was then new exploratory laparoscopy to determine whether her not getting her period was a symptom of a larger problem. They found no abnormality, and soon after, Andie began to menstruate. She remembers her mother's anger following what Andie gathers was the doctor's shrugging, "Well, I guess that [surgery] was unnecessary." But unlike her mother, Andie did not regret that later surgery: "I can remember, *I* wanted to do this. *I* wanted to know." She wanted to know whether she was— or could be—a "normal girl": "I had these questions about my sex, my sexuality, and I was burning with some question—it was really all about my sexuality." This burning question with which she struggled for most of her adult life was, she explains, the question she was really asking when she was eight and was the reason why she did not resist the genital surgery she had at that time. This struggle also explains, she reflects, the thank-you note she had written her doctor and discovered in her medical file almost forty years later: "It says 'thank you for'—and I had written something like, 'thank you for making me feel like other girls,' and I had crossed out the word, 'feel,' and put 'look,' then I crossed out 'look like'—I was obviously having struggles with the fact that I wasn't like other girls." "When I was eight," she continues, "I felt like, if I have these surgeries, I wouldn't like girls anymore. And that's what I wanted. And so when I wrote this letter to him, about feeling like other girls, I knew that that hadn't gone away. [I knew] in those months after, that [the surgery] hadn't magically cured my brain. So, you know, I just never felt like all the other girls."

The message that she was "different" was conveyed in a number of ways as she was growing up, not least through the multiple visits to the doctor she made with her mother throughout her childhood. Having salt-losing CAH meant that her health needed to be monitored closely, and the medical records she sought as an adult document the frequent visits and consultations her doctor conducted with his colleagues. They confirm, too, Andie's sharp memory of the frequent genital checks to which she was subjected, including the one at eight she remembers so clearly communicated—Andie thinks explicitly, but can't be sure—"that 'you don't look—' or 'you're not really a girl.'" Andie worked very hard for most of her life to appear "like all the other girls." While she never had any doubt that she was loved by her parents, she did have the sense that certain subjects—such as her body and her desire for girls—were dangerous and so off-limits.

Throughout her telling of her story, it seemed that there was a close connection between Andie's perception of her anatomical difference and her desire for other girls—one of the reasons, it appears, that normalizing surgery was, and perhaps continues to be, recommended.[5] Without anyone's saying so, these differences were for Andie of a piece; she thought that changing her body could also change her desire and that she must do her part to make her desire align with the normalized body the surgeons had created when she was eight. The doctors and her parents both assured her that now she was normal and that "it would be okay." When she went to college and learned for the first time that there were other women who desired women sexually, she was amazed. But she "steered clear [of them] because, she insisted to herself, '*I* was definitely normal,'" even if she had to work at it.

> It became like a discipline for me. Even though I was in college, and there were a lot of lesbians around, I really kept along the other path, because I just knew that I wasn't normal, and that was what I wanted to be. There was a part of me that—I didn't know what to do with it, but it was that I knew: All of this [medical treatment] had been done so that I would be normal . . . I was bound and determined to be normal, to be that kid that my parents wanted.

With equal parts of pride and rue, Andie insists, she *was good* at appearing normal. She married, started a successful business, and had the children—now teenagers— she adores. But at thirty-eight, when she realized "that everybody was really happy with my life but me," she ended her marriage and came out as lesbian.

Andie is one of the lucky ones, she believes. Unlike every other one of the contemporaries with CAH she has encountered in the last ten years or so, she was spared clitorectomy or what her doctor recorded as the "amputation" that a consulting urologist suggested she have at fifteen. It is for this reason, she thinks, that she did not suffer the social isolation and inability to form intimate relationships she has seen in her peers with CAH. She wishes now that she had not had the clitoral recession to which she attached hopes of normalcy as a child. It makes her more self-conscious than she believes she would have been had she not had surgery, and she does experience some of the discomfort that made the procedure fall out of favor after the late 1960s.[6] Nevertheless, she is aware of how fortunate she was to have had extraordinary medical treatment throughout her childhood.

It is Andie's fervent hope that efforts she has made to spur medical reform will mean that medical care will be based on genuine need and not motivated by the fear that she so adeptly internalized. In assembling the pieces of her story over these last few years, she has come to understand how little her parents really grasped about the treatment of her atypical sex anatomy and has had to accept how little they remember now. She understands why her doctors and parents made the decisions they did and sees these decisions as products of a time now past. In seeking to raise awareness of the terrible harm that has come from fear of difference, and, as she sees it, of prejudice, she has shared her story with medical students and seeks now to help physicians focus on attending to the health and well-being of all those with CAH, children and adults, to normalize the treatment of a threatening lifelong disorder, and not the atypical genitals they may have.

"It Wouldn't Have Been a Consideration": Ethical Judgment in Patient Care

For Andie, who was raised in a secular Jewish family, her doctors' being Orthodox Jews was a curious detail of her medical history. Listening to her recount her story, I was struck by the fact that her treatment differed so significantly from that of most other women with CAH at this time, and I began to wonder if her physicians' observance of Jewish law could have played any role in their treatment decisions. The medical record she retrieved as an adult demonstrates that her doctors were cautious about surgical normalization. Aside from a notation regarding her "circumcision" at two (contrary to her mother's memory) and clitoral recession performed when she was eight, her doctor had recorded the exchange he had with a consulting urologist who would perform the surgery Andie had at thirteen.[7] In addition to the laparoscopy, the urologist had expressed his hope of performing a number of exams and procedures, including the recommended clitoral amputation. Her physician's rejection of nearly all his colleague's suggestions is tersely noted in her record: "Only examine under anesthesia . . . [,] leave clitoris alone."

In *Women and Jewish Law,* Rachel Biale provides a helpful treatment of Halakhic regulation of marriage and sexuality. Pursuant to the rules of Halakha, men are obligated to provide food, clothing, and *onah,* a broad term that explicitly encompasses the right of a woman to sexual pleasure (see Biale 1984, 121–126). Halakha is not an ethics, understood in philosophical terms, but a body of law drawn first from the Torah (the first five books of the Hebrew Bible), from rabbinical law, and from custom. I wondered if it was possible that Andie's Orthodox physicians had engaged in a kind of Halakhic reflection regarding the "dilemma" presented by her body that was also an *ethical reflection* on her role—and theirs—in her treatment. The Halakhic proscription against bodily mutilation may well have provided some basis for caution in the performance of surgery in the absence of medical necessity.[8] But there is also the distinctive place that ensuring a woman's pleasure, including erotic pleasure, occupies as an integral component of the fulfillment of a husband's duties under Halakha. Might we find in her doctor's approach a model or framework that could provide resources in ethical decision making today?

Thus my interest in speaking with her doctor lay not in the effect of any particular (or general) religiosity, but rather in whether there was a set of ethical guidelines at work in his medical practice. My efforts to find existing resources was frustrated by the fact that I cannot read Hebrew, the language in which most scholarship on Halakha is carried out. Existing scholarship in English concerning these questions in the context of Halakha is scant; the little work in the literature is focused not on the questions of harm and bodily integrity that seemed salient to me, but instead on questions of gender assignment, a function, it appears, of the popular conflation of DSD and transsexuality, which makes DSD a problem of gender in so many discussions today (see Gray 2012). But at the time of Andie's treatment, and in her particular case, gender assignment was not in question; instead, concern was focused on whether or not she "looked like a normal girl." If I wanted to know what had occurred to make her treatment unique, it was clear that I needed to talk to Andie's doctor.

After a long and distinguished career, her pediatric endocrinologist had died. But his brother, the pediatrician with whom Andie had remembered her doctor consulting over the years, and who had been present at the exam that resulted in normalizing surgery when she was eight, remained in practice and agreed to speak with me. He remembered his former patient, to be sure. He knew how old she was now and asked how she was doing. I then asked him whether he thought his brother's Jewish observance might have had any influence on the treatment decisions he made in Andie's case. Her treatment, I told him admiringly, was exceptional, and I wondered if there could be some connection between his brother's medical practice and his understanding of the requirements of Halakha.

"I can reassure you," the doctor began, that "my brother [made no decisions on the basis of Jewish law] because he would have done what he—regardless of any advice from the rabbis—thought what was best for the *patient*." In response to my earnest efforts to determine if perhaps the laudatory caution his brother demonstrated in the medical record and in Andie's reconstruction of events could have any source in his and his brother's upbringing, the pediatrician emphatically repeated that "religious reasons" could have had no bearing on any decisions his brother made in the clinic. It was concern for the child's *normality*, which was for him identical with her well-being, that provided the sole criterion for the girl's treatment. When I importunately pressed the point, reminding the doctor that Orthodox Jews are concerned with erotic desire and with sexual pleasure (which may be tied to fertility not only for men but also for women), he said, "Yes [that is important]."[9] But after a pause, he added, "At the time, [erotic sensation] wouldn't have been a consideration. The consideration would have been whether we thought that the repair . . . would have led to better development psychologically . . . To have a big clitoris . . . would . . . make her be out of the ordinary . . . [My brother] would have advised repair." In our conversation it was clear that for this pediatrician, as for the brother he spoke for, the best interests of their patient were paramount. "Looking normal," something that was critical for the patient's psychological well-being and her prospects for marriage and children, for a normal life, were more important, he affirmed, than the possibility of impaired erotic response. Just as evident, however, was the strong exception he took to my forthright suggestion that an ethical commitment might have played a role in the care of his patient. It may be that, consistent with Andie's memory, the suggestion that "religious observance"—that is to say, Jewish observance—had any role in the modern life of postwar America was threatening somehow, that it could be construed as being in tension with the requirements or prevailing views that governed standard medical practice of the day. He wanted me to understand that if there was anything distinctive about the treatment Andie received, it was only because she was fortunate enough to have as her physician one of the nation's most capable pediatric endocrinologists, a leader in the field who sought to provide his patients with state-of-the-art care.

I did not doubt the pediatrician's representation of his brother's decision. I was disappointed that my hypothesis regarding the rationale for Andie's uncommonly good treatment could not be substantiated, but I was also troubled by what seemed to me his adamant denial that Jewish law, arguably a resource for ethical decision making, could have any bearing on treatment decisions, as if such an influence would itself constitute an ethical violation.[10]

I could not shake the impression of the offense I had provoked in my suggestion to Andie's pediatrician that his brother's observance of Jewish law had influenced judgments he made in his care of a patient. I sought guidance from another physician, Dr. Linden, a specialist in a field wholly unrelated to DSD care. He is an observant Jew who has been a leader in medical ethics, including Halakhic ethics. I relayed to him my experience with the pediatrician and the pediatrician's insistence that Halakha had no role in any aspect of his medical practice. Dr. Linden provided his own analysis of the "case" before him; in his view the treatment that Andie received would be wholly in line with Jewish law. The intention motivating cosmetic surgery could not be construed as the prohibited "mutilation" for its own sake, but the psychological well-being of the girl, including, of course, the prospect of a loving marriage and children. Dr. Linden took the pediatrician's denial of the connection between the treatment Andie had received and her doctors' religious commitments as a statement that in this case there were no conflicts between the aims of the standard of care and the requirements of Halakha. But, like me, he puzzled over the pediatrician's implying that there could be a tension between the observance of Jewish law and the best interests of a child.

I understood the possibility that the pediatrician might be sensitive to the charge that "religion," popularly cast in the United States at this time as a matter of personal, individual beliefs, had played some inappropriate role in the practice of medicine, particularly in the care of someone who did not share those beliefs. Furthermore, anyone knowledgeable about the anti-Semitism of the post–World War II years could appreciate why an observant Jewish physician practicing during this period would maintain even today that his religious values or beliefs had had no bearing on his professional judgment or commitment to his patients. But for me there remained a troubling sense that where the treatment of children with atypical sex was concerned, it was not only religion that physicians believed had no role to play but also that ethical reflection itself could have no place.

Seeking Moral Sanction

In response to my questions concerning what seemed to me the tension expressed by Andie's pediatrician between patient care and ethics, Dr. Linden told me, "Excellent patient care is the ethical thing to do. There is no tension [between the two]."

There are, of course, dilemmas that arise in the conduct of medicine, as the physician noted, including those involving a conflict between two ethical imperatives—for example, when forced to choose between the life of a pregnant woman and that of her fetus, or the ethical quandaries surrounding the decision to maintain someone on life support. Such dilemmas—where conflicting demands of moral actors are obvious—are the mainstay of courses in medical ethics. But most physicians do not necessarily confront ethical questions in the routine practice of their profession; the aim of their practice, understood as the promotion of the health of their individual patients and of the population, is unquestionably a good and so invites no further interrogation.

While Dr. Linden rightly sees the continuity between "good patient care" and ethics in medicine, the imperatives defining each are not the same. It is worth asking whether the imperatives that have guided care of children with DSD have, or currently do, make individual "patient care" the focus or whether the aim of treatment might more precisely be characterized in terms of the ends of "good medicine," what appears in the case of DSD care to amount to the promotion of "normality." In distinguishing the ends of medicine from those of morality, I follow the distinction introduced by Immanuel Kant—whose moral theory shapes the framework of bioethical principles—between "imperatives of skill" and "moral imperatives." With respect to imperatives of skill, Kant writes, "there is absolutely no question about the rationality or goodness of the end, but only about what must be done to attain it. A prescription required by a doctor in order to cure his man completely and one required by a poisoner in order to make sure of killing him are of equal value so far as each serves to effect its purpose perfectly" (1964 [1785], 82–83). An imperative of skill is concerned simply with the end to be achieved. Its value, its success, is bound to this end. A moral imperative, for Kant, is not good "for" some purpose, as are imperatives of skill; it is good in itself: "This imperative is *categorical*. It is not concerned, not with the matter of the action and its presumed results, but with its form and with the principle from which it follows" (83–84; original emphasis). Juxtaposing these distinctive imperatives may help us to better appreciate why physicians may see ethical reflection to lie outside the practice of medicine and why, to the extent that medical practice involves not simply outcomes, but flesh-and-blood individuals whose well-being is bound to those outcomes, ethical reflection and moral action are, at the same time, essential to that practice.

Efforts to normalize children's atypical anatomies more generally have a long history that demonstrates the intertwining of these distinct imperatives of skill and morality. The thread we may trace throughout this history—or multiple histories—is initial faith in the goodness of the end sought (namely, normalization), followed by reform spurred by revelations of harms unintentionally committed in these attempts to promote individuals' well-being. The reconstruction of missing or incomplete fingers in children (S. J. Kessler 1990, 125–127) and in craniofacial repair for infants and children with cleft lip and palate (see, e.g., Mouradian et al. 2006) are examples that follow this pattern. These types of reconstructive surgeries go on, and continue to be refined; what has changed is the psychosocial support offered to parents and children, as well as developing appreciation of the decision-making capacities of children and the responsibilities of parents to support that decision making (see, e.g., Alderson 2006). Other normalizing practices in medicine that have been shown to be risky or even life-threatening, such as the prescription of the synthetic estrogen diethylstilbestrol (DES) to stunt the growth of tall girls, have all but entirely ceased.[11] The feminist movement has broadened the conception of what is acceptable—what counts as normal—for girls; changes in standards for boys have not kept pace. The questionable use of human growth hormone, particularly to increase height in shorter boys, continues in the United States (see, e.g., Dreger 2011) despite opposition to use of DES for girls. Whether in the past or ongoing, these efforts to normalize children's bodies have seemed at some point a self-evident good, both medical and moral, and physicians' endorsement of these practices has served not only to instill confidence in parents that a normalizing intervention is warranted but also to convey that withholding such an intervention might itself constitute a wrong, as many specialists in DSD care have claimed over the years.[12]

What parents and physicians alike have had to learn as each normalizing technology arises is that this confidence in its goodness is not one grounded in evidence that a particular intervention will produce the flourishing or happiness it promises and that this confidence may serve—indeed, appears repeatedly to have served—to conceal from physicians and parents the possibilities of harm. Today most specialists in DSD care generally seem to maintain a sense that the benefits of normality—for the child and also for the parents—justify the risks of the interventions. Like Andie's doctors more than fifty years ago, most do not respond directly to questions, challenges, or doubts that have been raised or that they may themselves have. What philosophers would recognize as moral justification for normalizing surgeries was largely absent through the twentieth century. But to the questions that had been raised at this time, one physician sought, and believes he has found, conclusive evidence to support the standard of care, thereby settling any outstanding "ethical questions" concerning that standard.

Working in collaboration with colleagues in South and East Asia, Australian Garry Warne, a pediatric endocrinologist, claims to have found in the experience of children with DSD in developing countries proof of "the burden of the condition" (Warne and Raza 2008, 227) that, in his own country, would be "relieved" by surgical intervention. In "Intersex East and West," Warne and his colleague Vijayalkshmi Bhatia describe the impasse they understand to have occurred in the conflict between physicians and "activists" over what the authors characterize as the remaining ethical questions concerning normalizing surgery, questions, they clarify, of "when" and "how" to perform surgery (2006, 183; see also Warne and Mann 2011, 662). By contrast, in the Asian countries where the authors have worked and studied, there is no question of when and how to perform normalizing surgery, because in those places, "children born with ambiguous genitalia grow up with their original anatomy," exactly as do all children with the variety of "deformities and disabilities" for which treatment is unavailable. How, these authors ask, do these children do without cosmetic modification? "Are they treated with the respect and dignity that would allow them to grow up with intact self-esteem, and are they thereby empowered to make their own decisions about when to undergo surgery, or whether they need surgery at all?" (Warne and Bhatia 2006, 183). Rather than respond to this question (which appears to have been a rhetorical question, given that this care is not available), the authors provide a detailed discussion of their experience treating children in India, Vietnam, and Australia. They address the role of culture in shaping parents' expectations and acceptance or resistance to surgeries (and sometimes sex reassignment) in children seen in clinics by visiting physicians and document the outcomes in the children treated.

Warne and Bhatia suggest that examination of what they deem to be the terrible consequences of social stigma attaching to individuals with DSD who cannot benefit from Western medical intervention can afford special insight into our own culture and serve to clarify the imperative for normalization that is enacted in the West. To appreciate the nature of the imperative they seek to identify, we must reckon with Warne and Bhatia's understanding of the stigma they regard as a matter not so much of culture—as stigma has been figured from Erving Goffman (1963) forward—but of nature. Where cultural values vary from India to Vietnam to Australia, stigma attached to individuals with DSD, they argue, is the constant. The prospect of letting children be—as the authors suggest we may witness in the cases of India and Vietnam, where surgery is unavailable or grossly inadequate— "leads to greater unhappiness" (Warne and Bhatia 2006, 203) than the relatively positive outcomes they recorded in Australia, where, as in other developed countries, surgery is the standard of care.

I should acknowledge that Warne has done important work in bringing attention to what all regard as the critical medical needs of children with various forms of DSD. In a 2008 essay Warne wrote with Jamal Raza, the authors address the genuine health challenges associated with some DSD—for example, the scarcity of inexpensive and proven medicines to help manage the potentially fatal hormonal imbalances in children with salt-losing congenital adrenal hyperplasia. Warne and Raza rightly call attention to the exclusion of such medicines from the World Health Organization's Essential Medicines List (medicines that the WHO recommends should be available to affected populations) (Warne and Raza 2008, 233–234). Even though the imperative of such care (and the risk of cancer that accompanies some conditions) figures among the concerns that Warne and Raza enumerate, the obvious priority the authors assign the social implications of DSD suggests that the motivation for their concern about the care of children in the global south is not principally one of medical health, but of the consequences of the social stigma that they believe attaches to those individuals who cannot benefit from Western medical intervention.

In making their case for the "natural" imperative of normalization, Warne and his colleagues ignore substantial anthropological evidence that in cultures where there is a high concentration of a particular DSD—such as in the Philippines (Howell and Paris 2011, 92), in the Dominican Republic (Imperato-McGinley et al. 1979), and in Papua New Guinea (Abramson and Pinkerton 1995)—the stigma Warne and his colleagues guarantee is not actually present. Rather than critical insight into their own practices and the understandings that make sense of or justify those practices, it appears that Warne and Bhatia aim instead to confirm what they take to be the a priori goodness of the prevailing rationale for normalizing surgery. Casting their inquiries as a response to what they term the "ethical" questions that have been posed about the standard of care—a standard that all agree historically violated every accepted principle of bioethics—Warne and his collaborators seek to identify a unique sanction, a natural imperative in the difficulties that individuals with DSDs and their families face in underdeveloped parts of the world. They argue that in impoverished countries where cosmetic surgery is not available, or made inaccessible by prohibitive cost, the stigma is not refigured by the community but remains stable, even across distinctive cultural contexts. The claim that underlies the work of Warne and his colleagues looks like this: in parts of the world, such as India and Vietnam, where Western "ethical" standards are not a factor in the care of children with DSD, we find a glimpse into the natural order of things and identify an imperative that medicine should heed. Critics of the standard of care have forcefully and persuasively identified ethical problems entailed by the standard of care, and have argued for the elimination of cosmetic intervention for non-consenting infants and young children. Rather than reconsider the standard of care in light of these challenges, Warne and his colleagues tell us instead that this so-called ethical challenge, which would put off normalizing surgery in non-consenting children, results in a violation of a physician's oath to do no harm, for without normalization, children and their families will be inescapably subject to the stigma—the natural, and so universal, stigma—that attaches to those with atypical sex.

Ethics, as most trained in the Western tradition will understand it, is thus rendered invalid. Genuinely ethical practice, Warne and his collaborators hold, is grounded in what is natural, which is identical with what is true. In other words, where the ethical principles grounding bioethics distinguish between the descriptive and the normative, what is and what ought to be, Warne and his colleagues urge us to see that, at least where the treatment of DSD is concerned, what "ought" to be is already present in what "is."[13] In a reversal of the deontological terms that form the basis for bioethical principles today, the moral imperative is shaped not by reason, but by nature; that is, the imperative emerges in what Warne and his colleagues claim is the natural abhorrence of atypically sexed bodies, together with the (also natural—what Kant would thereby characterize as "necessary," or what might in this context be characterized as "inevitable") exclusion or isolation that revulsion supports.

Seeing the case in favor of ethical surgery framed in this way, I was able to more precisely identify what so troubled me about the discussion with the pediatrician who had participated in Andie's care. His insistence that no ethical framework had played a role in her care might not simply be a function of his response—whether deliberate or not—to prevailing cultural expectations or constraints, but might instead be continuous with the position outlined by Warne, what I take to constitute a naturalistic rejection of ethics. It seemed that if for Andie's pediatrician "ethics"—that is, a kind of enactment of a religious or philosophical commitment—had played some role in treatment decisions, the soundness of those decisions as medical decisions—decisions whose imperative is not, as the physician told Kessler, grounded in how things ought to be, but rather how they are—would be compromised.

The Cultural Problem with Ethics or the Ethical Problem with Culture?

"The problem" of intersex has been taken to be a problem of the individuals whose bodies somehow defy the clear distinction between male and female. In chapter 3 I proposed that we relocate the problem from the bodies of those with atypical sex and find it instead in "the rest of us," that is to say, in the problem of societal intolerance. Effecting such a shift in moral perspective might seem a daunting task. It will be particularly daunting, I believe, if we see this challenge to require a transformation of our understanding of gender, a transformation of our understanding of the basic division of society into men and women, boys and girls.

Among the most important "lessons from the intersexed," according to Suzanne Kessler, must be acceptance of the category of gender as "*always* constructed." No longer should we understand the construction of gender to apply only in the cases of those children who have had "reconstructive (which is not to say cosmetic) surgery." In this view the refusal to view genital ambiguity or other manifestations of atypical sex as a sign of the cultural construction of gender as a whole has resulted in the imperative to normalize children's bodies. "Accepting genital ambiguity as a natural option," Kessler famously wrote, "would require that physicians also acknowledge that genital ambiguity is 'corrected,' not because it is threatening to the infant's life but because it is threatening to the infant's culture" (1990, 25; 1998, 32).

I suspect that one reason that normalizing surgeries continue to be cast today as an imperative—and those few parents who have delayed or declined surgery taken to be unusual or even exceptional, together with the small number of physicians who recommend against such surgery—is that the category of gender is a fundamental organizing structure of our social world, a privileged "structuring structure" (Bourdieu 1990 [1980], 53). So fundamental is it that we may say that gender—or, more accurately, sexual difference—is the primary structure through which we make sense of the world and the world makes sense of us. For this reason I believe that understanding the problem of atypical sex in the terms that Kessler first proposed, the terms that have guided so much critical discussion in the two decades following—that is, as a problem of the "misrecognition" of sex as a social production—has functioned not to promote reform in care, but to justify ever more powerfully a standard of care that is intended to afford a child what are thought to be the considerable benefits of normality.

Framed as a conflict between opposing views of gender or sexual difference— where, on one extreme, many physicians subscribe to the view of intractable "natural" division and, on the other, feminists see a deeply embedded cultural production, "an act of constitutive uncertainty" (Morland 2011, 150), the ethical problems presented by the urgency to "fix" children in ways that have been demonstrated to promote harm, rather than flourishing, recede from view. The task is not a matter of making a good argument against the standard of care (as philosophers might want), but may require instead that we consider more carefully why it is that what appear to be sound arguments against the standard of care have failed.

I want to propose that in the work of Garry Warne and his colleagues we may find unlikely direction for developing the sort of understanding that makes sense of the force of normalization that effectively resists the sound and logically powerful arguments that have repeatedly challenged it. Recall that in their work, particularly in the essay Warne authored with Bhatia, the authors claim to seek insight into Western cultural practices by examining non-Western practices. "It may be difficult for us to discern cultural influence on our decision-making from 'inside' our own culture," they write, "but stepping 'outside' may give us a glimpse of our culture as others see it" (2006, 183). Rather than look at the purportedly terrible outcomes of children with DSD in other countries who do not have the access to surgical normalization, however, we might consider instead the remarkable similarity between the motivations for maintaining rites of "traditional" genital cutting that have occurred over centuries in much of Africa and parts of the Middle East and those that have supported the performance of normalizing surgeries in the United States and Canada as well as throughout Europe and Australia since the 1950s.

The 2012 statement by the Public Policy Advisory Network on Female Genital Surgeries in Africa is particularly instructive in providing a basis for this comparison. In an effort to promote more enlightened and informed discussion of female genital modifications in Africa, the statement criticizes the inflammatory, "one-sided" characterizations that have proved polarizing and calls for greater accuracy and understanding that can promote genuine dialogue (19). In place of the term "mutilation" or even "cutting," the authors use the term "surgery," thus identifying what have been presented as "cultural" (ignorant, primitive, uncivilized) practices associated with genital cutting in the south with those "medical" (beneficent, scientific, modern) practices performed by physicians in the north. The network nowhere makes specific reference to normalizing surgeries for atypical genitalia in its statement. Including such surgeries would have reinforced the network's argument that genital surgeries wherever practiced are motivated by what they characterize as cultural "conceptions of a normal body and appropriate gender development" (20).

In her comparison of normalizing genital surgeries for atypical sex anatomies with "traditional" practices of genital cutting in *Lessons from the Intersexed*, Suzanne Kessler observed that both practices aim "to reduce variability within each gender and to increase differences between the two genders" (1998, 119). Amplifying the appearance of sexual difference, members of the network confirm, "is a significant feature of genital surgery from the point of view of insiders who support the practice."

> In the case of male genital surgeries, the aim is to enhance male gender identity by removing bodily signs of femininity (the foreskin is perceived as a fleshy, vagina-like female element on the male body). In the case of female genital surgeries, the aim is often to enhance female gender identity by removing bodily signs of masculinity (the visible part of the clitoris is perceived as a protruding, penis-like masculine element on the female body). (Public Policy Advisory Network 2012, 22)

The social reward for compliance with genital modification is high. The authors note that participating in normalizing practices can mark one's inclusion, or sense of belonging, in a social group. Furthermore, individuals who have had such surgeries see them as a route to "cosmetic beautification, moral enhancement, or dignifying improvement of the appearance of the human body" (21).[14]

But if the rewards described by the authors of the statement resonate with the rationale for normalizing atypical sex anatomies in children, so do the risks of noncompliance: "cosmetically unmodified genitals in both men and woman are perceived and experienced as distasteful, unclean, excessively fleshy, malodorous, and somewhat ugly to behold and touch" (21), which is to say, such genitals provoke disgust. Contesting the view that such surgeries are regarded as mutilations by "insiders," the authors remind their readers that aesthetic norms governing genital appearance in Africa are beginning to take hold in Europe and

North America, where "the ideal of a smooth and clean genital look" has made clitoral reduction and labiaplasty "one of the fastest growing forms of cosmetic surgery in those regions of the world" (23).

As presented in the statement by the Public Policy Advisory Network, there are important similarities between rites that have been practiced for centuries among communities throughout Africa and those that are emerging in Europe and North America. There are nevertheless striking differences between the two. Where those practicing genital modification in Europe and North America would regard these as elective cosmetic enhancements, those in Africa may regard these practices, together with the elaborate rites that comprise initiation, as fundamental to the constitution of one's personhood. As anthropologist Fuambai Ahmadu documents in her ethnographic study of initiation among Sierra Leone's Kono, the men's and women's "societies" charged with carrying out these rites are "responsible for the 'creation' of female and male sociocultural beings from the raw material of nature, young children" (2000, 288). Rather than the "natural fact" that sexual difference is generally taken to be in the West, the Kono regard sexual difference as a "cultural creation" (288). Rites of initiation are practices that not only shape what might otherwise be taken to be a natural capacity for procreation but also function as the condition for political participation, for "legal rights and dignity" within these communities (309).

Examining global practices of genital modification as a matter of producing gender, one might characterize the differences in the meanings between the practices Ahmadu describes and the surgical normalization of genitalia in children with DSD as differences of degree rather than kind. Among the significant differences is the fact that among peoples like the Kono, all "legal" members of their society partake in these rights; that is, the work of creating meaning is a collective endeavor that requires the sacrifice of all. In the West the work of maintaining a coherent notion of sexual difference appears to require the sacrifice of a few.[15] Until recently, this sacrifice was completely shielded from view. Interventions to normalize atypical sex anatomies have been regarded as private not only because they concern parts of our bodies culturally regarded as intimate but also because the difference these anatomies mark is regarded as shameful. The secret— the "open secret"—of Kono initiation is not, or has not historically been, maintained as a mark of shame, but rather one of pride in exclusive membership as an adult in a respected community.[16]

While the differences are marked and the histories apparently divergent, there is a point in the mid-twentieth century where the histories of genital modification in Africa and the surgical normalization of children in North America converge. In their 1966 article, Drs. Robert Gross, Judson Randolph, and John Crigler, three of the pioneers of normalizing surgery for atypical sex anatomies at the Children's Hospital Medical Center at Harvard Medical School (the chief competitor in this area to the group at Johns Hopkins, discussed in chapter 1), sought to reassure those who might be "reluctant to advocate excision of even the most grotesquely enlarged clitoris." The doctors attribute this reluctance to "the belief that the clitoris is necessary for normal sexual function [in women]." But this belief "is no longer tenable," they write, for "there are a number of sound studies which demonstrate normal sexual response in females who have undergone clitoral extirpation" (1966, 307).

Among the studies to which the authors refer is one from 1955, conducted by psychiatrist Joan G. Hampson of six previously anorgasmic women, five of whom "reported normal sexual gratification" following clitorectomy. But perhaps more compelling is what the authors describe as "evidence that the clitoris is not essential for normal coitus." This evidence was garnered from the data of "a number of African tribes" that customarily "excise the clitoris and other parts of the external genitals at pubertal ceremonies." Despite clitoral amputation, the authors state, "normal sexual function is observed in these females" (Gross et al. 1966, 307). The "personal communication of unpublished data" by one P. H. Gulliver, "a visiting lecturer in sociological anthropology at Harvard College, 1958" (308), provides the evidence for this assertion. Having established the safety of excision through the example of African women (as anecdotally reported by a single, Western observer)—an irony given the vitriol of Western criticism that currently takes issues of safety and sexual unresponsiveness as central to arguments promoting prohibition of these practices—this moment of convergence of the histories of genital modification in Africa and the surgical normalization of children in North America, occurring during a period of rapid development of the standard of care for DSD, has been forgotten. The history that is more often recounted—the account that usually begins with John Money but is more accurately located in the work of Lawson Wilkins—marks a discursive division of the contemporary history of normalizing surgeries, Western and non-Western: "medical" practices must be distinguished from "traditional" practices, "modern" from "primitive."

In her criticism of Australian laws prohibiting what are referred to as "folk" customs of genital cutting that distinguish these practices from, and so defend, medically sanctioned normalization of the bodies of children with atypical sex anatomies, Nikki Sullivan asked, "In what sense is intersex surgery (at least when it is not essential to save the life of a child) *not* a 'folk custom' that is particular to our time and culture?" (2007, 403; original emphasis).[17] Taking the question Sullivan poses seriously requires that we ask whether normalizing interventions are what we usually take to be a medical or surgical "fix" akin to, say, repair of a defective organ like a heart, or whether this intervention is one intended to shape identity and one's place in the community. Physicians have been quite clear that the intention of such interventions *is* cultural and, as such, has significant consequences for an individual's health and well-being. For this reason, we should attend far more closely to the question of how these practices might work to shape a sense of one's self as a sexed, and sexual, being.

In an article addressing the difficulty Western feminists have in understanding the experience of African women who have been circumcised, anthropologist Janice Boddy argues that bodily experience is "not simply culture's natural base" but is itself "produced *through* culture." It may be that in realms other than sexuality we may more easily accept that "desires and pleasures can be culturally and historically specific" (2007, 58; original emphasis). While Boddy's aim here is to challenge Western feminists to critically examine the frame through which they read the experience of cultural "others," her point is one that seems especially important when we consider the implications of the medical management of the bodies of children with atypical sex anatomies; it is important, in other words, to take that critical perspective she offers not only to reconsider how we see the practices of "others" but also to look at practices that are indigenous to our own culture. It may be especially helpful to look once more to the practices that Ahmadu and others discuss for this purpose.

Initiation into Kono society, Ahmadu observes in a 2009 interview with anthropologist Richard Shweder, also marks the beginning of a process of sexual education.

> Bondo [female society] elders believe and teach that excision improves sexual pleasure by emphasizing orgasms reached through stimulation of the g-spot, which is said to be more intense and satisfying for an experienced woman . . . [attaining these] must be taught and trained, requiring both skill and experience on the part of both partners (male initiation ceremonies used to teach men sexual skills on how to 'hit the spot' in women . . .). (Shweder 2009, 16)

Physicians and parents in North America and Europe may resist the notion that, however intended, normalizing interventions function also as a kind of sexual education, a formation of knowledge about oneself as a sexed and sexual being. And yet acknowledgment of harms effected by repeated visual and manual genital examinations and by medical photography in the meetings of the U.S. and European endocrinological societies in 2005 (Hughes et al. 2006) indicates physicians' growing awareness that these practices have worked not to better integrate children with atypical sex anatomies but to inculcate in them a sense of their stigmatic difference.[18] Seen in the light of the comparison with the practices Ahmadu describes, we can better appreciate the implications of the harm of clinical practices that have frequently accompanied the normalization of sex in children. For example we can begin to come to terms with how repeated displays or exams during childhood might function to shape an individual's sexuality. If cultural imperatives are at work in the normalizing interventions in the West, then we must recognize that there are at the same time cultural imperatives that militate against these practices.

In his 1996 essay on the challenge presented by reform of established cultural practices of body modification, political theorist Gerry Mackie wrote, "Female genital mutilation is a self-enforcing convention, nearly universal where it is practiced, persistent, and practiced even by those who oppose it." It is seen as necessary for living the good life and is for this reason "an obviously compelling tradition" (1996, 1010). No matter that such practices may be described as violations of human rights or that they might be cast as accommodation to custom or tradition; indeed, Mackie identifies such characterization as an additional barrier to change, a point echoed in the Public Policy Advisory Network's statement (2012, 26). But perhaps the most daunting obstacle in the way of achieving reform, Mackie writes, was the failure to recognize that genital cutting, "transmitted by women," as all acknowledged, was performed not from malice but out of mothers' love for their daughters (1996, 1003).[19] The blueprint for change that Mackie outlined, garnered from the campaign to end the centuries-long practice of foot binding in China, describes a strategy of resistance to such practices that is not understood as imposed from without but that is crafted within the terms of the culture; it is a design for change grounded in a given culture's commitment to community and to individuals' love of their children.[20]

By gazing into the mirror of those cultures in the global south who continued to practice genital cutting in the face of arguments to end it, perhaps we may better appreciate why it is that sound arguments against normalizing surgery in the North have not resulted in the change that activists anticipated in the first years of their work to raise awareness, as Alice Dreger recounts in "Intersex and Human Rights: The Long View" (2006a, 73). We may understand why "when doctors see a clash between a child's body and the social body and they choose to address that clash by changing the child, they are in effect saying the social body cannot, will not, or should not be changed" (78). In the face of deeply held beliefs about the conditions for social acceptance and belonging, and for individual flourishing, arguments framed in terms of abstract ethical principles come to seem like an imposition. Such imposition may take the form of punitive laws that appear to draw a line between "some bodies as socially viable, and others as 'repulsive' and as a threat to the common good" (Sullivan 2007, 403), as Sullivan writes in her criticisms of the Australian legislation prohibiting "folk" practices of genital cutting. Resistance to the imposition of values regarded as alien appears in Western physicians' indignant rejoinder to the possibility that children with atypical sex anatomies be "left as they are": such children, they insist, would be rendered social experiments in sex ambiguity.[21] From whatever direction, calls for change taken to come from "outside" a given community—even, and perhaps especially, when those calls come in the form of punitive legislation—have (see, e.g., Thomas 2000; Johnsdotter 2007) often resulted in resistance and effective reinforcement of cherished beliefs perceived to be under attack.

The members of the Public Policy Advisory Network on Female Genital Surgeries in Africa are right to see in the practices of genital modification in Africa a similarity to Western commitments bound by culture and the rules that govern it. Their work to assert the legitimacy and importance of cultural norms is helpful for encouraging a more productive and respectful discussion of practices of genital cutting in Africa. Their identification of these norms with those in Europe and North America may prove revelatory to those who may wonder why there has been so little change in the practices governing the standard of care for atypical genitalia in the West; in both cases we see how the rules of culture, or what we might see as the operation of a "popular morality," guiding cultural practices may be distinguishable from what we may understand as abstract ethical principles, as well as how popular morality could be in apparent tension with ethical principles. Perhaps it is because, for the members of the network itself, the practice of ethical reflection is itself a cultural matter, their analysis—published in a leading journal of bioethics—is silent on the question of where ethical analysis enters the discussion of genital modification. Such a question may not be entirely out of place, however.

The practice of genital cutting in Africa has raised questions over the centuries of its practice. Despite the fact that it predates Islam, genital cutting is asserted to be, and accepted as, a requirement of Islam in a number of places (e.g., Johnson 2007). What is important here is not the specific recourse that is made to a religious authority in this case; rather, I want to point to the fact that when questions are raised about what are taken to be everyday practices of popular morality, appeals to some metaphysical source of truth and the good—that is, to moral law—are frequently sought to settle such questions. It is not only proponents of genital cutting who have looked, for example, to the Koran and its legal commentaries (see Ali 2006, 97–111) to support the practice. Those seeking to end the practice of genital cutting have also sought a ground for their opposition in Islamic law (e.g., Abusharaf 2001, 118). Even as such an authority is essential for settling disputes regarding the practices of everyday morality, however, the authority must be recognized as such within a given culture; it cannot function effectively if it is regarded as alien to the context in which a given practice is in question.

In this light, hostility to arguments against genital cutting made in the language of "human rights" begin to look a lot like the hostility to claims concerning the "contingency of gender" by those supporting normalization of atypical sex anatomies of children in the West. Insistence on the goodness of cultural practices on the basis of tradition or religious law bears a striking resemblance to the appeals to "nature" made by Warne and his associates. Despite the salience of such appeals in critical discussions of these practices, however, it is important to recognize that appeals to authority are in fact only intermittent, and, as we see in both "traditional" and "medical" genital modifications, these appeals are ineffectual as well, regarded as irrelevant. Practices that have been well established are not the result of careful and repeated reflection, but instead are a matter of repeated enactment of cultural values, in rituals that have shaped and function to reinforce these values. No wonder, then, that arguments in favor of resisting the standard of care, cast as a response to the weak or wrong reasoning maintained by proponents of that standard, have little traction on the ground, in the decisions made by distraught and worried and confused parents and by physicians eager to ease their pain. Despite, or perhaps because of, the insight to be gained by closer consideration of the cultural imperative for normalization, we may notice that in the case of atypical sex anatomies the rules governing popular morality do not lead inexorably to normalization. If there is a strong impetus to normalize the bodies of these children, there is also increasing awareness that the customary practices violate what we might see as the everyday values that guide our practices and our understandings of them. We can see the extent to which such understandings are in flux when we consider that it was only in 1997 that the American Society of Bioethics and the Humanities first sponsored a panel about ethical questions raised by the medical management of atypical sex. More remarkable, however, was the bewilderment of one ethicist who later approached presenters Alice Dreger and Cheryl Chase and said, "I don't think you understand; there isn't an ethical issue here because these children are abnormal" (Dreger, pers. comm.). We can credit the work of activists and academics in promoting increasing recognition on the part of physicians, which has already resulted in significant changes. Whether, or to what extent, these changes pass muster by the standards of morality—popular or abstract—requires further investigation.

6 Neutralizing Morality

Nondirective Counseling of Parents of Children with Intersex Conditions, 2006–

Among the most significant changes in the standard of care for children born with sex anomalies has been the definitive move away from what Cheryl Chase characterized in the late 1990s as a "concealment-centered model" of care for children with DSD (Chase with Dreger 2000). Before the publication of the Consensus Statement in 2006, physicians cautioned parents against open discussion of a child's condition with extended family or friends in order to protect the child from potentially harmful comments that could damage her psychosexual development. The risk posed by such comments was understood as a threat to the "concordance" a child ought to experience between the appearance of her body and her assigned sex. It was for this same reason that parents were also advised not to discuss the child's condition with the child herself (B. Wilson and Reiner 1998, 363). Today there is little question that the revised standard requires physicians to honestly and forthrightly discuss with parents the nature of their children's conditions. The paternalism that prevailed during most of the second half of the twentieth century in the experiences of the families I discussed in chapter 2 is increasingly a thing of the past.

Having accepted that ambiguous sex is not the emergency it was taken to be twenty years ago, physicians' understanding of their role has changed considerably. Prevailing practice does not entirely satisfy the requirements detailed in Bruce Wilson and William Reiner's "Management of Intersex: A Shifting Paradigm" (1998), an essay that marks the inauguration of a new view on the standard of care. Much of Wilson and Reiner's proposal, particularly with regard to the necessity of a mental health practitioner as a member of a treatment team (365), and the participation of the child in the treatment plan as he or she matures (366), has not been realized, although their proposal that parents be included as members of the team (365) could be understood to have been incorporated to some degree. Where in the past, surgery was undertaken by physicians who understood themselves to be acting in response to a crisis and indisputably in the best interests of the child, these same surgeries are performed today because physicians report that this is what parents want (e.g., Rebelo et al. 2008, cited in Zeiler and Wickström 2009, 360). Physicians' justification of surgery as fulfillment of parents' wishes is not new, though its salience in these decisions appears novel. Reflecting the views of specialists in the care of children with intersex working in the 1980s, Suzanne Kessler wrote in her 1990 essay "The Medical Construction of Gender" that "physicians 'psychologize' the issue [of genital correction and reassignment] by talking about the parents' anxiety and humiliation in being confronted with an anomalous infant . . . [they] talk as though they have no choice but to respond to the parents' pressure for a resolution of psychological discomfort" (25). A decade later Cheryl Chase recounted a conversation with an endocrinologist who said "he had never in his career seen a good cosmetic result in intersex genital reconstructions, but 'what can you do? The parents demand it'" (1999, 150).

Doctors practicing today would not likely see parents as members of the medical team precisely, but they do see parents, and not themselves, as the primary decision makers when it comes to normalizing interventions. Rather than clear advice or the sort of outright prescription we expect in just about every other aspect of medicine, doctors working with parents of children with ambiguous genitalia report an increasing use of a kind of consultation that has come to be called "nondirective counseling." A nondirective approach involves the provision of information a health-care provider believes to be important for weighing various possible interventions in a given medical situation and what is known of the outcomes without directing the person counseled to make a particular decision. Nondirective counseling was first employed in the psychotherapeutic context following the Second World War and was adapted in the late twentieth century in the new field of "genetic counseling" (S. Kessler 1997, 166). Under the model of nondirective counseling, decisions regarding treatment rest ultimately with the patient and not with the health-care provider.

Because I wanted to understand how treatment decisions regarding care of children with atypical sex anatomies were being made following the 2006 Consensus Statement, I spoke with ten specialists in the care of children with DSD over the course of 2010–2011. I asked each of them how decision making had changed over the last decade. While all of the doctors with whom I spoke had demonstrated, in publications or by reputation, some degree of criticism of the prevailing standard of care, only a few might characterize themselves as forceful proponents of "letting be" a child's atypical sex anatomy, at least in the clinical context. Rather than strongly directive in their advice to parents, their approach tended to reflect the nondirective approach established in the field of genetic counseling.

On its face, nondirective counseling appears to resolve the ethical questions that have been raised with respect to past treatment of children's atypical sex anatomies. Putting decisions in parents' hands marks a departure from paternalism and toward patient (or proxy) autonomy. Rather than a resolution of the ethical problems raised by the prior standard of care, however, the adoption of a "nondirective" approach appears to raise new questions concerning the management of DSD in young children. In developing this analysis, I draw on bioethicist Arthur Caplan's criticism of the goals of "neutrality" in genetic counseling (1993), the field in which the nondirective approach originated in medical practice and continues to be refined. Genetic counselors may understand nondirectiveness as a "moral" approach that promotes the autonomy of those counseled; empowered to make decisions by virtue of the wealth of information counselors provide, parents (or prospective parents in the case of prenatal counseling) can come to decisions that will be shaped by their own values rather than those of the counselor or some other interested party, such as the state.

In discussing the exchange I had with the pediatrician who treated Andie in the last chapter, I focused particularly on what I took to be his unsettling claim that the application of ethical principles could be at odds with the practice of good medicine. What might be characterized as variations of this view emerged in many of my discussions with specialists in DSD care practicing today. The prevailing belief was not that of Andie's physician, whose perspective could be characterized as an assertion of the importance of seeing religious obligations as distinct from civil obligations that bind us in a pluralist society. What I encountered instead was the idea that good medical care—which is to say, care in the best interests of a child—could be in tension with the kind of care to which accepted ethical principles of their profession would direct them. So obvious did this idea appear to them that there was little more to say. Where treatment of children with atypical sex was concerned, many of the physicians with whom I spoke suggested that, for their colleagues and sometimes for themselves, acting from what they took to be an "ethical" perspective could constitute a standard incongruous with good medical care. In other words, physicians suggested that putting a child's interests—that for physicians might favor surgical normalization—second to an abstract ethical principle might not be in the best interests of their patient and would therefore be a bad medical decision. Framing the discussion in terms of what physicians presented as a conflict between respect for the principle of autonomy on the one hand, and the concrete interests of the child's place in her family and culture, on the other, doctors suggested that subordinating an individual child's interests to abstract principles would also constitute an ethical violation.

The notion of making a child suffer to satisfy the demands of an abstract principle is certainly disquieting. Whether acknowledged or not, it is a real problem that all parents face in raising children. Parents may have to make decisions in raising their children that involve inequitable distribution of resources not only within their families if there is more than one child but also involving their participation in a larger community. In the United States, for example, parents' responsibility to their own children's needs may come into conflict with their felt responsibility to be good citizens, which may entail attendance of neighborhood public schools. While such decisions have implications for one's community, these decisions are typically understood in our own cultural context as "private" matters of conscience or deliberation that are not the concern (or business) of "professionals" or of the government. And indeed in the cases of some other physicians with whom I spoke, there was less of a sense that there might be a violation in "imposing" an ethical perspective; for them, the issue could more precisely be the idea that the promotion of ethical reflection would exceed the requirements of good medical care—that is to say, it was not their place to promote ethical reflection in the parents of the children with atypical sex anatomies they treat, and they saw nonurgent medical decisions as properly the parents.'

It is easy to appreciate, perhaps especially in the United States, why doctors would want to avoid genuinely difficult issues of value, both familial and cultural. And yet my conversations with doctors led me to question the extent to which the counseling they provided was in fact nondirective. Following Caplan, we must ask whether in the case of atypical sex, the putatively neutral counseling that many in the United States claim to provide is not only "non-moral," as Caplan might put it, but unethical as well. The ethical violation cannot be characterized readily in terms of the bad intention of the moral agent—whether the doctor or the parent—but is instead a failure to appreciate the moral character of the decision facing them.

Nondirective Counseling and Its Discontents

As it was conceived after the Second World War, the field of genetic counseling aimed to distance itself from its early twentieth-century origins in eugenic science (Marks 1993, 15). Sheldon Reed, the geneticist who coined the term "genetic counseling," envisioned the ways this new practice could assist families in making reproductive decisions and adjusting to genetic problems within families. As Elving Anderson (2003), Reed's student and then successor at the Center for Human Genetics at the University of Minnesota, explained in a tribute to his teacher,

> [Reed] insisted that the presentation of this genetic information "must be compassionate, clear, relaxed, and without a sales pitch." He believed that the counselor also could help to alleviate some difficulties associated with genetic problems: quarreling between husband and wife as to the "blame" for an abnormality in their child and a sense of shame owing to the social stigmas that often accompany hereditary diseases. Maternal guilt is an emotional reaction that should be watched for. On the other hand, one usually *can* explain to parents the chances of another abnormal child, so that they can adjust well to the facts. (original emphasis)

Nondirectiveness as a goal seems to capture Reed's concern with "avoiding a sales pitch." In his own "Short History of Genetic Counseling," composed after almost thirty years of practice, Reed recounts that he understood his work with families beginning in the late 1940s to be nondirective and was well aware of how important it would be for the emerging field of genetic counseling to be practiced in a way that would clearly distinguish it from its immediate past. His own institution, the Dight Institute for Human Genetics, founded in 1927 by a eugenicist physician, was originally intended "To Promote Biological Race Betterment"; it was to be a center where individuals and families could seek counsel and advice as "to their fitness to marry and reproduce" (Reed 1970, 334). Though from the start the institute's focus was individual counseling, Reed observed that before his tenure this counseling was, as he put it, "bound in eugenic shackles." In 1927 he remarked, "[Eugenics] was a reasonable concept," but after the Second World War the work of the institute would not be for the benefit of improving society, as eugenic science had promised, but for the benefit of the individual families who sought counsel (334).[1]

In the years since, there has been a good deal of criticism of nondirectiveness in practice, particularly in the prenatal setting, where most genetic testing occurs (White 1999, 14). Nondirective counseling aims to provide neutral "facts" about various disorders for which a fetus may be at risk, without the provision of opinions on the part of the counselor as to any difficulty entailed by, or stigma attached to, a given disorder or disease. If a disorder or other abnormality is positively diagnosed in the fetus, genetic counselors are to lay out the facts of the diagnosis and follow the lead of the parent or parents with respect to any course of action. If, for example, a parent or couple is determined to terminate a pregnancy with a fetus diagnosed with a genetic disorder, the counselor's role is not to discourage the parent(s) in any way (including by providing additional information about the condition or facilitating opportunities to meet individuals with, or families affected by, the disorder), but to support them in carrying out their decision to end the pregnancy. The same would be true of those families determined to carry to term a pregnancy following identification of a genetic disorder: Rather than counseling parents about the consequences—to themselves, existing or future siblings, and the child to come—of bringing to term a pregnancy of a child with severe disabilities, for example, the genetic counselor's role would be limited to providing whatever contacts or referrals may be at her disposal. While some provision of support for individuals' decisions may be offered in this setting, the absence of any challenge to prospective parents' decisions or their deliberations is consistent with what Arthur Caplan describes as the "purely factual environment" (1993, 150) in which nondirective counseling has been understood to optimally take place.

What is meant by the term "nondirective counseling" has been contested over the last fifteen years or so, with some major proponents, such as psychologist Seymour Kessler, arguing that the characterization of this counseling as "purely factual"—a model that has seemed to discourage discussion and critical engage-

ment from the counselor (e.g., asking questions, suggesting different possible responses)—is badly out of date. For Kessler, what defines nondirectiveness is the
absence of coercion, which he considers identical to the promotion of autonomy
(e.g., S. Kessler 1997). Notwithstanding his criticism of what nondirectiveness entails, it seems that for the most part nondirectiveness as a method continues to
be characterized in terms of the neutral position of the counselor. The counsel-
or's neutrality serves the dual purpose of promoting patient (or in this case, parental) autonomy, a fundamental tenet of bioethical practice, and safeguarding
the profession from any "confusion with, and moral contamination from, the eugenics movement" (Elwyn, Gray, and Clarke 2000, 135).

Today bioethicists take as axiomatic the point that eugenic goals are at odds
with an ethical perspective. Since the end of the Second World War, human "betterment" of the sort associated with state efforts to "improve the [human] race" has
become synonymous with moral violation, not to say evil. Questions concerning
whether or to what extent individual desires for, and pursuit of, "enhancement"
may be identified with eugenics are a matter of controversy in the bioethical literature generally and appear in the literature on prenatal genetic counseling as
an ever present danger.[2] If eugenic aims, identified with directing families in a
coercive manner to bear offspring without disorder or defect, are widely taken to
be unethical, it makes sense that the imperative to be nondirective in counseling
parents would be "ethical." Or would it?

Challenging the ethical claim of nondirectiveness is one of the aims of Caplan's essay "Neutrality Is Not Morality" (1993). Caplan's title already indicates the
complex problem he identifies with respect to the presumed morality of nondirectiveness. His central concern is to disentangle the claim to neutrality from
the matter of ethical practice altogether and to provide a more robust reflection
on what is meant by these claims, both to "neutrality" and to "moral neutrality."
It is "not obvious," he writes,

> that a shift away from an ethical stance favoring the prescription of eugenic
> or preventative goals toward one favoring respect for the autonomy of client
> decision making is in any way morally neutral. On the contrary, the shift to-
> ward an ethic that elevates client or patient autonomy above all other values is
> highly value laden and prescriptive. (1993, 159–160)

Caplan's concerns are both abstract and material; that is, he is concerned with the
soundness of the claims to ethical neutrality made by proponents of nondirective counseling, and he links this concern with the practical (and moral) impact
that nondirective practices have in the decision making of those counseled. Chief
among these concerns is the worry over what Caplan suggests is a misguided "belief that the client's autonomy can be allowed to flourish only in certain environments" (160), a belief held and promoted by genetic counselors who, Caplan per-

suasively argues, unintentionally infringe on clients' autonomy by shaping these environments and limiting precisely the kinds of exchange and interrogation that mark autonomous decision making. Drawing on empirical studies, Caplan details specific ways in which the goals of genetic counseling are at odds with the practice. Being inundated with information, what he vividly terms "truth dumping" (160), can promote frustration in patients rather than the capacity for autonomous decision making. Absent genuine discussion and exchange, receiving the news that one's fetus is "different" or that parents are carriers of an atypical genotype can influence reproductive choices in ways such information might not were other kinds of exchange and information allowed or encouraged as well.[3] In other words, methods intended to be nondirective can turn out to be powerfully directive, but directive in ways that can be difficult to identify.

While Caplan was indubitably concerned with the moral status of nondirective counseling as it was understood in the early 1990s, his primary aim was to provoke further reflection about how genetic counseling should be understood going forward. The questions he raised about the unanticipated limitations and perils of a putatively value-neutral approach have continued to promote conversation in a growing field that has seen increasing sophistication, investigation, and analysis as it attempts to keep pace with advances in genetic medicine (see e.g., Bernhardt 1997; Oduncu 2002). As a result, "directiveness" is no longer uniformly regarded as identical with coercion or eugenic aims, and the language of "shared decision making" more frequently appears in descriptions of the goals of genetic counselors (Elwyn, Gray, and Clarke 2000; Shiloh, Gerad, and Goldman 2006). But while increasingly nuanced reflection characterizes discussions of nondirectiveness in the context of genetic counseling, it appears that the less reflective understanding of nondirective counseling that prevailed in genetics through the early 1990s has been adopted by some physicians outside the context of genetic medicine.[4] Although it is difficult to determine exact prevalence, anecdotal evidence suggests that in the last few years such practice has become commonplace in the counseling of parents faced with decisions concerning normalizing surgery for children with atypical sex anatomies.

Nondirectiveness Refigured: The Case of DSD, 2006–

From the 1960s through the early 1990s, specialists in the care of children with atypical sex anatomies based their recommendations for treatment on the strong conviction that a child's health and well-being would be threatened if there were too great a disparity between the child's sex of assignment and the appearance of her body. Their certainty and confidence in this belief was such that in many quarters it would have been regarded as inappropriate, or even malpractice, to suggest that a child might thrive with genitals that appeared "ambiguous," which is to say, neither clearly male nor clearly female.[5]

After the revelations of the harm that "managed" individuals had experienced, and the recommendations for greater caution in sex reassignment and normalizing surgery in the 2006 Consensus Statement, the issue of counseling has become a critical one in DSD care, particularly with regard to surgical decisions made on behalf of infants and young children. There is a marked absence of evidence that normalizing surgery benefits patients; limited studies and substantial anecdotal evidence attest to the physical and psychosocial harm that such surgeries may effect. Rather than strong recommendations against normalizing surgeries, however, many specialists in DSD care increasingly have allowed parents to make decisions regarding cosmetic procedures without informing them of these risks and outcomes. Parents technically have always had the authority to consent to normalizing procedures—or for that matter any medical intervention—on behalf of their child. What is novel in this case is that physicians have come to understand their roles in guiding parents as more in line with the tradition of nondirectiveness that has been most closely associated with the field of genetic counseling.

The recourse that specialists in DSD care have made to a nondirective approach seems to be a well-considered response to concerns such as those articulated by pediatric surgeon Jeffrey Marsh, a specialist in craniofacial care. In his contribution to *Surgically Shaping Children,* Marsh observes that in cases for which appearance-normalizing procedures may be considered, surgeons don't always know that surgery will alleviate the problem(s) it seeks to address. He calls upon surgeons to "recognize and distinguish between consequences [of delaying or forgoing surgery] that are well documented in peer-reviewed literature and accepted by the medical profession in general [as in the cases of craniofacial anomalies, for example] and those that are speculative." Appreciation of this distinction, he writes, "should temper the authority with which the surgeon advocates surgical management" (2006, 117). A nondirective approach would seem to honor the lack of clarity in cases where a benefit of having normal-appearing genitals has been established to be a matter of speculation or supposition. One might expect an approach such as this to result in the performance of fewer surgeries. Parents would be informed about the risks as well as the lack of evidence of success of surgeries, the assumed necessity of which had also never been established clinically.

This, at least, was my understanding before I began in 2010 to ask specialists in the care of children with DSD what was happening in their practices and in their clinics. I was surprised to find that in their judgment no significant change in the number of surgeries performed has occurred. In the face of what appeared to be significant change in the counseling of parents faced with decisions about normalizing surgery, I wondered why there was so little change in performance of surgeries. The long acknowledged paternalism that preceded the more recent changes made implausible the idea that physicians had simply been telling parents what they wanted to hear, namely, that normalization was in their children's best interests, no matter the cost. Was this because the influence of physicians who continued to believe that normalization was in the child's (and parents') best interests still could be felt, despite the apparently nondirective form that counseling now took? Or was it that the compelling appeal of normality went unchallenged?

In my efforts to understand what was happening in these cases, I spoke with physicians, including pediatric specialists in surgery, endocrinology, genetics, and psychiatry, who had demonstrated, in their published work or by reputation, a critical perspective on surgical management. I did not seek out obvious proponents of surgery in medical management of atypical sex; these physicians, it seemed to me, would be more likely to direct parents to a surgical outcome and would provide little information about the new developments that I found puzzling. The varied discussions I had with specialists over that year confirmed that, almost without exception, normalizing surgeries continued to constitute the standard of care for all practical purposes, if not by published consensus. While doctors, including most of those with whom I spoke, maintain that the impetus to perform normalizing surgeries comes more from the parents than the doctors, their accounts of discussions with parents—discussions in which they themselves had participated, as well as discussions among their colleagues to which they were privy—indicate that, paradoxically, at least some degree of the urgency that parents feel may be a result of the formally nondirective methods of providing information to parents.

Of the ten physicians with whom I spoke, only a few had expressly thought about what nondirective counseling entails. The physicians who were less familiar with the principles of nondirective counseling likely would not have characterized their approach to counseling in the ways that genetic counselors do but nevertheless asserted consistently that parents were the primary drivers of decisions regarding their children's care—something they did not say of other kinds of treatment they would, or in fact did, prescribe children with DSD. Those who were most critical of the performance of early surgery in the absence of medical necessity—where surgery may be understood as a matter of cosmetics rather than function—took a nondirective approach to be ethically wrong, much in the spirit of Caplan's criticisms. However, most of these physicians admitted their own uncertainty regarding decisions to forgo normalizing surgery, expressing concern about the risks of looking abnormal. One surgeon explicitly named his concern that parents would be unable to bond with a child assigned female whose genitalia appeared masculine. Without making this specific claim, others alluded to parents'—and sometimes grandparents'—inability to tolerate such difference, or their projection of this intolerance onto others such as babysitters or day-care providers. In the position one physician ultimately took to support normalization of a girl's genitalia, he pointed to the considerable risk to a mother's mental health as being at stake in the decision to normalize the appearance of her daughter's genitalia. For nearly all of the physicians with whom I spoke, what is best for the patient is no easy matter, and for good reason: the problem of atypical sex anatomy is not generally a problem of medical risk to health. It is instead a familial or cultural problem that, like any number of "cosmetic" issues, has been managed in the West by medical professionals.

The recourse to nondirective counseling in DSD care is enacted in quite different ways. Individual physicians' accounts of what occurs in their clinics suggest that these differences are closely tied to matters such as the institutional context (e.g., whether the clinic is part of a university hospital, or whether it has an established center for DSD care that includes a commitment to ongoing research); the background and training of the colleagues with whom they work is another important factor. Dr. Willow explained that some centers without formal teams, such as the one in which he works, have so few cases that busy surgeons are disinclined to treat children with DSD differently from how they would treat what they would regard in other contexts as a straightforward case of "repair."[6] If, for example, a senior urologist has had few occasions over a thirty-year career to consult with his colleagues regarding patient care, he may be disinclined to believe his clinical opinion should be taken to be other than decisive. Dr. Birch was involved in such a case in a hospital like Dr. Willow's. Called in for consultation, Dr. Birch was concerned that the surgeon's recommendation for surgery for this particular patient was too strong; in response he sought to provide the parents a counterbalancing caution against surgery in an effort to provide what he described as a kind of "net neutrality" that would enable the parents to make an informed and autonomous decision—the goal of much of genetic counseling. As Dr. Birch put it, "It's almost like we have to advocate for a particular position [against surgery], knowing that already that patient has come under a certain influence [to consent to it]."

This concern with providing a ground for parents' autonomous decisions was a refrain in the reflections of many of the doctors with whom I spoke. Dr. Cedar, another physician accustomed to offering parents the "alternative" view of delaying surgery as part of a team that tended to promote it, found himself faced with a couple who vehemently refused his colleagues' forceful recommendations for normalizing surgery for their daughter with CAH. In their case, he explained, he attempted to provide the most sympathetic perspective on surgery, perhaps with a view to preparing parents for a future in which their daughter might seek it. But on this point he could only offer to the parents a possibility he could imagine, as there is little data concerning cases in which older children or young adults have themselves sought normalizing surgery; given that the standard of care in cases of genital ambiguity in infants has been, and for the most part remains, normalization, it may be especially challenging for physicians to support parents in considering what possibilities there might be for addressing needs that an atypical anatomy can pose apart from immediate normalization.[7] The dominance of pediatric specialists in the field of DSD care raises a question posed by the one specialist in adolescent surgery with whom I spoke. She suggested there could be a "conflict of interest for pediatric surgeons . . . if they don't do the surgery now, then they lose the child to who-knows-who." We might ask whether, or to what extent, some of the "urgency" that may be experienced by the physicians or parents may stem from the division of specialization between pediatric/adolescent/adult.[8]

What we might term the temporal outlook of physicians or parents turns out to be a matter of some complexity that bears further examination: in what ways, precisely, are doctors or parents truly thinking about the child's future? Of his role in a better organized DSD team as a nonsurgical specialist, Dr. Cedar gestures toward this problem of the time to which parents are directed to focus in making decisions on behalf of their children.

> Often what I'm left doing in the group is [providing] the "uncovering the assumptions" speech, saying, "Okay, the surgeon is telling you . . . that surgery will create genitals that look normal, that there will be no complications, or few complications." There's also the assumption that no one will desire someone with atypical genitals, which the surgery will fix, and that fixing the genitals will also fix all sorts of other anxieties both at the level of the family and of the child as he or she grows up. So I try to make parents understand that [this view] is based on a number of assumptions that have not been proven. The problem I'm facing [in counseling parents] is that the surgeon speaks in the present and I speak in the future. Parents want solutions in the present and they don't project into the future. You can engage in all the arguments you want, but in the end, you know, you have the choice of an apparently easy fix versus no fix and an uncertain future. So it's a sort of a no-brainer from the parental perspective.

It is easy to appreciate the appeal of a "fix," an intervention that will finally cure a condition rather than manage, contain, or control it. We cannot discount, as pediatric endocrinologist Dr. Spruce cautioned, the enormity of the distress, the panic so many parents feel when they learn that their child has a DSD: "They are suffering; they are really frightened; they are very confused; they tend to feel very guilty." Presented with the possibility of a genuine resolution—or, better, dissolution—of those feelings that surgery promises, it may be difficult for parents to find genuine succor in the alternatives offered by other physicians. As one psychologist, Dr. Cypress put it,

> My ability to have meaningful discussions with parents is directly related to what the other team members say to families . . . If another member of the team says, "Well, I'm sure you're feeling stressed, [so] let's move forward [with surgery]," and I think, no, no, let's not rush—if you're feeling urgency, that is not the moment to make decisions. I can relate to parents here. They have a daugh-

ter who [has a male karyotype], with testes, her clitoris is enlarged, and [the parents] want to take care of it. They want the testes out. I say, well, this is not urgent medically, and my colleague says the parents feel urgency, and now is the time to address it. Delaying becomes a hard sell when somebody [else] is saying, "I can take them out tomorrow. When do you want to come in?"

The apparent ease that practiced surgeons in this field display and the confidence they inspire in parents seeking relief of the anxiety provoked by diagnosis of their child's abnormality may be attributable more to the personalities and dispositions of these doctors than a genuine measure of the relief that parents are assured surgery will bring.

As a specialization, surgery "attracts the fixers," Jeffrey Marsh observes, "those who have already known the personal pleasure of manual labor associated with problem solving or creation. These individuals are interventionists: they need to be the active agents in resolution of situations to obtain personal satisfaction." Together with their military-like resident training, which Marsh describes as unique to specialization in surgery, "these factors combine to make most surgeons proactive, positive, enthusiastic individuals who strongly advocate the treatment they perceive to be the best. Not surprisingly, that treatment usually is surgery" (2006, 121). Dr. Willow, also a surgeon, echoes Marsh's observations, remarking on what he experienced himself as a kind of "cultural adjustment" as he came to understand that some decisions might warrant input from colleagues in other fields, such as psychiatry:

> I think, hey, this person has this interesting disease, and I get excited about the medicine and the physical findings, and it takes talking to people and seeing how to look at [the situation] differently. It's how we [surgeons] think; it's how we've been trained; it's who we are. We go into these fields because we [look at things] this way.

Focusing laser-like on treating or correcting the disease or the condition, rather than taking into account the care of the whole person, appears to be part of the training that Dr. Willow points to—something most of us who have needed surgical treatment have welcomed in their surgeons who "need to detach from the emotions . . . if they are [to] cut open their patients" (Mouradian 2006, 131).

In addition to the ways that the training of surgeons may shape their dispositions, there is a crucial aspect of that training on which Marsh does not remark, one that raises the possibility of a conflict of interest, namely, the fact that medical training requires that physicians "make use" of children's conditions, if not directly for research, then for training of the next generation. Gesturing toward the surgical fellow present during our conversation, Dr. Willow noted, "We all feel that conflict; I'm training [this fellow] and I want her to get more exposure [during her time here]; I want her to see these [rare] surgeries." In pointing out what physicians would consider an obvious point, I do not mean to raise doubt that surgeons genuinely believe that their work will bring the normalization they promise. Nothing said by any physician with whom I've had contact would challenge Marsh's claim that surgeons recommending normalizing interventions are motivated by the desire to conceal, and so ameliorate, the (still) stigmatic difference of atypical sex. Many have nevertheless expressed regret that they remained unaware for so long of the consequences of what, according to Dr. Pine, they now see as "mistakes," such as the routine sex reassignment of 46,XY males with what physicians took to be insufficient penis size, for example (see, e.g., Skoog and Belman 1989; S. J. Kessler 1990).

Sex reassignment of this kind was among those interventions specifically criticized in the 2006 Consensus Statement, which reports that "available data support male rearing in all patients with micropenis" (Hughes et al. 2006, 556). Physicians describing cases of gender "self-reassignment" have amply documented evidence of the failure of what for many years stood as the standard of care in cases of micropenis or aphallia, that is, where a penis was atypically small or absent (e.g., Reiner 1996; Phornphutkul et al. 1998; Phornphutkul et al. 2000). In addition, there is now documented evidence that clitoral reduction and vaginoplasty have not been successful in all the ways doctors had once taken them to be.

The first outcome studies involving clitorectomy began in the 1970s, but rapid advances in surgical technique—particularly with regard to what are known as "nerve-sparing" surgeries—have meant that many surgeons regard data from these studies as irrelevant to decisions facing parents now. Rather than certainty of a poor outcome, most surgeons, and many specialists outside surgery, believe that surgical outcomes are greatly improved, though the evidence in both directions generally remains anecdotal.[9] Perhaps it is this wide agreement among physicians concerning the improvement in surgical outcomes that accounts for what appears to be only a minor diminution of normalizing surgeries. Because the United States does not maintain national records of such procedures, it is impossible to determine with certainty whether the number of surgeries performed there has been significantly reduced, or what effect the 2006 Consensus Statement has had in this respect.[10] It is plausible that the improvement of technique and the increasing numbers of trained specialists in the field has had the effect of broadening access to such interventions to areas of the country where they might earlier have been less common.

Given the wide acknowledgment that change in clinical counseling practice has occurred in the last ten years, I was genuinely surprised that only a small proportion of the physicians with whom I spoke reported what they perceived to be even a modest decrease of surgeries in the hospitals in which they worked, although they did note differences in the delivery of care. These differences appear to reflect a movement toward comprehensive and team-based care that is comparable to that developed in the field of craniofacial repair. Perhaps for this reason, changes that have occurred in the care of children with atypical sex anatomies are not reflected in the rate of surgery so much as they are in the ways that recommendations for surgery are conveyed. Absent evidence that surgery is beneficial to the patient, doctors no longer appear to make recommendations for intervention without qualification. Even among those physicians who had demonstrated a perspective critical of the standard of care, however, only a few of the physicians with whom I spoke believed it was appropriate to indicate anything but full support for parents seeking normalizing surgery on behalf of their children.

Having completed interviews with most of the physicians over a year, I was struck in particular by the differences between the counseling physicians described providing to parents of girls with the salt-losing form of "classic" congenital adrenal hyperplasia beginning in the 1960s (like that of Ruby, which I described in chapter 2) and the counseling provided to parents today. Girls with this form of CAH, like boys with CAH, must be closely monitored; much is now known about how to properly regulate levels of cortisol for a child's health.[11] Instructing parents of children with CAH on the necessity for vigilance in administering appropriate levels of medication, as Dr. Elm, a pediatric endocrinologist, acknowledged, is much like the instruction of parents of children with type 1 diabetes, formerly known as "juvenile diabetes": "You're saying, 'You need this for life, and you'll be sick if you don't take it.'" But cosmetic surgery for girls with CAH who have larger than typical clitorises is something that has shifted significantly. Where atypical genitalia was previously regarded as an emergency needing urgent correction, and regarded as continuous with other aspects of medical management of CAH, physicians now readily acknowledge that decisions to perform normalizing surgeries are distinct from, and bear little resemblance to, decisions regarding aspects of care that genuinely entail disease and even the loss of life. As Dr. Elm succinctly put it, "You're not going to get sick if you don't have genital surgery, whereas you are going to get sick if you don't take cortisol."

And yet it appears that most physicians—though by no means all—who are counseling parents will not challenge those parents who want to pursue normalizing interventions, even when physicians acknowledge the possibility of harm to their children. It is difficult to ascertain why it is that most doctors do not challenge parents and why the majority appears to condone, or even actively promote, surgical normalization. Dr. Elm seems representative of the particular group of physicians with whom I spoke in the obvious ambivalence he describes with respect to treatment recommendations he makes to parents. In considering the prospect of putting off or forgoing surgical normalization, he observes, "It takes guts to hold off on therapy . . . to hold off and see what happens," he says. Describing normalizing surgery as "therapy"—a term usually used to describe a known treatment of a recognized disease—may indicate that Dr. Elm feels something stronger than sympathy for the parents he counsels. On the other hand, he is critical of parents who are so concerned about a baby's appearance that they may focus on these problems at the expense of appreciating or addressing truly serious matters of a child's health. "People are expecting their baby to look perfect," he says, and if a baby doesn't, "they want it improved. I have had babies with all sorts of terrible malformations on the inside and the family wants to have some kind of cosmetic surgery done on the face because something doesn't look right." Dr. Elm's remarks suggest the salience of a narcissistic investment in anxieties over a baby's appearance. Most parents, in this doctor's experience, are concerned that "if I don't [pursue surgery for my child], there will be [some] problem" down the line, and surgery is an attempt to keep that problem (and its attendant anxiety) at bay. Dr. Elm reports that he is "more comfortable" than he once was "with waiting on surgery," particularly because in the case of CAH, "if [the disease] is well managed medically, the phenotype gets milder or more feminine." Even as he notes changes in his own perspective on the urgency of early surgery, however, he sees his role in counseling parents in this case as fundamentally different from the role he assumes when counseling on other matters. While talking to parents about the regulation of cortisol or normalizing surgery—both of which require careful "listening to the parents" and coming to understand their perspective—his job in the first case bears no ambiguity: it is to bring the parents to an understanding of the medical perspective that will optimize the child's physical health:

> I think the practice of [pediatric] endocrinology—and here is the reality of it—and I tell my students this: half my job—or maybe a third—is figuring out what the problem is here; the other two-thirds is actually getting the people to do what is in the best interest of the child. [Parents] have to be on board with [the treatment plan]. And the way to have them on board is to have them come to the conclusion that "my child needs cortisol." I mean that isn't very hard, but every now and again you have someone who has diabetes who doesn't think they should take insulin.

But if the matter of taking cortisol or taking insulin is straightforward and requires a clearly directive approach, decisions regarding the normalization of genitalia are another matter entirely. In this case, Dr. Elm says, "you have got to understand where [the parents'] heads are . . . and bring yourself to where they are . . . and [not] expect them to be where you are." He may be better able to follow parents who are not seeking surgery "without fear that I am making a big mistake," as he might have before, but he does not see his role as challenging parents in their "need" to change their children's bodies as he might in cases that do not involve genitalia. For Dr. Elm—whether he speaks of his own intolerance or disgust or that which he sees operative in culture, is not entirely clear—there is something about atypical genitalia, or the treatment of atypical genitalia, that is unlike other matters he confronts in his medical practice, and the adjustment he has made in the counseling he provides reflects that difference. It is not only that this physician sees his role to be different where normalizing surgery is concerned; parents, too, are put in the position of making decisions on behalf of their children that differ significantly from those they may be called upon to make with respect to other matters of medical care.

In the wake of the vociferous protests of intersex activists who brought to light the suffering they experienced as a result of efforts to normalize their bodies, many specialists have embraced nondirective counseling. "What I've been observing," explained Dr. Cedar, "is really a sea change in the attitudes of the surgeons mainly when they discuss [options] with families. There's more caution. I can't prove it, but I think it's motivated by fear, more than any other possibly ethical or reflective reason." Dr. Pine explained his approach this way: "I think the main thing we acknowledge is that there are people who feel that there are different opinions about whether surgery should be done and when it should be done." Before intersex activism, Dr. Pine recounted, he and his colleagues saw their work differently. The infant or young child parents brought to his clinic, he says, "had a birth defect that [the parents] wanted to have corrected . . . they came from the endocrinologist to see me to have a vaginoplasty and that's what they wanted, so you would give them a talk about what it involves and what the risks were, how it's done, what to expect, and that was it." But now, he continued, his aim is to "have the parents understand as best as they can that there are options and [that] the option they choose is what they're entitled to—it's *their* decision."

In this surgeon's characterization of his approach, there's a good deal of equivocation on the question of nondirectiveness. On the one hand, he emphasized that the decision was the parents' and that his role was to present options, "like a buffet almost." But almost immediately after, as he was thinking out loud about his impression of the way nondirectiveness had been adopted by some of his colleagues in oncology—in cases of prostate cancer, where evidence and outcomes are also a fraught business—he was frankly dismissive of what he characterized as a kind of throwing up of one's hands and leaving it to the patient: "You're coming to the doctor because . . . you trust that person and want their advice." And this, he finally concludes, is what he aims to give his patients. He presents the available options and also provides his sense of what is right in a particular case, which for this physician, who is most often referred cases by his colleagues in endocrinology, would mean surgery.

The sometimes conflicting ways that Dr. Pine characterized his counseling of parents during our discussion recalls a kind of dry and cautionary observation Dr. Cypress made to me when I shared with him, as I did with all of the physicians, the questions concerning nondirectiveness that I was trying to understand. "There's a relatively modest correlation between what [clinicians] say they do, what they believe in, and what actually happens," he instructed me. It is clear, though, that physicians who specialize in the treatment of DSD often report that parents aggressively seek normalizing surgery for their children no matter what cautions their doctors offer or assurances that most surgery can be delayed. What few say directly is that many physicians, both surgeons and non-surgeons, believe that, except in the mildest cases of genital anomaly, surgical normalization is in the best interests of the child.[12] There remains little evidence to support Money's theory that for their psychosocial health, children's phenotype must correspond with their gender of assignment. And yet surgery is motivated still by what doctors describe as a desire to promote a positive body image in children. As Dr. Willow put it, "We don't know the effects of being very [genitally] ambiguous in the long term." Perhaps because of this uncertainty—what doctors and parents alike take as the biggest unknown—it does seem clear that doctors feel they cannot recommend strongly against normalizing surgery. However skeptical one might be about this particular uncertainty, it is clearly because of the lack of evidence of the success of surgeries—not only physical success but psychological as well—that physicians can no longer strongly recommend surgeries or, rather, that they cannot do so outside the closed doors where parents and physicians speak about the problem of a child's atypical sex.[13]

Situating Parents' Decisions

From my discussions with doctors, it seems that the choice with which many parents of children with atypical sex are confronted is this: *do something* about your child's condition, or *do nothing*. I don't know of many parents, presented with options concerning what has been identified as a problem, a defect, or a disorder in their child, who would opt to "do nothing" when there is the possibility of aggressive and active medical intervention intended to secure a child's well-being. "Correcting" a feature of a broader disorder in the case of girls with CAH may be particularly attractive to parents who have learned that their children will have to live with a congenital disorder for which there is no cure. This problem, they may believe or be led to believe, is one aspect of this disease that they have the opportunity to set right.

The frustration or sense of powerlessness parents may feel in the face of the news that a child has a problem that they cannot somehow fix is obvious and hardly unique to the case of atypical sex anatomies. The asymmetry between the options presented to parents is not only a function of which option may appear to offer the prospect of improving the chances of a child viewed as beginning life at a disadvantage, together with the assurance that parents are actively pursuing their child's best interests; one must wonder how often the option of "doing something" is accompanied by an express promise of ongoing support and attention by medical professionals not only to the child but also to the parents themselves. Precisely because the issue of atypical sex anatomy is not visible, precisely because it is marked as "private," parents may, in their own struggles have to come to terms with their own understanding of, and feelings about, atypical sex anatomies and, without the promise of ongoing support by those professionals with whom they can speak openly and honestly, be unable to see that they have any other place to turn.

The construction of parents' choice in terms of doing something versus doing nothing is not only reductive, but it also obscures a host of questions that the situation raises concerning what most parents would take to be ordinary obligations to their children. These are the sorts of questions that Dr. Alder tries to bring into focus for the parents he counsels. In speaking with parents faced with decisions about normalizing surgery, he seeks above all to emphasize

> that we are speaking about a real live human being, a child—a person in the making. Meaning, we don't know who the child is yet. So I start out by pointing out that we are talking about a person, not a set of genitalia or a set of arms or a set of fingers or anything else, because I think it's very, very important to get the parents' anxiety off the genitalia and back where it belongs—on the child.
>
> All parents have a lot of anxieties in raising children. Raising children is very anxiety-provoking. You can get overly focused and really home in on some abnormality, especially genitalia. I try to point out the fact that their child, like all children, is an unknown, but that that isn't a reason to be anxious in and of itself . . . I try to teach parents that they need to be good observers because they want to do the best for their child . . . Doing the best for their child partly requires them to figure out who their child is . . . And ultimately ask the child in some way. And I also point out that there's nothing ambiguous about their child's genitalia from the child's standpoint. Those are that child's genitalia—whatever they look like.

Dr. Alder's approach differs from that of many of his peers. In his discussions with parents, he works to move their attention away from a view of "the problem" as an anatomical abnormality that requires immediate attention. He asks that parents focus instead on the lessons of parenting he himself has come to appreciate as a father of grown children, namely, to see one's obligation to children as bound to the particular needs and interests and desires of each child that a parent must come to know. If doctors' emphasis—explicit or implied—on the importance of a child's "normality" in general terms accords strongly with what appears to be most every parent's desire for the easier life that normality promises, there is every reason to believe that parents will advocate strongly for medical intervention "taken" or "understood"—as Bourdieu would put it—to be crucial for their child's future. Understanding that new parents, who cannot yet know their child, may be torn about this decision, Dr. Alder adds, "I end up, of course, trying to be neutral on the point of surgery, but pointing out that you don't want to remove things you can't put back . . . they might need it."

Dr. Alder's discussions with parents, like those described by Dr. Cedar, are an effort to help parents recognize that, where normalizing procedures are concerned, it is best to cast the options before parents not so much as a matter of taking action or not taking action—a choice that more accurately describes some of the other physicians' presentation of the options as they see them—but instead to try as far as possible to provide support to parents who must endure a kind of crash course in appreciating what this daunting long-term project of child-rearing entails. Most parents are granted a less hurried education in parenting as their children grow. While few would describe the work of parenting as easy, parents are generally eased into their roles and the multitude of requirements over a more extended period; by contrast, new parents of children with DSD— in particular, first-time parents—are not likely to have had a chance to reflect on what parenting may involve over the long term. These parents are not only faced with the challenge of considering the immediate and abundant needs of an infant or young child, but they also must take into account—that is, they must already anticipate—the complex and no less critical affective needs their child will develop, needs that require a different kind of parental attention.

Because the decisions involved in the medical management of a child with DSD are complicated in this way, the matter of counseling is one that a number of the specialists with whom I spoke had reflected upon with considerable care. In thinking about this matter of "patient—or parent—choice," Dr. Spruce suggested that counseling of parents in cases such as these should be understood in a larger context concerning what he describes as a "crisis over issues of patient autonomy versus providing support for parents for the last twenty to thirty years." More doctors, he suggests, are addressing this crisis by presenting to patients "a menu of options" from which patients will choose. Such an approach, he believes, "allows physicians to relinquish their obligation to provide care." In the case of DSD, he continued, that obligation involves more time than many physicians are willing to take and certainly more hours than any insurance company will be willing to provide compensation for.

> The idea that a baby with DSD could be born and a physician could deliver care without spending somewhere around three to six hours just talking to parents I think is ludicrous. *That's how long it takes.* Figure out how you are going to spend that much time with them, because you are not going to get anywhere in thirty minutes. And it's going to have to take place over the course of multiple days, because people need a chance to absorb information and reflect and talk

with one another. So when you say, "Here's an array of options," it's an invitation for somebody to make a decision quickly. You don't think about alternatives in that way if you're not trying to be efficient with time.[14]

Such an interest in efficiency, Dr. Spruce suggests, could contribute to an understanding of why it is the case that even today the majority of parents opt for surgery. The dearth of evidence positively supporting normalization appears to have had little effect in checking parents' desires for it, especially when it appears it is presented as "the best choice." As Dr. Cypress observed of parents he sees in his own clinic, "I haven't encountered any of these cases in which families are saying they don't want [surgery] when it's recommended."

Parents faced with decisions about normalizing the bodies of their children with atypical sex seek comfort in the terms that are most familiar to them, that make sense to them in the face of a situation that appears to interrupt their hopes and expectations for their children. What it means to be a good parent is to take action to relieve the suffering—here the projected suffering—of their children. Casting decisions about normalization in these terms, we may also appreciate why for many physicians the decision might not require much time. Additional reflection could, as Dr. Spruce suggests it should, entail clearer recognition of the nature of the decision facing parents. Like any truly difficult decision parents must make, it is a decision they may have to reckon with over many years, if not over the life one shares with their children. Presented as a false choice between doing something and doing nothing—a choice that can be characterized in parents' experience and, it appears, in the judgment of the majority of physicians practicing today, as a decision between "choosing normality" and "choosing abnormality"—it is easy to appreciate why physicians, and so parents (or perhaps why parents, and so physicians), continue to decide in favor of normalizing surgeries. Nondirective approaches employed today do not—perhaps cannot—provide a ground for the kind of reflection that would provide an alternative to surgery. Perhaps, then, we could understand the nature of the ethical violation in precisely this way, namely, as physicians' refusal to acknowledge, and so, to recognize their participation in, the moral reasoning parents must engage in to make decisions on their children's behalf.

7 Practicing Virtue
A Parental Duty

Rᴇᴄᴀʟʟ ᴛʜᴇ ᴘᴀɪʀ of studies presented by Suzanne Kessler in her 1998 book, *Lessons from the Intersexed,* discussed in chapter 2. In one study, college students were asked to imagine that they had been born with an atypical sex anatomy and to consider what they would want their parents to decide on their behalf. In the other study, students were asked to imagine that they had a child born with atypical sex and to consider what they would decide for their children. In their responses to the first study, students strongly opposed surgery on their own behalf while nearly 100 percent of students participating in the second study would support normalizing surgery for their own children.

On the one hand, it is easy to make sense of these studies. Responses to the question posed in the first study confirm how unappealing the prospect of compromising erotic response for the sake of cosmetic enhancement appears to be. Responses to the question in the second study support the idea that as parents we want what is best for our children and, if it is possible, to spare children stigma, particularly that associated with atypical sex. Certainly, this study seems to say, we parents should do what we can to defend our children against any harm we imagine could result from such a difference. But, on the other hand, even if we can understand the students' responses to the individual studies, bringing them together demands, once more, that we ask how it can be that parents would consent to procedures on behalf of their children that they would decline for themselves.

Beginning with an examination of parents' own "derivative" dependency as parents (Kittay 1999, 42), my aim throughout this project has been to gain a better appreciation of the conditions that make surgical normalization appear, from a parental position, to be the good—even the obvious—choice. If those imagining themselves as parents in Kessler's study make the same choices as those parents who decades ago agreed to normalizing surgery for their children, and those parents who still ask for—or even demand—such surgeries, this near universal impulse seems to suggest that the choice is perceived to be required in order to fulfill parents' fundamental duty to protect their children.

If, from the perspective of those who imagine themselves as candidates for such surgery (as well as from those who actually underwent such surgeries as infants or young children), this choice does not seem at all obvious but, on the contrary, wrong and a violation, then we must understand the ethical challenge presented here to involve closing the distance between these two positions that are not only far apart but also fundamentally different.[1] The commitments each entail conflict in ways that should signal the presence of a greater risk than has been acknowledged by proponents of normalizing interventions for DSD.

Those supporting the current standard of care identify a "stalemate" resulting from critics' challenges to both the standard of care and physicians' and parents' support of that standard (e.g., Warne and Bhatia 2006, 183). (Though, given what we know from the twentieth-century history of the medical treatment of atypical sex anatomies, it appears that "checkmate" more accurately describes the state of the conflict.) They recognize the irreconcilability of the two positions as most understand them—precisely in the terms in which Kessler's studies were designed. Instead of seeing in the difference between the positions of parents and children the difficult challenge of how to bridge the gap between them, proponents of the standard of care seem to see in critics' demands an unreasonable and irresponsible call that parents abandon their parental role by adopting the perspective of the child. I want to begin by proposing that we identify proponents' defense of the standard as a recognition that parents' practice of their duties as parents often involves just the kind of conflict illustrated by Kessler's studies and that parents' firm, insistent, and loving occupation of this position vis-à-vis their children requires parents to maintain their position as parents, that they not "switch sides."

Let me be clear that I do not think that critics of the standard of care are asking parents to abandon their positions as parents. It has been difficult to articulate criticism of the standard of care in ways that are not susceptible to proponents' characterization of the alternative to normalizing surgery as "doing nothing." To many pediatric specialists in DSD care, and to the parents they advise, "doing nothing" is regarded as a poor alternative to intervention aimed at normalizing a child's atypical anatomy. Misunderstandings of critics' demands have so far served to reinforce the standard of care that usually results in surgical normalization, even if in more refined and seemingly satisfactory ways.

My aim in this chapter is to propose an approach to closing the distance between the positions of the parent and the child that takes seriously the integrity of each position and the commitments and duties particular to them. At the center of my analysis are the recommendations of the Bioethics and Intersex Group, a subgroup of the German Network DSD/Intersex that aims to balance what appear to be the conflicting commitments of parents and children. The group outlines compelling reasons to exercise caution in consenting to normalizing surgery. Ultimately, however, the group argues that parental rights to make decisions on behalf of their minor children must be respected; parents' rights, they argue, are constitutive of the human right to "familial privacy."

Appearing to set aside the relevance of the principle of autonomy in medical decision making in cases of DSD, the Bioethics and Intersex Group effectively relocates the doctrine of respect for autonomy from the individual, to the family. However, my interest in the statement by the Bioethics and Intersex Group is not based on an interest in the issue of autonomy in the narrower ways it is taken up in contemporary bioethical discussions as a matter of how to ensure that patients are able to make informed decisions regarding their health care.[2] Instead, I am concerned with how the group's focus on autonomy—applied in their analysis to families rather than individuals—distorts the notion of parental duties the group takes to be threatened by criticisms of the standard of care.

I think most would agree that parents of children with ambiguous genitalia who agree to, or even insist upon, normalizing surgery do so because they seek above all to protect their children, a duty that familial privacy is intended to safeguard. The parents I call Sonja and Elias, parents of a girl with ambiguous genitalia born a year or two after the publication of the 2006 Consensus Statement, would no doubt agree. But as my discussion with them suggests, they would identify in the German group's analysis a fundamental misunderstanding of the characterization of this duty, perhaps better understood in ethical terms as a virtue.[3]

In Kantian terms, duties are those acts the moral law obligates us to perform as rational beings—for example, telling the truth or keeping our promises. We must tell the truth or keep our promises even if we have some interest in doing otherwise. Reading Kant, we might take moral action to be characterized by constraints on desires that pull us to act contrary to the moral law. Faced with a situation where duty commands that we keep a promise when we might want very much to do otherwise, Kant's *Groundwork of the Metaphysics of Morals* provides a compelling standard for ethical judgment and action. The conflict between what we should do (reason) and what we desire (inclination) makes plain where moral obligation lies. When considering more complex or nuanced ethical action less readily characterized as fulfilling (or violating) the moral law, however, Kant's moral philosophy may prove limiting at the outset, encouraging a sort of thinking that reduces ethical reflection to answering only the single question of which act is right and which is wrong.[4] Even if we finally see the protection of our children as a duty—and consider the manner in which that protection is offered as important for how we conceive of this duty—Kant's moral philosophy does not provide effective means of building a picture of this duty and a guide to its fulfillment. Virtue ethics provides much better tools for these.

Like most philosophical concepts of virtue, the practice of virtue that I explore here is rooted in Aristotle's *Nicomachean Ethics*. While the ancient Greek concept of virtue is not precisely at odds with the conception of duty that is conventionally identified with the prevailing approaches in bioethics (an approach on which the Bioethics and Intersex Group relies), an emphasis on ethical virtue nevertheless moves us to reconsider some of the ways that ethical questions regarding consent have been formulated. Returning to ancient conceptions of virtue can help us understand, for example, how parents and physicians are motivated by a conception of the good that may be mistaken. Errors in moral judgment take many forms, but perhaps most salient among such errors with respect to questions of normalization are those that, in the terms of philosophical ethics, mistake the "is" for the "ought": they mistake assumptions or observations about what people do or how they behave for guidance in ethical judgment, that is, what people *ought to* do, or how they *should* behave. But this distinction between what Kant calls "anthropology" and "morality" (1964 [1785]) is one that has come to be understood, in bioethics and perhaps in other realms, as a matter of intellectual understanding of moral "rules," which may not offer meaningful guidance to individuals and families lacking the fortitude, or perhaps even the luxury, that would enable them to comply with such rules. It may be that the expectation that individuals should comply with moral principles is a standard "too high for humanity," as John Stuart Mill put it (2001 [1861], 18). Emphasizing virtue and the ancient tradition that grounds it serves to remind us that, however it may appear in some professional contexts, ethics is not merely a legalistic tool for distinguishing "right" from "wrong" but is first understood as a way of living and of promoting human flourishing.

Ethical Arguments for the Normalization of Atypical Sex

Beginning with the work of John Money and his colleagues in the 1950s, the "optimal gender of rearing policy" guided physicians' recommendations in favor of normalizing surgery for children with atypical sex anatomies. As we have seen, strong challenges to the evidence supporting the wisdom of this policy did not have a significant impact on the frequency of the performance of surgery; although few physicians now explicitly invoke the optimal gender policy in their continued support of the standard of care (see, e.g., Meyer-Bahlburg 1999; Meyer-Bahlburg et al. 2004), the rationale for the optimal gender policy may nevertheless be understood to continue to prevail in the medical management of atypical sex. Physicians no longer rely explicitly on the optimal gender policy to justify normalizing surgery; instead, they present the therapeutic value of normalizing surgery (if not sex reassignment) in terms of the seemingly obvious rewards of normal appearance, the imagined tolls of abnormality, and the assumed difficulties parents would experience in bonding with their children if normalizing surgery were to be delayed.

Physicians recommending and performing normalizing surgeries since the late 1990s maintain that their practices are in the best interests of their patients, a belief all physicians would be expected to hold with respect to any intervention they undertake. But the significant questions that have been raised by the standard of care call for justifications for interventions that no one today characterizes as urgent and that many charge are not only unnecessary but also pose a genuine risk to children's health and well-being. We have seen one response to this need in the work of Garry Warne and his colleagues, who head off ethical challenges to the standard of care by asserting the primacy of a "natural" imperative over any ethical imperative—what amounts to, as I suggested in chapter 5, an invalidation of ethical reasoning, at least with respect to the treatment of children with atypical sex. Though I would like to think that even the staunchest proponents of the standard of care would find suspect the argument advanced in the work of Warne and his colleagues, the identification of standard medical practice with "the good" nevertheless captures the prevailing sense of physicians who continue to recommend and perform normalizing surgeries. Public criticisms of the standard of care since the late 1990s are numerous and have been made by affected individuals and their parents, as well as professionals in law, the humanities and social sciences, and even members of the medical community. Arguments in favor of normalizing surgeries have usually taken place in the private settings of physicians' offices in compassionate discussions between physicians and families, and in informal communications among doctors themselves. The medical literature generally takes for granted the value of intervention; while particular articles might allow that genital normalization is "controversial" or "sensitive," articles or textbook chapters treating this issue generally focus on the details of the performance of a particular intervention, just as they would any other technical matter of medical treatment.

The tensions that characterize the standard of care today are best illustrated by the 2005 consensus meetings convened by the U.S. and European endocrinological societies, and the resulting Consensus Statement published in 2006. Even as the resulting statement heralded significant changes in practice, it failed to provide a reasonable rationale for the normalizing surgery expressed in the statement's continued, if qualified, support. That failure is especially startling in light of the statement's unprecedented acknowledgment of conspicuous problems that had characterized practices since the 1950s. In addition to the new nomenclature of disorders of sex development that replaced variations on the term "hermaphroditism" (Hughes et al. 2006, 554), participants agreed on a number of changes to the standard of care. Physicians should make clear to parents that DSD "is not shameful"; candor in the provision of information to parents about their child's condition is now understood to be essential (555), as is providing age-appropriate information to children (557–558). The statement also recommends against sex reassignment of 46,XY males with micropenis and makes preservation of fertility in males as important as it has consistently been for those assigned female (556). Recommendations for clitoral reduction are now tempered (557), but the statement acknowledges forthrightly the trauma that has resulted both from repeated examinations of children's genitals and from medical photography (558).

In the context of these fundamental shifts in practice, the failure to challenge some types of normalizing surgery—particularly for girls with very large clitorises—as a standard of care suggests a refusal to investigate the assumptions that made the optimal gender policy so convincing over the decades preceding the consensus meetings. The Consensus Statement provides no argument in favor of normalizing surgery apart from the assertion that it "relieves parental distress and improves attachment between the child and parents." The authors' admission of the absence of evidence to support this "feeling" (557) indicates the need for considered reflection upon a standard of care that no longer stands on the once apparently unassailable ground that Money's theoretical work provided.

In 2009 the working group Bioethics and Intersex responded to this need for more extended ethical reflection on medical management of atypical sex and developed what the lead author of the resulting paper elsewhere describes as "an exhaustive catalogue of ethical recommendations" to support the care of children with DSD (Wiesemann 2010, 2). The work of the Bioethics and Intersex Group is not the first effort to craft an ethical approach to the medical management of children born with DSD,[5] but it is the first that takes as its ground the authority of parental decision making that it endorses. The importance of this focus is easy to overlook. In the care of children with atypical sex, the role of parents, even in recent memory, has often been regarded as inconsequential ("doctors' orders!"). When the standard of care was firmly established in the last century, parental authority was cast as an obstacle to be overcome in ensuring that children receive optimal care.

In "Ethical Principles and Recommendations for the Medical Management of Differences of Sex Development (DSD)/Intersex in Children and Adolescents," authored by three of the sixteen members of the German Network DSD/Intersex working group, we find not an evasion of ethical reasoning such as that offered by Warne and his colleagues, but a genuine and unique effort to "develop, discuss, and present ethical principles and recommendations for the medical management of intersex/DSD in children and adolescents" (Wiesemann et al. 2010).[6] There can be little doubt that the reflection in which the working group engaged, and arguably seeks to promote, is vitally needed; the principles it adumbrates provide a promising ground for ethical reflection. Identifying the productive tensions between the project of the main paper and the work of the paper's addendum, attributed to the working group as a whole, directs us to attend to the gaps in reflection on practices and understandings that not only continue to shape the medical treatment of DSD but also are reproduced in the selected principles on which the main paper focuses.

In setting out its project, the main portion of the 2010 paper acknowledges the significant ethical violations entailed by the optimal gender policy. Four of these are now well known: (1) the policy required some degree of deception regarding not only affected individuals but also families; (2) the policy was itself grounded on evidence that was falsified to degrees we may never fully know; (3) even aside from the falsification of data, it involved obvious violations of ethical and scientific standards in the conduct of the research; and (4) the collection of meaningful data on outcomes in line with prevailing ethical standards has been difficult precisely because of the original conditions under which care was administered.[7] For these reasons, it is not surprising that the authors of "Ethical Principles and Recommendations" conclude that the "optimal gender policy has lost its attractiveness as a comprehensive and successful strategy for managing DSD" (Wiesemann et al. 2010, 673).

One might wonder about the narrowness of the criticism of the optimal gender policy presented in the paper; Claudia Wiesemann and her colleagues do not challenge its central premise that conditions a successful psychosocial adjustment on conformity of one's physical appearance with one's sex assignment. For half a century, physicians relied on the protocols developed at Johns Hopkins to justify the standard practice of normalization that would support the successful psychosocial development of a child's sense of self. But now it appears that the emphasis on shaping genitalia to match a child's assigned sex functions to ensure that *others'* sense of who the child is will not be disrupted. Among the majority of specialists in the care of DSD, the importance of this goal is now taken for granted, and challenges to the importance of "normal appearance" are ignored.[8] Uncritically accepting this assumption, the authors of "Ethical Principles and Recommendations" cannot but locate the focus of the question they pose on the problem of the ethical justification for parental consent to normalizing surgeries.

This focus emerges from the three principles the authors identify as "relevant to decision making in DSD." The first is the well-being of the affected child and the adult she will become; the second is respect for "the rights of the patients to self-determine decisions that affect them now or later"; and the third is the fostering of "family and parent-child relations." While Wiesemann and her colleagues understand that the principles may "often conflict" (675), ultimately they argue for an obligation to respect parental authority. Such authority, they aver, should be recognized as constitutive of the right to familial privacy that is recognized in the major declarations of human rights of the twentieth century, namely, the Universal Declaration of Human Rights, as well as the U.N. Convention of the Rights of the Child (674).

The right to privacy, and the authority associated with this right, however, are "not unlimited." The exercise of this right, they acknowledge, has to comply with the ethos of parenthood determined by the larger cultural context, not just by the individual parents themselves. This almost universal ethos demands both a caring and encouraging human relationship between parent and child and respect for each and every child. The way in which parents are expected to live up to this ethos has to be socially negotiated in line with social, cultural, or religious attitudes. (674)

Wiesemann and her colleagues do not remark on the specific social, cultural, or religious attitudes that can cast normality as an imperative, but the working group's characterization of atypical sex as a "psychosocial emergency" (677) may indicate that at least some of its members regard atypical sex in the monstrous terms that evidently continue to shape the standard of care.

As an adumbration of "Ethical Principles and Recommendations," promised by the title, the main paper falls far short of its promise to "provide a comprehensive view of the perspectives of clinicians, patients, and their families" (671), though the more numerous principles detailed in the addendum may be read to correct in some measure for the limitations of the main paper. There is nevertheless no genuine attempt to take on the ethical test presented by Suzanne Kessler's studies, to reckon with the revelation that, imagining ourselves to be in the child's position, the overwhelming majority would not have wanted their parents to consent to normalizing surgeries of the sort Kessler describes. To the extent that the analysis presented by Wiesemann and her colleagues can address this issue at all, it does so only in terms of the problem of consent and what the authors describe as the doubt that has been cast "on parental surrogate decision making" by critics of normalizing surgeries performed in infancy and early childhood. Specifically, the authors of the main paper are concerned with responding to the (unattributed) claim that in the absence of medical necessity it is wrong to make irreversible decisions on behalf of children when the desires of infants or very young children cannot be known. "Although appealing in its simplicity," they write,

> [this argument] is flawed: it does not sufficiently distinguish between the interests of the child, particularly the small one, and those of the future adult . . . According to the maxim of postponed informed consent, only the adult would be truly able to determine the best interests of the child he or she was in a former time. But this child no longer exists, and its interests, thus, can no longer be respected. (673)

Although this criticism may be persuasive on its face, the authors' characterization of opposition to proxy decisions in favor of normalizing genital surgery fails to represent the fuller articulation of those objections found in the earliest published arguments against it. These include criticisms the working group cites elsewhere in their report, including that of Kenneth Kipnis and Milton Diamond, whose call for a moratorium on normalizing surgeries in a 1998 essay is based not on the question of consent the group takes to be primary, but on the possibility of harm resulting from unnecessary surgery.[9]

According to Kipnis and Diamond, the "presumption has always to be against surgery unless two types of evidence are at hand." This evidence includes how other patients have fared having undergone surgery and whether those who have not had surgery have suffered for "going without."[10] "Because this evidence is lacking," Kipnis and Diamond write, "the surgical assignment of sex remains an experimental procedure: one in which the results cannot be properly assessed until at least 20 years after the intervention" (1999 [1998], 406).

Contrary to the representation of Wiesemann and her colleagues, criticism of early surgery in the literature has not focused on an epistemic problem as they have defined it, that is, as "knowing" what a particular child would want (though certainly objections have been raised, as the working group notes, with respect to the irreversibility of decisions made in the absence of medical necessity). The fundamental problem that Kipnis and Diamond identify instead is that *the consent sought from the parents cannot be informed consent.* In other words, as Kipnis and Diamond put it, "Doctors can't tell parents what the long-term risks and benefits are because they haven't done the studies and don't know" (406). Given the priority they assign to parental rights to proxy consent, it is curious that Wiesemann and her colleagues do not consider the substantial constraints on the information parents have in making decisions about surgical normalization. Erecting a straw man in their treatment of criticism of early surgery not only gives short shrift to consideration of the perspective of the children the working group claims to represent, but it also fails to consider meaningfully the challenges facing parents in their decision making. Some physicians may claim that improvements in surgical technique substantially mitigate the problems outlined by Kipnis and Diamond. But rather than address the fundamental problem of consent that the two authors identify, it appears from physicians' accounts that they "resolve" that question by frankly acknowledging the absence of evidence and by putting the decision in the parents' hands.[11]

However, far more important than demonstrating the reductive treatment of objections to early surgery in the terms offered by Wiesemann and her colleagues is what strikes me as their failure to address the divergent moral intuitions demonstrated in Kessler's studies. Where those imagining themselves as parents support normalizing surgery on behalf of children with atypical sex, the overwhelming majority of adults asked to imagine that their own parents had been faced with the decision of normalizing them say that they would have opposed it. Perhaps because the authors of the main paper narrowly focus on clarifying the principles that support parental consent, they do not develop the principles limiting parental discretion that they gesture toward at the end of the essay. These principles, they write, should be outlined "in accordance with commonly shared beliefs of the good parent on the one hand and of the child's human dignity and bodily integrity on the other hand" (Wiesemann 2010, 674). But perhaps the problem here is in the construction—in seeing shared beliefs about good parenting and those concerning children's human dignity as fundamentally in tension with each other. If we examine more closely the question of parental duty, I believe we may see how the tension the group assumes—precisely the tension with which physicians grapple—is the result of an uncritical valuation of the principle of autonomy, literally, the capacity to be "self-governing," which is generally taken within bioethics as the rights of patients to make informed decisions in their care.

The Duty to Protect

If it seems obvious that individuals would not have wanted their parents to consent to normalizing surgeries, one reason is owing to the long association of autonomy with human dignity. Whether explicit (in our legal codes, both domestic and international) or implicit (in what psychoanalysis casts as a kind of inevitable fantasy), autonomy figures as an incontestable good.[12] Indeed, I would suggest that the question of autonomy is central to the Bioethics and Intersex Group's understanding of what they also take to be the dilemma presented by the prospect of normalizing surgery. Infants and toddlers are not autonomous in the sense that they lack the capacity to make informed decisions on their own behalf. Parents are able to make these decisions for themselves and extend that capacity to make decisions on behalf of their dependent charges. But as Kessler's studies suggest, the decisions that an individual would make in the one case may be very different from the decisions she would make for her own children.

Let us focus, then, on the distinctive position of parents and the characteristic difference that sets their position apart from that of children. Here I think we gain greater insight into what moves parents—and when I speak of parents I also mean those imagining themselves to be parents, as the students in one of Kessler's studies did—to favor normalizing surgeries. Granting that the answer to the question of whether to allow or seek normalizing surgery for a child will vary according to the historical and sociocultural context in which particular parents find themselves, I think that today most would agree that parents presented with the option of normalizing surgery for children with atypical sex agree to, or even insist upon, this intervention because they seek above all *to protect their children.*

A wide variety of the normalizing practices in which parents frequently engage are intended to protect children, socially and medically. Alice Dreger writes that she teaches her child "when to say 'please,' 'thank you,' 'you're welcome'" and how to use pronouns appropriately in speech. She works to encourage him to eat nutritious food and has agreed to vaccinations to guard against infectious disease. The motivating force of these practices is continuous with that expressed by parents of children with atypical anatomies, whose "desire to normalize [their] child can be especially strong."

Most children with unusual anatomies are born to parents who do not share the unusual trait, and so parents' reaction often involves fear, shame, guilt, and distress, even while those feelings are tempered by relief, excitement, and joy at the birth. The parents often can't imagine living "that" way. They flash back to the worst teasing they ever experienced when they were young, and imagine it being infinitely worse for this child. They remember how difficult it was to make friends and how much personal appearance counted, and they worry that this child will always be alone. They know how important it is not to feel alone. (Dreger 2004, 55–56)

Identifying the continuity between the desire to normalize children and the desire to protect them suggests that parents feel a kind of compulsion that can be understood in terms of what Immanuel Kant calls in his moral philosophy "inclination."

For Kant, an inclination is a feeling of desire or need that is definitive of humans' animal nature. "Inclination" is a term that in this context might strike one as failing to capture the force of the impulse or instinct to protect one's child from harm. But such feelings are exemplary of the "nonrational" aspect of our humanity: these are the whole range of needs and desires to which we are, in Kant's terms, subject as beings who are rational, but not purely rational, as he takes divine beings—God, or angels—to be.

In the *Groundwork of the Metaphysics of Morals,* Kant writes that moral "imperatives" apply only to rational beings endowed with reason who are also subject to the law of nature. In other words, imperatives apply only to creatures who have the capacity to make choices or exercise judgment in the face of desires that may pull them in a direction at odds with what reason would command. For this reason, imperatives have no role in determining the activity of nonrational creatures (e.g., plant life, or nonhuman animals, according to Kant). Imperatives also have no place in the determination of a purely rational will such as "the *divine* will [or] in general . . . a *holy* will," he writes, "because '*I will*' is already of itself necessarily in harmony with the law. Imperatives are in consequence only formulae for expressing the relation of objective laws to the subjective imperfection of the will of this or that rational being—for example, the human will" (1964 [1785], 81; original emphasis). That is not to say, however, that every "natural" impulse that humans have is at odds with the "moral law." The decisions motivated by inclination and those commanded by the moral law may—and frequently do—coincide.

Even as we may identify parents' protective instinct in what Kant calls the "natural" aspect of ourselves that we share with nonhuman animals, we may also understand that at the same time, protecting children is a duty of the sort that is worthy of ethical (and legal) defense, as the German Bioethics and Intersex Group would appear to agree. Characterizing a parent's impulse to protect a child as a duty, however, cannot be sufficient to sanction normalizing surgery for a child, because it assumes too much about the protective qualities of normalizing surgery, on the one hand, and not enough about the potential of that surgery to result in harm, on the other. However, if we see the protection of children as a "perfect" duty in Kant's terms, it is a duty that must be exercised in very different ways depending on a variety of factors, the understanding of which relies on practical wisdom acquired by experience and education.[13] A parent's duty to protect her child, I propose, is one better cast as a virtue.

Back to Aristotle

For Aristotle, a virtue (*aretê*) is not fixed. Virtues, or "excellences," must be learned and practiced so that one is disposed to acting in ways that promote humans' ultimate good, namely, "happiness" or "flourishing" (*eudaimonia*). In philosophy an Aristotelian approach to ethics is generally contrasted with a deontological, or Kantian, approach. For Kant, the goal of ethical understanding is not conceived as happiness or flourishing so much as it is acting from duty, and discerning what actions are necessitated by duty. Where "virtue" in Kantian terms may be understood to be a matter of constraint (and especially constraint on pleasure), virtue—or virtues—for Aristotle, constitute "excellences" to master, precisely in order to promote flourishing. Virtues are never "finally" learned, but are exercised over one's life. It may be that describing parents' obligation to protect children as a duty leads us to see the duty to protect our children "in an unqualified way," as Aristotle puts it. Yet, for Aristotle, we must understand ethical virtues in terms that involve how they are exercised and specify "the manner in which they should or should not [be practiced], or . . . the time [at which] they should" (1984, 1104b). They are not given by nature, but are learned over a period that permits the development of one's habitual exercise of them. In the *Nicomachean Ethics*, Aristotle offers any number of examples that illustrate the kinds of knowledge and experience necessary for the proper exercise of virtues such as courage, generosity, and high-mindedness so that our actions are appropriate at the moment of their performance, neither in excess nor in deficiency, but achieve "the mean."

In Aristotle's terms, the sort of education that results in this achievement is not what readers of Kant would take to be the mark of moral character, that is, an education to promote "resistance" to one's natural impulses in fulfillment of the requirements of duty. Instead, the cultivation of virtue is intended to develop an individual's inclination to act in ways that are consistent with the achievement of the mean. In Aristotelian terms, "overprotectiveness" would be an excess of protection, while a failure to protect a child—neglect, in the legal parlance of the United States—would be a deficiency. For Aristotle, the mean is not a matter of arithmetic, but instead is determined relative to the subject and to her circumstances. When we consider what is necessary for ensuring the safety and well-being of our children, a fixed notion of protection cannot capture the sort of finely tuned adjustments parents must make as a child grows and as we learn to be parents of the particular children for whom we are responsible. The protection of newborn children is primarily concerned with making sure they are fed and clean. New parents often fret about getting these "right," that is, in ensuring that their practice aligns with the mean, and the natural consequences of excess or deficiency of nutrition or hygiene—from finding ourselves covered in spit-up to encountering a baby's glowing and angry backside—teach us soon enough that we must adjust our practices. Quickly this knowledge becomes superseded by the need for increasingly complex understandings of a child's needs. Where protection in infancy may involve keeping choking hazards out of reach, those impulses to safeguard a child from all hazards must soon be tempered by the child's developing needs to learn. Take walking, for example. When babies are learning to take their first steps, a parent's impulse may be to keep them from falling. But the disappointment or surprise or discomfort of falling, as a grandparent might need to gently instruct a new parent, is essential for the child's learning to walk; falling down promotes the gross motor skills important in the process of learning to walk, such as developing a reflex of cushioning her own fall with her hands, to pick herself back up, and to try again. There are other lessons a parent might need in this case, too: a child with a more reserved disposition might need to be encouraged to take risks, a sensitive child to see that falling is not so terrible, an overly bold child to understand the consequences of running before walking. And if someone is not acquainted with other children, it may be hard to know where one's child fits in these schemes and the degree or kind of protection one ought to provide. At the same time that we endeavor to be good observers of our children, we rely on the guidance of extended family, friends, teachers, pediatricians, as well as on books, articles, and, increasingly, on those we encounter virtually, to gain the kinds of knowledge, insight, and attention our children require of us.

Understanding parents' desire and duty to protect their child as a virtue helps us to see that an unqualified promotion of parents' desire to safeguard their children from all pain cannot be in their best interests. We can at once appreciate a parent's desire to protect her child from the pain of abnormality—and the correlative desire for normality—and see that that desire is one that a parent is obliged to temper. This is the difficult lesson with which the parent I call Sonja has been grappling since the birth of her daughter a few years ago.

Sonja's Story

The experience of Sonja and her husband, Elias, after the birth of their child was very similar to those of parents of children with atypical sex over the last fifty years. It was not immediately clear that Shai was a boy or a girl, but genetic testing soon confirmed that she was a girl with the salt-losing form of CAH. Once her health had been stabilized, the medical team initiated discussion about normalizing surgery. Doubts Sonja and Elias already had about the urgency and value of normalizing surgery were only deepened by what the couple recounts as the farcical effort to convince them of the value of surgery during their first meeting with the medical team. The pediatric urologist who proposed to do the surgery said he understood their anxiety about the prospect of surgery, because he had recently recovered from cataract removal. And he was going to retire soon, so really, now was the time to take advantage of his considerable expertise. "It's laughable now," Sonja says, "but when he said that, I looked at Elias, and he looked at me, like 'What the hell?' Why would we let someone with failing eyes operate on our child?"

Skeptical of the need for surgery at the outset, Sonja and Elias did understand that their daughter might require vaginal surgery if there was a structural problem that might inhibit function, and they accepted that an exploratory procedure to determine the existence of such problems was important. Another member of the team, who saw that the parents' trust in their surgeon was compromised, suggested that they might consult specialists in other parts of the country. They declined the appointment of one surgeon after the receptionist exclaimed that they should immediately schedule clitoral reduction, saying, "It's what everyone does!"

As their search went on, their questions became more sophisticated. In considering the possibility that their daughter would require vaginal surgery, they asked another surgeon whether he could do so while leaving their daughter's clitoris intact. He told them, "Oh, no, I don't do [surgery] à la carte." Throughout this process, they were fortunate in their confidence in the pediatric endocrinologist who would manage the delicate business of maintaining their daughter's health. She provided no advice on the question of normalization except to remind them that if they did pursue surgery, she would need to be consulted to ensure that Shai was medicated properly to deal with the physical stress of anesthesia and postsurgical recovery. They settled finally on a well-regarded surgeon who was a strong proponent of normalizing surgery and who made clear his opinion that, like his colleagues, he thought they should permit the surgery to go forward but nonetheless told Sonja and Elias the decision was theirs. Aside from the "scope," they told the doctor, he was to do no cutting. Having determined that Shai had no genuine malformation but, rather, a narrower vagina than was typical, and which she would be able to expand herself later on as she decided would be necessary, they returned home to their jobs and to their new lives as a family.

Sonja and Elias's recounting of the narrative of the first year of Shai's life makes absolutely clear that they were preoccupied by how best to care for and protect her. But this protection was not directed against the imagined stigma of her physical difference so much as it was focused on safeguarding what they talk about as her sense of agency, her capacity to be a critical thinker, equipped to meet the challenges that life brings. They can anticipate some of these challenges, certainly, since their daughter has a chronic disease that requires vigilant management, particularly in childhood. And already they imagine a number of scenarios in which her atypical anatomy could be challenging for future romantic partners (though they believe it possible that it might not be); they know that decisions not to alter her surgically might be something with which she struggles later on, that decisions they made on her behalf could be a source of conflict or gratitude, and that she might experience each sequentially or simultaneously over her life. Still, not only did "fixing" her, as so many advised in her first year, carry considerable risks to her capacity for erotic sensation, and perhaps even her sense of self, but there were also broader risks for Shai that Sonja immediately recognized in a podcast she had tuned in to when her daughter was a toddler.

The podcast was called "Do You Feel Pulled Hither and Thither by Each New Bit of Parenting Advice That Comes Your Way?" (Mom Enough 2011). The featured child psychologist, Linda Budd, provided a compelling commonsense notion of parenting. Sonja recalled how Budd decried the way that parents are increasingly "reactive" rather than "proactive" in their childrearing. In their efforts to make their children's path through life easier, they provide quick fixes and so fail to provide children opportunities to develop the skills that they need in order to become "caring, competent, and contributing adults." This notion—together with the "mission statement" that the psychologist described as essential for realizing this goal—provided language to describe the aims Sonja recognized in the discussions she and Elias had had about their priorities for raising their child. They had begun these discussions even before Shai was born. When they learned, shortly after her birth, that their daughter had CAH, and that they would need to think through a good deal of the sense of their mission well before they might otherwise have done, Sonja and Elias already had a firm basis for thinking through what their commitment to their child's development entailed.

Sonja was particularly struck by Budd's invocation of the image of the "curling mom." Curling is the winter sport that the world outside of Minnesota and Sweden becomes aware of during broadcasts of the Olympics. One may recall how players look at once frantic and focused as they brush aside ice and snow, clearing and shaping the path of the stone to guide it to its destination. The "curling mom" captured for Sonja precisely the image of the parent she did not want to be. Like its counterpart, the "helicopter parent," who anxiously hovers near her child to provide direction and assurance, the curling mom's aim is to smooth and direct a child's way. "That's fine if you're curling," Sonja says, "but it's no good if you have a kid and you have to teach them how to go over obstacles." That is not to say that the temptation to clear the path is not a strong one; Sonja experiences this temptation still and acknowledges that "the curling mom does [these] things out of love; a helicopter mom hovers, out of love." Resisting that impulse, affirming her commitment to her daughter's future competence, maintaining a clear vision of her "mission" as a parent responsible for facilitating her daughter's development as a competent, caring, and contributing adult, is one that Sonja feels obliged and challenged to practice every day.

The Practice of Virtue and Care of the Self

Cultivating the attitude that enables a parent to avoid the temptation to sweep obstacles aside for her child is no easy task. The immediate rewards of being a curling parent are substantial. For example, there is the child's feeling of safety or success, as well as the parent's own sense of accomplishment or sense of control. There are also considerable and immediate disincentives for resisting this desire that we encounter, in the child's or parent's frustration or disappointment, perhaps especially in the uncertainty that the work of growing up entails for children and their parents. To restrain this urge, to practice continence, as Aristotle terms it, requires deliberation (*boulêsis*). For Aristotle, as for Plato before him, "good deliberation" helps us to identify the good toward which we should aim (Aristotle 1984, 1142b). While we may truly believe that our actions aim at a good, whether momentary or lasting, our experience, together with reflection upon this experience, as well as our interaction with others, can help us to see that we can be—and indeed often are—mistaken in our evaluation of the good toward which we aim.

All those assembled at the home of Callias agree when Socrates asserts in the *Protagoras,* "No one goes willingly toward the bad, or what he believes to be bad." But if one is "forced to choose between one of two bad things," Socrates observes that "fear or dread . . . an expectation of something bad" (Plato 1961a, 358d-e) can lead one to make a bad choice, one grounded not on a bad intention but on the failure to recognize where the good lies. Fear or dread is often the result of ignorance, or "false belief" (358c), and can impede a true understanding of what such a choice entails. Virtue lies here in the courage to overcome one's fear, but this courage requires knowledge (539d). Indeed, Socrates goes on to conclude that courage itself should be defined as *"knowledge of what is and is not to be feared"* (360d; emphasis added). Such knowledge—which may require good deliberation—is essential in the cultivation of virtue.

Sonja's understanding of the difficulty of the choice she and Elias have made echoes the characterization of virtue we find in ancient Greek philosophy. Parents fear the consequences of the obstacles they project to lie ahead for a child with a body that is "not normal," and Sonja lives with the keen awareness of this fear. "I *really* understand parents who have surgery for their babies," Sonja says, "because they were not told different, and they have a different experience, and they love their little girls so much that they would plow all the snow out of their paths." Those who choose normalizing surgeries for their children, Sonja believes, are making choices out of ignorance and do not have available to them the knowledge that would provide them the means—that is, the courage—to do otherwise. It was her own mother's belief that cosmetic surgery would make Sonja more appealing, and so enhance her chances for flourishing, that led to the rhinoplasty she underwent as a teenager. Sonja knows that her mother wanted only the best for her, and she also remembers how "susceptible" she was at fifteen or sixteen, how fragile her self-esteem, when her parents proposed that she have a nose job. As an adult, Sonja appreciates that her parents had themselves so thoroughly internalized a cultural conception of beauty that they felt it important that she undergo cosmetic surgery; she can understand their actions as motivated by their care and concern for her. But she also remembers how much it hurt her that they felt it necessary to change her body, and how they were thinking not only of her future but also of their own—as grandparents to the beautiful grandchildren Sonja would bring them with her enhanced opportunities to attract an appealing son-in-law. This last point was one her father made on a number of occasions, though Sonja thinks being reminded of that remark now would cause him pain, as he must regret what he said. Sonja laughs when she thinks of her parents' visions of her future husband, so unlike Elias, whom her parents cherish, and of their head-turning toddler, who enchants the grandparents who nevertheless still ask whether Sonja and Elias should consider that normalizing surgery after all.

Sonja believes her own experience as a teenager planted doubt about the prospect of changing her own daughter's body. But the knowledge that guides her decisions as a parent is not only a matter of having had the experiences she has had but also the result of deliberation, of critical reflection upon her experience. This is the examination that grounds the pursuit of the self-knowledge that Plato's Socrates famously casts as the condition of the good life.[14] When I first discussed the implications of Suzanne Kessler's juxtaposed studies in chapter 2, I asked what could account for parents' failure to ask themselves the question on behalf of their children that it appears they would ask of their own parents: why would they agree to a surgical procedure they would likely refuse for themselves? There I detailed the obstacles to the caring identification that would allow parents to ask how their children might view parents' decisions to normalize their bodies. Following Sonja's lead, perhaps we should understand those obstacles as stemming from a broader problem, one that twentieth-century philosopher Michel Foucault points to in his work on what he called "the care of the self." "The idea that one ought to attend to oneself, care for oneself (*heautou epimeleisthai*)," Foucault remarks, "was actually a very ancient theme in Greek culture," an "imperative" (1988 [1984], 43) that is not only present in the works of Plato but is also a focus of Epicureans and Stoics alike (46–47; 1997 [1984], 284). This is not to say that self-examination, and the resulting knowledge, is the same across the work of the different thinkers and the philosophical schools with which they were associated (Foucault 1988 [1984], 63). Foucault nevertheless sees across these thinkers' work a "common goal," namely, to promote active attention to the "relation of oneself to oneself" (64), to take the "path by which, escaping all dependencies and enslavements, one ultimately rejoins oneself" (65).

The emphasis on the control one must learn to exercise over oneself and one's impulses might resemble a kind of abnegation, but the ancient notion of the care of the self, Foucault writes, "is also defined as a concrete relationship enabling one to delight in oneself" (65), not only to feel a kind of ownership of oneself, what we might better understand as a kind of "self-possession," but also directed one to take pleasure in the acceptance of oneself, including in the recognition of both one's capacities and one's limits (66). Foucault explains that during the rise of Christianity this concept of the care of the self became "somewhat suspect . . . at a certain point, being concerned with oneself was readily denounced as a form of self-love, a form of selfishness or self-interest in contradiction with the interest to be shown in others or in the self-sacrifice required" (1997 [1984], 284) by an ethical relationship to others.[15] The identification of a concern with oneself with a kind of selfishness that would interfere with a parent's—perhaps particularly a mother's—obligation to care properly for her child resonates with the sort of worries that are pervasive today.[16] Recognizing the conflicting views of parenting that direct us to "do everything" for our children and yet to practice the restraint in our parenting that will enable children to achieve for themselves the self-possession necessary for the practice of ethical virtue (which we especially hope children will be able to exercise when they are out of our sight) should move us to clarify the ethical problem facing parents of children with atypical sex anatomies.

Reimagining the Object of Protection

In the terms of the tradition on which Foucault draws, what is necessary for a parent such as Sonja, who sees as her ultimate aim, as the measure of her success, "putting herself out of a job," is a relationship to herself that allows her to resist the temptation to extend protection to her daughter in ways that will disable Shai. The source of such temptation may be found in a number of factors, singly or in combination. The temptation could be a function of ignorance, a lack of knowledge of what a child needs to learn to grow and succeed. It may also come from a concern about what others will think about one's child. Certainly this is the motivation that has figured explicitly in the standard of care for management of atypical sex anatomies. As has been evident in the recent history of medical management, the concern about what others will think has not been limited to what one thinks about one's child, but is concerned correlatively with how others may judge one's parenting.

Conceptions of parenting have been integral to the organization of medical management of atypical sex anatomies in children, but such understandings are mostly of the sort that are taken for granted. Recall that although parental response was consistently understood to play a central role in the standard of care, for decades there was but a single article that discussed parents of children with atypical sex in the medical literature. "Divergent Ways of Coping with Hermaphrodite Children" (1970) presents two case studies intended to support physicians in their efforts to help parents accept "the medical decision of sex assignment" and to promote in parents "a feeling of complete conviction that they have either a son or a daughter" (Bing and Rudikoff 1970, 77).

The article juxtaposes the stories of two families. The "Wests" were white and upper middle class; the "Torres" family was large, uneducated, and of Mexican descent. Both families had genetically female children with genitalia that appeared more masculine than feminine; the immediate response of the parents from both families, we learn, was "extreme shock." Following the initial distress and confusion shared by both families, however, their responses sharply diverged. Where the Wests' education and background had resulted in their "faith in medical science" that allowed them to become full partners in their child's treatment, the Torreses' stubborn adherence to the superstitious view that "there are many things which only God can know and perhaps the physicians made a mistake" marred the parents' relationship with the child's physicians and compromised her sex assignment. Rather than accept the recommendations of the physicians who prescribed a course of treatment in line with the model developed by Money and the Hampsons, the Torreses "coped with the intersex problem . . . by accepting the ambiguity of the situation and . . . actively implement[ed] it by giving the baby a neuter name (the name of a warlike tribe)" (Bing and Rudikoff 1970, 80).

Bing and Rudikoff are clear about the aim of their essay: for physicians to succeed in the work of sex assignment, cultural differences such as those displayed by families like the Torreses must be taken into account to ensure what the authors take to be the best care for children with atypical sex anatomies. Rather than working to understand how physicians might support parents in the "coping" the authors purport to address, Bing and Rudikoff cast the problem as one concerned with overcoming obstacles to the success supposed to be guaranteed by the optimal gender policy that was virtually unchallenged at the time. This policy was itself grounded on, and promoted, a particular view of sex and gender; it also conveyed prevailing social expectations of parenting with which these categories are supported and through which they make sense.

While the optimal gender policy no longer figures in the standard of care—or at least not explicitly—the conception of parenting contained there continues to demonstrate currency in the statement by the Bioethics and Intersex Group more than forty years later. The ethos guiding parents' responsibility is represented visually in the arresting portrait that appears on the cover page of Bing and Rudikoff's article, a black-and-white reproduction of Mary Cassatt's *Mother and Child* (see figure 7.1). In Cassatt's painting, a young girl, perhaps two or three years old, sits naked on the lap of her mother. One of the mother's hands rests lightly on her daughter's shoulder in a steadying gesture. The other hand holds a mirror to her daughter's face, which the girl's hands clasp awkwardly at the bot-

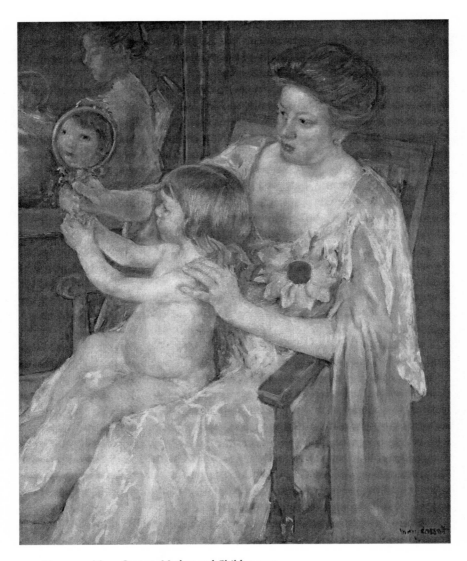

Figure 7.1. Mary Cassatt, *Mother and Child*, c. 1905.

tom of the handle. Both faces turn toward the mirror as mother and daughter regard the effect of her mother's work. The mirror reflects the face of the child; her eyes look directly at the viewer.

The portrait is an eloquent statement of an important dimension of maternal practice, namely, the role of the parent in the development of the child's identity. In holding the mirror to the child's face, supporting her as she reaches both hands to position it just so, the mother instructs her daughter in the ways of self-consciousness, that is, to see herself the way that others see her. The focus of the painting's viewer may be on the child, whose intent gaze meets the viewer's in the hand mirror, but the portrait's focal point is not singular. It includes the mother, whose own image is, like the child's, doubled. The viewer is directed to look at the mother not only because the mother's body is turned toward the viewer as she holds the child but because her body also appears in the mirror adjacent to the chair in which the two are seated. The viewer's eye is drawn to the reflection, positioned as the backdrop of the child's face in the hand mirror. In the story the portrait tells, the mother's work is directed not only at the child but also at herself, in her role—her own identity—as a mother.

That the mother's identity would be bound up with the development of the child's is not in itself remarkable. The shaping of identity is not only individual but also cultural, and it is this conception of identity and its development that grounds the rationale for the Bioethics and Intersex Group's argument in favor of preserving familial privacy as a "human right." From Sonja and Elias's understanding of their responsibilities as parents, we might form an image that differs from the Cassatt portrait, one that provides a critical perspective that is nevertheless consistent with the values the Bioethics and Intersex Group aims to uphold in its recommendations.

In place of the mother holding the mirror to the child's face, let us envision that child perhaps two or three years later. She holds a self-portrait she has drawn. She is not looking at her own portrait, but instead at her mother, to whom she is showing the portrait she has made. In Cassatt's painting the parent is portrayed as bearing responsibility for the development of a child's sense of self. The movement of identity creation flows here in a single direction, from the parent to the child. In the alternative I propose, this development is not entirely reversed, moving from the child to the parent, but is, as Gail Weiss puts it, "intercorporeal." In showing the parent a picture of herself—itself a product of interaction with her parents and others—she offers her parent the opportunity to learn something about the child as well as a chance to learn about herself as a parent. Even as this image tells a different story from the one that Bing and Rudikoff appear to see in Cassatt's painting, it is not a story at odds with cultural views that value autonomy, whether applied to individuals or to families.

It is a serious flaw in the German Bioethics and Intersex Group's reflections that we cannot find resources for the understanding Sonja demonstrates, which, I argue, is exemplary of "the ethos of parenthood determined by the larger social context." In the ethical perspective Foucault brings from the ancient Greeks, we may find a resolution to what might otherwise appear as a tension between the right of parents to make decisions on behalf of their children and the "limiting conditions" for parental discretion, which include, as the group says, respect for "the child's human dignity and bodily integrity" (Wiesemann et al. 2010, 674). If the "protection" that parents seek to extend to their child with atypical sex is an effort to "clear an easier path for the child," it must also be understood as an effort to diminish the vulnerability of the child to what parents and doctors see as the inevitable consequences of a stigmatized anatomical difference.

The tradition of virtue ethics from Aristotle to Foucault provides an important foundation for understanding the conditions of the possibility for closing the gap between the differing views presented in Kessler's paired studies. If the work of parenting entails a variety of ethical commitments and obligations, we must acknowledge that fulfillment of those commitments, and the meeting of those obligations, requires careful deliberation. The work in which Sonja and Elias have engaged as parents illustrates the shortcomings of the vague notion of familial privacy to which the German Bioethics and Intersex Group makes recourse in its endorsement of the permissibility of normalizing surgeries. Sonja and Elias's thinking directs us to consider, too, how we are to understand the "human rights" that the Bioethics and Intersex Group claims to safeguard in its support of this privacy. The responses by prospective parents in the second of Kessler's paired studies seem to support the concept of human rights promoted by the group, and yet this notion of rights seems to directly conflict with the conception of rights expressed by those responding as children in the first study. This conflict suggests that the grounding notion of human rights within the field of bioethics requires closer consideration.

8 Protecting Vulnerability
An Imperative of Care

BIOETHICAL REASONING TAKES respect for autonomy as its grounding principle; human rights discourse focuses on the principle of dignity. These forms of ethical reasoning have begun to intersect as prevailing understandings of human dignity have increasingly been cast in terms of autonomy, emphasizing the capacity for rational decision making. This intersection is evident in the recommendations of the German Bioethics and Intersex Group (Wiesemann et al. 2010), which grant priority to what the group identifies as parental rights—rights conceived in terms of parental autonomy—to make decisions on behalf of their minor children. Such rights, they argue, are constitutive of a human right to "familial privacy." As they present it, this right serves to protect the cultural and religious commitments of social groups and functions to protect individuals within these groups. Focused on familial autonomy and parental rights, there is scant attention in the recommendations to what we might expect to be the more salient consideration of the place of moral *obligation* in making irreversible and potentially damaging decisions on behalf of children in the absence of medical necessity. The construction of the question raised by normalizing interventions for atypical sex anatomies by the Bioethics and Intersex Group exemplifies the power of the concept of autonomy in bioethical reasoning; its constricted view of the moral problems presented by the standard treatment of children with atypical sex anatomies illustrates, too, what moral philosopher Onora O'Neill (2002) famously identified as a fundamental flaw in the formulation of bioethics, namely, the failure to investigate more thoroughly the grounding principle of autonomy.

I follow O'Neill's criticism of the role of autonomy in bioethics generally in asking whether the principle of autonomy as it functions within the reasoning of the Bioethics and Intersex Group is a sound or sufficient principle to ground ethical reasoning, specifically regarding interventions for children with atypical sex anatomies. Further, as the group appeals to the concept of autonomy in the discourse of human rights, I turn to an important development in that discourse that occurs at the beginning of the twenty-first century. In *Contesting the Politics of Genocidal Rape: Affirming the Dignity of the Vulnerable Body*, philosopher Debra Bergoffen details the significance of the landmark decisions crafted by the International Criminal Tribunal for Rwanda (ICTR) and the International Criminal Tribunal for the former Yugoslavia (ICTY) that "resignified women's legal status and reconstituted human rights law" (2012, 1). The recognition of wartime rape as a "crime against humanity," Bergoffen argues, established "a human right to sexual self-determination [that] recalibrated the meaning of dignity and integrity that human rights protocols are created to protect" (1). Where before the verdict human dignity had been cast in terms of autonomy, the decisions, first by the ICTR and then by the ICTY, shifted the location of human dignity to our embodied vulnerability.

Bergoffen's work on genocidal rape may seem an unlikely source for criticizing the argument set forth in the German Bioethics and Intersex Group's "Ethical Principles and Recommendations for the Medical Management of Differences of Sex Development (DSD)/Intersex in Children and Adolescents" (Wiesemann et al. 2010). In one case we are dealing with a criminal offense; in the other, a moral wrong. But however different the cases, we are nevertheless confronted with the issue of human sexuality and the meaning of the sexed or gendered body. Though the actions that demand our attention—and the intentions guiding those actions—are not comparable, we will see that the reasoning by which the wrongs of these actions are identified is the same. The evaluation of the moral reasoning demanded in both cases entails a judgment about the principle of autonomy.

In what follows I argue that Bergoffen's discussion of human dignity, and the salience of vulnerability in the constitution of human dignity, provides a critically important corrective to what has been the prevailing ethical rationale for normalizing atypical sex anatomy in children. My interest, in other words, is in exploring the implications of the reconsideration by the ICTR and the ICTY of the principles that underlie our conception of human dignity for reevaluating the principles that have been used to justify the cosmetic normalization of children's atypical sex anatomies. Following Bergoffen's analysis, I argue that normalizing surgery is not only a violation of the child's vulnerability, understood as a desire for intimacy, community, and love, but of the parents' vulnerability as well. For these reasons the putative aim of normalizing interventions to promote bonding between parents and children is misguided from the start.

After reviewing Bergoffen's presentation and her analysis of the implications of the decisions that privileged embodied vulnerability rather than autonomy as the ground of human dignity, I turn to what is generally taken to be the source of our thinking about human dignity in the context of both human rights and that of bioethics, namely, the ethical theory of Immanuel Kant. Where autonomy—understood in terms of rationality—has been taken to be the unassailable ground of dignity in Kantian ethics, closer examination suggests that dignity in Kant's work cannot be attributed solely to the capacity for autonomy, but should instead be understood as a property of those beings who constitute the distinctive blending of rational capacities and animal natures that is humanity. Recognizing the importance of protecting the dignity of the humanity that is shared by children and their parents, I conclude, requires that we reconsider the questions we ask concerning the ethical care of children with atypical sex anatomies.

Recasting Human Dignity: The Decisions by the International Criminal Tribunal for the Former Yugoslavia

For parents who seek the best means of safeguarding their children's capacity to become self-legislating moral agents, it may already be clear, as I argued in chapter 7, that the object of protection might not be best conceived in terms of autonomy, which, according to the Bioethics and Intersex Group, can only be afforded children by means of their proxies. Here I pursue this critique by showing how the ethical questions we pose with respect to the care of children with atypical sex anatomies would change if the principle of human dignity were framed not as a matter of protecting autonomy, but rather, as Bergoffen has proposed, in terms of protecting "the humanity of our embodied vulnerability" (2012, 2). Bergoffen's argument for understanding human dignity in terms of our embodied vulnerability challenges the traditional grounding of human rights in the principle of individual autonomy. While the notion of human dignity remains central to the understanding of human rights in the judgments concerning wartime rape by the ICTR and ICTY, the decisions crafted by the courts nonetheless transformed our understanding of the locus of that dignity.

As Bergoffen recounts, the tribunals' recognition of wartime rape as a crime against humanity was hailed as groundbreaking. Prior to the creation of the category of crimes identified as crimes against humanity, rape was recognized as a war crime in international law. It was nevertheless an ignored crime. Prosecutions were rare and convictions even rarer. But the evidence of the calculated use of public rape and sexual enslavement in Rwanda led the ICTR in 1998 to link wartime rape and genocide for the first time (Bergoffen 2012, 6). The campaign of ethnic cleansing by the Bosnian-Serb soldiers against Bosnian-Muslims civilians that made women's bodies "weapons of war" (12) made it impossible to continue to treat wartime rape as a negligible crime. It moved the ICTY in the 2001 case of the Bosnian-Serb soldiers Dragoljub Kunarac, Radomir Kovač, and Zoran Vuković (known as the Kunarac case) to affirm the ICTR finding that sexual violence is a crime against humanity, and also to reconsider its own understanding of the principles of human dignity that the laws of human rights were intended to affirm and to protect (7).

The new category of crimes against humanity filled a gap in international law that had previously allowed for prosecution of war crimes only between enemy combatants across international borders and not for crimes committed by a state against its own inhabitants. It would no longer be relationships between those recognized as "alien" to one another by virtue of national citizenship that set the scene of the crime. In introducing the notion of crimes against humanity, the Nuremberg court, in the mid-twentieth century, made possible the recognition of war crimes committed by a nation against its own inhabitants (17).[1] In her discussion of the harm identified as a crime against humanity, philosopher Hannah Arendt described the effort to exterminate whole races—"an attack upon human diversity as such"—as a violation of "the very nature of mankind" (1994 [1963], 268–269).

Prior to the ICTY ruling, wartime rape was classified as a species of torture. Like torture, it was considered to be a crime against humanity because it inflicted "severe bodily pain." In the ICTY, lawyers for the accused challenged this assumption, arguing that the rapes with which the defendants had been charged could not be considered crimes against humanity, because rape "is not in itself an act that inflicts severe bodily pain" (Bergoffen 2012, 23). Absent evidence of the experience of such pain or the perpetration of obvious harm, defense lawyers claimed, the charge could not be sustained in that court. "Given accepted legal definitions of rape and crimes against humanity," Bergoffen observes, "there was nothing amiss in the defense lawyers' logic" (23). The court ultimately rejected the defense attorneys' arguments but not because they took the lawyers' reasoning to be flawed; instead, the court took issue with the lawyers' understanding—that is to say, the prevailing understanding—of what constitutes a violation of human rights.

> Without discounting the matter of physical and psychological suffering, the court found that the crucial issue in a crime against humanity charge is the matter of human dignity. The women's testimonies convinced the court that sexual integrity and human dignity are too tightly intertwined to be separable. Violating one violates the other. (23)

The transformation effected by the court in this ruling is in the recognition of the place that sexual self-determination must have in the discourse of human rights. This recognition, in turn, requires significant reconsideration of our understanding of human dignity.

Before the ICTY decision, human dignity had been presented in the discourse of human rights in ways that identified it with individual autonomy and in universal (and ostensibly gender-neutral) terms. While the court's recognition of a right to sexual self-determination could be seen as continuous with a form of autonomy now extended to women, this right also necessarily differs from other kinds of rights that might be understood to belong to an individual, such as the right to bodily integrity. Unlike the right to bodily integrity, the violation of which is obvious in the case of torture, for example, Bergoffen argues that sexual self-determination must entail a conception of a self "existing in relationship with and vulnerable to others" (80). For this reason, the court's decision displaced understandings of dignity predicated solely on autonomy—what Bergoffen describes as a fantasy born of "a desire to escape the risks of being vulnerable" (74–75)—and recognized that our dignity should be understood to reside instead in our shared human vulnerability. The violation of a right to sexual self-determination recognized by the ICTY, then, cannot be narrowly understood as a right "inhering within individuals," but should be reconceived as a kind of right that is located "between" individuals (80). Thus, the vulnerability to which the right to sexual self-determination points, and which its recognition should safeguard, would be understood from two directions: first, because it necessarily implicates a body in relation to another, and, second, because it constitutes a vulnerability each of us has in common with other human beings. Following the logic of the court's decision, Bergoffen argues that the crime of wartime rape is a specific violation of the shared vulnerability that is the basis of the intimacy and connection that make our lives worth living.

In making the shift from autonomy to shared vulnerability, the ICTY had to reconsider the criminality of wartime rape. As detailed in the Geneva Conventions, prior to the proceedings at the ICTY and the ICTR, rape was taken to be a crime against individual women whose dignity—and vulnerability—was seen as particular to them as women. Women's "unique" vulnerability as women, under this rubric—a vulnerability that identified them with children rather than with adult men—required special protection. For this reason, rape could not be regarded as a violation of a "universal" dignity (Bergoffen 2012, 25). But wartime rape, understood in terms of special protection and honor, was not seen as a violation of the woman's "personal dignity"; rather, a "raped [dishonored] woman's body [in this context] implicates her people, specifically its men, for it is the men who are charged with protecting and guaranteeing 'their' women's dignity. Her honor cannot be separated from theirs" (25). What Bergoffen terms the "special criminality" of rape committed as an intentional stratagem of war was predicated on this understanding of women's bodies as community property, whose violation was an assault on the honor and dignity of her people's men.

Where the Geneva Conventions were concerned with protecting women's honor, the ICTY saw this protection in terms of their vulnerability, a vulnerability that was neither concerned with honor nor unique to women, but was instead a particular instance of human vulnerability women shared with men. Bergoffen's discussion of how this change affected the meaning not only of a raped woman's body but also of a raped man's body is illustrative in conveying the significance of this change.

> Instead of a raped man being stigmatized for "allowing" himself to be used like a woman, his rapist is now criminalized for violating his victim's right to the dignity of his sexual integrity. According to the law, then, being a woman no longer carries the stigma of being a vulnerable body. The shame of rape is nei-

ther the shame of being exploited because you are a woman nor the shame of being treated like a woman. It is the shame of being alienated from your humanity. (2012, 27)

In its decision the ICTY did not deny the particular vulnerability of women's bodies to rape, but the court radically recast this understanding, asserting a *human* right to protection of the vulnerability that the court saw as constitutive of our nature as sexual beings.

It is perhaps unfortunate that recognition of the atrocity of genocidal rape was the catalyst for a reconsideration of the ground of human dignity as constituted by our shared human vulnerability. But recall that the lesson in the overlapping histories of human rights and bioethics teaches us that innovative theoretical insights such as this one have often occurred only as a result of confrontation with what was before unthinkable. Furthermore, Bergoffen's analysis suggests that despite the fact that our embodied vulnerability had not been the explicit object of human rights protections during the pre–ICTR/ICTY era, one may see the dignity of this vulnerability as the implicit concern of what has long been recognized as a violation of human rights. While crimes against humanity must always be a violation of human dignity, Bergoffen details, phenomenologically, how different sorts of crimes already included in that category constitute distinctive assaults on that dignity *as that dignity is embodied*: slavery impedes what Merleau-Ponty calls the "I can" body, whose production is not one's own, and "sustains a world where I have no place." The devastating pain of torture threatens our humanity insofar as we value our "experiencing sensate body" and the richness of our sensory experience. The ICTY decisions may be understood, then, not as establishing a completely novel ground for human dignity, but as making explicit the centrality of our embodied vulnerability to a conception of human dignity that had previously subsumed this vulnerability under the principle of autonomy. But even as the ICTY decisions may be counted as another in a series of events that have marked changes in the history of the conception of rights, the inclusion of wartime rape as an assault on human, universal dignity is a significant development, Bergoffen argues, for it "directs us to consider the ways that the sensuous body and its desire for the other, for intimacy[,] and for community is integral to our humanity" (2012, 31).

Had the Bioethics and Intersex Group's "Ethical Principles and Recommendations" integrated this critical development in the understanding of human rights into their reasoning, I do not think they would have identified familial privacy (i.e., familial autonomy) as the privileged object of protection; instead, they would have seen that recommendations consistent with the understanding of human rights in the ICTY, together with what I argued in chapter 7 constitutes the ethos of parenting they ignored, require the protection of the dignity of the vulnerability parents share with their children. Bergoffen's analysis directs us to understand that the protection of familial autonomy stipulated in the conventions of human rights to which Wiesemann and her colleagues refer is better understood as the best means available to secure the protection of vulnerability within the terms of a discourse that takes autonomy as its guiding principle. That is to say, familial autonomy must be protected not because it is intrinsically precious but because it is the most common—though certainly not the only—means of protecting the dignity of its vulnerable members. This vulnerability is the condition of the meaningful relationships marked by our desire for love and connection.

Honoring the Dignity of Our Shared Vulnerability

To underscore the broad implications of Bergoffen's readings of the ICTY's decisions as I contend they should be understood with respect to ethical thinking regarding atypical sex anatomies in children, I propose that there is an illuminating analogy between the identification of the object of harm in cases of rape that preceded the decision by the ICTY and the "ethical" approach to the problems presented by atypical sex detailed in the recommendations by the Bioethics and Intersex Group. Comparison of the construction of the problem of wartime rape in the Geneva Conventions with what the Bioethics and Intersex Group identifies as the ethical problem in the normalization of atypical sex anatomy in children suggests that the reconstruction of the problem of wartime rape by the ICTY can enrich and complete the understanding of the ethical problems presented by atypical sex anatomies in children by the Bioethics and Intersex Group.

Recall that, according to Bergoffen, the Protocols of the Geneva Conventions acknowledge that rape and forced prostitution are crimes that may be committed against both men and women, and yet the protocols make clear that the "meaning of a raped woman's body is not commensurate with the meaning of a raped man's body." Rape of a woman, unlike the rape of a man, is an assault on the dignity of "her people, specifically its men . . . charged with protecting and guaranteeing 'their' women's dignity" (Bergoffen 2012, 25). In other words, the protocols recognize that rape may function as an assault by proxy. For this reason, Bergoffen observes, wartime rape is an effective weapon in the campaign of ethnic cleansing (26). In recognizing the relationship between the violation of the raped woman and her community's integrity, however, the protocols see the violation of wartime rape at a remove from women's bodies, from their humanity.

The Bioethics and Intersex Group sees the ethical problem posed by atypical sex anatomies in children as similarly removed from what critics of normalizing interventions take to be the objects of violation, namely, the bodies of children with atypical sex anatomies. While the practices that we might expect to be the focus of ethical reflection are those involving significant changes to children's bodies, and (as is presumably hoped) their identities or their sense of themselves, the group is concerned instead with the right of parents to make decisions on behalf of their children—a right they see as threatened by critics of the standard of care who have argued that surgeries in the absence of medical necessity have caused harm. Though the Bioethics and Intersex Group grants that parental authority must be qualified, the authors believe their recommendations to be defined in advance by the acceptance of a human right to familial privacy, and so by the rights of parents to make (autonomous) decisions on behalf of their children. In the same way that the Geneva Conventions see wartime rape as an assault on the dignity of husbands, fathers, or brothers of raped women, the Bioethics and Intersex Group takes the object of potential violation (and protection) to be the parents of children with atypical sex anatomies.

The decision by the ICTY appears to affirm women's "unique" vulnerability, but as Bergoffen demonstrates, the decision also "moved beyond the Conventions in saying that a human right was needed to protect this vulnerability, because *as sexual beings men and women are vulnerable to threats to their dignity by sexual abuse*" (Bergoffen 2012, 27; emphasis added). In other words, the court refused to see rape as a matter of women's (or their men's) honor, but characterized it as a matter of the dignity of their shared vulnerability. As Bergoffen describes it, this vulnerability resides in the ever present risk to the constitutive elements of our humanity from which we may be alienated and which are now recognized to include sexual integrity (27). That is not to say that the risk to sexual integrity is itself definitive of our vulnerability; rather, Bergoffen's inclusion of sexual integrity as both distinct from and yet integral to the other aspects of our humanity makes possible the shift from locating human dignity exclusively in our autonomy, to seeing our dignity in our embodied vulnerability.

Following Bergoffen's reading, the decision by the ICTY shifts the ground for human dignity from individuals' autonomy to a shared human vulnerability. This decision, she suggests, could "inaugurate a paradigm shift, where the subject of rights, instead of being understood in terms of the first person singular, autonomous 'I,' will be understood in terms of the first person plural corporeal, sexed, intersubjective and vulnerable 'we'" (80). With this reconceptualization of rights must come a correlative reconsideration of our obligation to honor the dignity of our embodied vulnerability. We can no longer see vulnerability as a state that uniquely or even especially applies to women and children, because, as the decisions make clear, it is on the basis of a genuinely shared vulnerability that the war crimes committed in the former Yugoslavia constitute crimes against humanity. But how might a recognition of human vulnerability in the discourse of human rights clarify the shortcomings of the recommendations made by Wiesemann and her colleagues?

Understanding the dignity of our humanity to lie not in our capacity for autonomy but, rather, in our embodied vulnerability, we can see the right to familial privacy as an attempt to protect a shared vulnerability that has been covered over by what feminists have described as a masculinist investment in autonomy, that is, a conception of autonomy that could be ascribed only to men (Pateman 1988). Understood in this way, I think we may characterize the Bioethics and Intersex Group's identification of the grounding principle for their recommendations in autonomy as a kind of category mistake. The group works within what it takes to be the prevailing ethical framework that shapes the questions it asks with respect to the limits they can or cannot impose upon parents, which ends up restricting the focus of their inquiry to the question of the permissibility or impermissibility of normalizing genital surgery.

In the same way that the decision by the ICTY may help us to reconceive the vulnerability of men to which the Geneva Conventions pointed, even if incompletely, I think we may also view the efforts of the Bioethics and Intersex Group as similarly in need of completion. If protection of the right to familial autonomy is taken to be an affirmation of our intersubjective vulnerability, then I think we should understand the questions raised by the birth of children with atypical sex anatomy not exclusively in terms of permissibility of surgery that takes "the problem" of ambiguous genitalia in children as a dilemma of conflicting interests (projected or imagined) of parents on the one hand and of children on the other, but instead in terms of our obligations to affirm the dignity of our shared vulnerability.

Dignity's Ground

The moral philosophy of Immanuel Kant would hardly seem the place to find support for the conception of dignity the ICTY relied upon in its decisions. After all, it is Kant's assertion of autonomy as "the ground of the dignity of human nature and of every rational nature" (1964 [1785], 103) that appears to be at the heart of the understanding of human rights that was recast by the ICTY.[2] And yet closer examination of Kant's work suggests that he does not understand the ground of this dignity of human nature as a property of personhood, or as a kind of human endowment, as we might expect.

Onora O'Neill's criticism of more familiar readings of Kant's moral theory are particularly helpful in explaining the difference between the concept of autonomy in political theory (and in bioethics) and that found in Kant's moral philosophy. Where the former takes a concept of individual autonomy as the foundation for a claim to "rights," autonomy is identified in the latter as the ground of obligation (O'Neill 2002, 74). At the center of O'Neill's challenge to conventional bioethical treatments of autonomy is her argument that Kant's account of autonomy is not an account that can support a notion of "individual" autonomy.

> [Kant] never speaks of an *autonomous self* or *autonomous persons* or *autonomous individuals*, but rather of the *autonomy of reason*, or the *autonomy of ethics*, of the *autonomy of principles* and of the *autonomy of willing*. He does not see autonomy as something that some individuals have to a greater and others a lesser degree, and he does not equate it with any distinctive form of per-

sonal independence or self-expression, let alone with acting on some rather than other sorts of preferences. (83; original emphasis)

The close identification of autonomy with dignity suggests that, like autonomy, dignity cannot first be understood as a property of individuals—something that individuals are said always to "possess," or something that is understood as a quality that inheres in them—but should be understood instead as marking the distinctive capacity to use reason to recognize and respect the moral law. One might want to insist that we "possess" such capacities, but a capacity marks only a potential to be exercised, one that can be compromised or impaired. Certainly, one would want to argue, the willful destruction of such a capacity would constitute an assault on human dignity. But the possibility of that destruction rests itself on the specific constitution of humanity, of which the capacity for autonomy is one integral part.[3]

In his exhaustive catalogue of Kant's ethical and political writings, historian of philosophy Dietmar von der Pfordten challenges the primacy of the concept of the "dignity of man," demonstrating, as O'Neill might have anticipated, that the notion of dignity more often appears in Kant's work in conjunction with terms like "duty," "law," or "rational being," and in fact does not figure centrally in Kant's ethical writings (Von der Pfordten 2009, 372). (Von der Pfordten also notes the "historical irony" that the twentieth-century notion of human rights, long attributed to a Kantian conception of human dignity, appears nowhere in Kant's "major work in political philosophy" [373].) Engaging in a technical reading of dignity and autonomy is not my intention; however, I think it is worthwhile to ask whether there is, in Kant's work, a genuine grounding for the identification of these terms that has made autonomy the privileged marker of human dignity in the field of bioethics. Although in most discussions of human rights the primacy of autonomy is taken to be a settled matter, closer examination suggests that the ICTY decision may not be at odds with a Kantian notion of dignity at all. In other words, while what appears to be a completely novel emphasis on vulnerability marked by the landmark decision of the ICTY identifying vulnerability with human dignity may constitute a significant transformation of the concept of human dignity in the discourse of human rights, that decision may nevertheless find unexpected roots in the very moral philosophy widely regarded as the foundation of the conception of human rights that has been identified with the principle of autonomy. As O'Neill argues, contemporary "Kantian" ethical frameworks, including those currently dominant in bioethics, rely on a certain concept of autonomy understood to reside in the self-legislating individual (and the dignity associated with this conception must also reside in this same individual). It is far less clear, however, that such a conception, as appealing or attractive as it might be, is well supported by Kant's own writing. Indeed, in one of the very few places that Kant identifies dignity with humanity explicitly, it appears that our vulnerability—a product, at least in part, of our animal nature—has some role to play in the constitution of "the dignity of man."

In the "Doctrine of Virtue," the second part of the *Metaphysics of Morals,* Kant writes,

> A human being regarded as a *person,* that is as the subject of a morally practical reason, is exalted above any price; for as a person (*homo noumenon*) he is not valued merely as a means to the ends of others or even his own ends, but as an end in himself, that is, he possesses a *dignity* (and absolute moral worth) by which he exacts *respect* for himself from all other rational beings in the world. He can measure himself with every other being of this kind and value himself on a footing of equality with them . . . hence he can and should value himself by a low as well as a high standard, depending on whether he should view himself as a sensible being (in terms of his animal nature) or as an intelligible being (in terms of his moral disposition). Since he must regard himself not only as a person generally but also as a human being, that is, as a person who has duties his own reason lays upon him, his insignificance as a human animal may not infringe upon his consciousness of his dignity as a *rational human being.* (1996 [1797] 6:435; original emphasis)

The notion of dignity that Kant elaborates here is one that seems consistent with O'Neill's treatment of autonomy as a capacity rather than as a property, because it is only insofar as he acts on the basis of the self-given moral law that a human being may be said to "possess dignity." It is only by acting autonomously—that is, on the basis of reason—that we can value ourselves as persons with dignity. But this dignity is a specifically human dignity and is due to the special nature of humans: for Kant, humanity marks the blending in our persons of the capacity for rational self-legislation (which we may be understood to share with purely rational beings such as we imagine to be exemplified by God or angels), together with our "natural" being (which we share with nonhuman animals as far as our desires or needs are concerned, and even in some important respects with plant life to the extent that we also have in common with this form a "vegetative" nature, as the ancients termed it). Nowhere, as far as I know, does Kant link divinity with dignity. It is, I would suggest, not only the special nature of humans as "mixed" creatures that makes morality necessary for us where it cannot be for God or angels (for whom no imperative is possible, according to Kant, since the divine will is always aligned with reason) or for nonhuman animals or plants (which Kant believes are determined wholly by natural necessity); it is also the special nature of humans that makes us *obligated* where these other beings are not.

Rather than an endowment or property, then, Kant's distinctive "dignity of man" is demonstrated in humans' capacity to act out of reason, that is, to obey a law of our making, even when our (natural) inclinations may pull us to act otherwise. Von der Pfordten points out that the notion of human dignity that is found in the discourse of human rights is most often associated with what is known as the second formulation of the categorical imperative in the *Groundwork of the Metaphysics of Morals,* which states, "So act that you use humanity, whether in your own person or in the person of any other, always at the same time as an end, never merely as a means" (Kant 1964 [1785], 96; Von der Pfordten 2009, 374–375). The right not to be treated as a mere means is another way of understanding the "human right" to the dignity that is violated, for example, in crimes against humanity. But as Von der Pfordten points out, "dignity" is not linked in Kant's work to this formulation of the moral law, but instead to the formulation of the "Kingdom of Ends," which emphasizes the exercise of reason.[4] This, I propose, means that the ethical imperative is concerned less with the object of (potential) violation and far more concerned with the self-legislating moral agent, that is, the agent whose obligation is born of this unique blending of characteristics that in Kant's view sets humanity apart from all other creatures and forms the basis for human dignity.

Recasting the Principle of Protection

Untangling the problems presented by the recommendations of the Bioethics and Intersex Group is no easy task. The group's claim that the human rights conventions of the twentieth century (Wiesemann et al. 2010, 674) must limit their question to the permissibility of parental decision making on behalf of their children may be challenged, as I have proposed, on the basis that they privilege the (legal) question of "rights" over and against the (moral) question of obligation, though the latter question is the foundation of the tradition of ethical reasoning in which they locate themselves.

From Bergoffen's analysis we learn that the idea of dignity originating in this early modern European tradition, and adopted in the discourse of human rights in the mid-twentieth century, has been, and continues to be, regarded as a living concept. The promise of its enduring value may be found in the possibilities it affords to reckon with violations to the dignity of humanity that could not have been foreseen. If the analysis I have been engaged in throughout this book is sound, we may see that the challenge of atypical sex anatomies in children poses just such a possibility, that is, that the nature of the violation the standard of care entails is one that is only now beginning to be recognized by those whose lives have not already been marred. The struggle of ethicists to accommodate the conflicting imperatives, "cultural" and "ethical," reveals the confusion on the part of doctors and parents who appear unable to distinguish the moral imperative from the admittedly pressing cultural concerns that have obscured it. The error that the Bioethics and Intersex Group makes in restricting its focus to protecting the rights of parents to make decisions on behalf of their children is characteristic of this confusion.

But I also want to propose another reading of the efforts of the Bioethics and Intersex Group that can direct us to see in its formulation of its central question—

a focus, not on the dignity of autonomy as they present it, but on a deeper, unacknowledged concern with the dignity of vulnerability. What if the protection of the autonomy of the family the Bioethics and Intersex Group seeks to support is an effort to protect the rights of those who are not typically marked as vulnerable, namely, the child's parents? Such a proposal might not be as far-fetched as it may first appear. Study of the rationale for normalizing surgery has long demonstrated equivocation on the question of for whom normalization of atypical sex anatomy in children is undertaken. If we take seriously the possibility that such interventions are for the benefit of the parents, we should investigate further the ethical implications of this rationale not only for children but for their parents as well.

Bergoffen's discussion of wartime rape as a crime against humanity might appear to be far removed from Eva Kittay's discussion of dependency, which I discussed in chapter 2. In asking about parents' vulnerability in the context of considering whether to accept normalizing surgery for their children with atypical sex anatomy, it is instructive to note the important elements Kittay's and Bergoffen's analyses share. Following Kittay's account, the responsibilities that caregivers have toward their dependent charges render caregivers themselves vulnerable. For Kittay, the necessity of their reliance on others to fulfill their obligations to another—a secondary or derivative dependency—grounds a moral obligation to those engaged in caring labor. Kittay's discussion of the particular vulnerability to which those who care for dependent others are subject calls attention to the ways that the history of medical management violated parents' autonomy as understood in the prevailing terms of bioethical reasoning (e.g., by lying to parents or misleading them). If today physicians acknowledge their appreciation of that violation, as my discussions with some of these physicians attest, their counseling of parents of children faced with decisions about surgical normalization does not adequately address the extent to which parents of children with atypical sex anatomies have been, and continue to be, placed in a situation in which their capacity to make decisions is compromised. Parents are not provided the opportunity to consider their decisions in the ways that parents like Sonja and Elias believe they ought to be considered. Parents are not provided the opportunity to see that the decisions they are asked to make are not as simple as it might appear, that making these decisions can entail, in the terms that Bergoffen has offered, an obligation to protect their children by respecting, and demanding that others respect, the dignity of their child's vulnerability.

What I think Sonja and Elias also appreciate, perhaps implicitly, is not only the obligation to affirm the value of their daughter Shai's vulnerability but also the obligation to acknowledge the value of the vulnerability they share with her. While I think most people would agree that being parents renders us vulnerable in ways we might not have been able to anticipate before we had children, it is easy to see how being a parent to a child who is in some way atypical can make that vulnerability seem overwhelming. Rather than grow into the role of parent as the child grows, those faced with decisions regarding normalization are asked to make decisions that may affect that child's conception of herself long before the parents have had a chance to get to know her and long before parents can learn, as most parents will learn, the importance of affirming—rather than protecting against—the child's vulnerability. It is this vulnerability that makes possible the connection that most parents desire, and that also creates the foundation for that child's loving connection with her parents and then with others as she grows. Bringing Bergoffen's analysis into conversation with Kittay's can help us see that parents of children with atypical sex may be tempted not only to fix what cannot be fixed—namely, their children's vulnerability—but also to ignore the attendant vulnerability that grounds those parents' own loving connection to their children.

Reconsidering the Vulnerability of Parents

Early in Lisa Hedley's documentary, *Dwarfs: Not a Fairy Tale* (2001), we are presented with the true story of Bob Heinemann, a middle-age man with achondroplasia, the most common form of dwarfism. We learn that the man, who has worked at a Connecticut inn most of his adult life and whose possessions include the few clothes he has in the small room he rents, was born to a wealthy and presumably educated family. Heinemann reports that when he was five he was sent to the Southbury Training School; he did not see his mother again until he was an adult.[5] He tells about an unannounced visit he made to his mother's address on the Upper East Side of Manhattan, describing her shock at seeing the now adult son she had abandoned at Southbury and her brusque command that he leave immediately. In a 2004 interview Hedley relates that it was her own encounter with Heinemann that inspired her to make *Dwarfs*. Herself the mother of a daughter with achondroplasia, Hedley reported that "she saw Heinemann walking on the street and jumped out of her car to tell him about her daughter. He got so agitated. He said, 'You're going to keep her, right?'" (FitzGerald 2004). In this same interview, Hedley says that in making the film she learned that it was parents' love and acceptance of their children that set Heinemann's experience apart from that of all the other individuals with dwarfism she featured, including Michael Ain, a pediatric surgeon at Johns Hopkins.

Following the narrative of Heinemann's life in the film, it is difficult to resist harsh judgment of the parents who abandoned him as they did. But the film subtly solicits of its viewers not only compassion but also more critical reflection through the story of Martha Holland, which immediately follows Heinemann's. Holland has a less common and more debilitating form of dwarfism than the others in the film. Martha's mother, Cathy, remembers that after her daughter's birth, physicians told her that her baby should be sent to an institution. An interview with Cathy Holland featured in a local Richmond, Virginia, article about the film's opening fills out the account of Martha's birth and makes the story all the more remarkable. Martha's legs were twisted in addition to being short, and she also had "a cleft palette, clubfeet, and no joints in her fingers." The swelling of her ears led her physicians to a diagnosis, several days after her birth, of diastrophic dwarfism.

The recommendation doctors made for institutionalization was based not on the problems associated with this kind of dwarfism, and which could all be addressed outside of institutional care, but on their mistaken diagnosis of deafness and a "degenerative brain disorder." It was a medical resident who told the Hollands he did not believe that Martha suffered either of these latter conditions but was merely fatigued from all the testing. "Take her home and love her like any other child," Cathy remembers he told them, "and she'd be OK" (Bredimus 2001). The insistent words of that young medical resident made possible the life that unfolds—a focused child playing piano despite her fused fingers and "floating" thumbs, a career as a wry middle-school teacher of "at risk" youth, and a storybook finale featuring a white-gowned Martha marrying her prince. In the juxtaposition of the stories of Heinemann and Holland, the film directs us to see not only the cruel and unnecessary limits that can be imposed on those whose different embodiment is stigmatized but also the pressures, fears, and, above all, the shame to which parents can be—and in the case of Heinemann's parents, likely were—subjected. The stories of the parents of children born with dwarfism, like the stories of parents of children with atypical sex anatomies, are mostly out of sight. Hedley's film is a vivid reminder that their condition—which necessarily includes the condition of the parents—requires far more careful ethical consideration than recourse to conceptions of "parental autonomy" can allow.

In *Better Than Well: American Medicine Meets the American Dream* (2003), philosopher Carl Elliott provides some helpful direction in understanding what that different kind of thinking will require. Among the stunning variety of ways that individuals consume technologies of "enhancement"—whether in taking pills or in pursuing body modification, ordinary and otherwise—Elliott sees in the motivation common to all a basic desire to fit in, to feel we belong to the communities in which we find ourselves or seek membership. Parents of children with atypical sex anatomies and the physicians who advise them appeal to this desire when they support normalizing surgeries for children.[6] But for Elliott, this fitting in cannot be reduced to the sort of conformity that we typically ascribe to such desire; fitting in, according to Elliott, is inextricably tied to a sense of identity that is not only about a sense of self—or, maybe better, it is also bound up with a sense of self that conditions the possibilities of identifying with others.

Elliott directs us to consider more carefully the operation of stigma in the production of our identities. On the one hand, the prevention or removal of stigma appears to make different kinds of enhancements appealing, such as cosmetic surgeries to make features less "ethnic" (Elliott 2003, 190–191). And yet any number of the identities we may claim with respect to racial or religious subgroups of U.S. American culture are "linked to marginalization or oppression" (199) and present opportunities for the kinds of "reclamation" of those identities that have become increasingly familiar. "If," as Elliott writes, "a marker of identity has been regarded as humiliating, limiting, or shameful . . . then the task is to create an identity in which the marker is seen in a more positive way" (200). Groups whose identities are rooted in histories of oppression, Elliott suspects, are less interested in connecting with these histories than in sustaining meaningful bonds with others. Recognizing the importance of such bonds, which are perhaps most often formed in the intimacy of family, helps us see that it is, as Elliott puts it, "the fragility of selves" (207) that we ultimately aim to safeguard, even if we misrecognize this aim in the name of autonomy, whether individual or "familial."

Following Elliott's discussion of identity and desire, we should ask if the fear of having children with whom we will not identify or with whom we do not want to identify—and who will not identify with us—might help us to better understand "the problem" of intersex over the last half century. The close association between atypical sex anatomy and homosexuality that John Money, together with his colleagues, promoted, and that has been sustained by their students and by the students of their students in the decades following, along with a small but visible movement to cast those with atypical sex as another "kind" of person, has likely contributed to the urgency that parents and their physicians feel to normalize children. If children with atypical sex are a kind of person unlike their own parents, normalization of children that is intended to secure their bond with their parents would seem justified. Indeed, such normalization would in one respect be understood as entirely ordinary, continuous, as I take it many physicians genuinely believe, with the kinds of normalization parents impose on their children as a matter of course. In this way we can make better sense of the Bioethics and Intersex Group's insistence on respecting parental authority, not because it truly legitimates the authority to consent to normalizing genital surgeries, but because in addressing and affirming the vulnerability that we must understand also to be the parents'—their deep wish to have children with whom they will feel connected and to whom they will feel bound—the Bioethics and Intersex Group assumes that we can only love, and be bound to, those who are like us. Seen in this way, the group's defense of parental authority may either be seen as an effort to conceal that vulnerability by invoking the discourse of autonomy or as an effort to normalize the ideology of like loves like.

Closing the Distance between Parents and Children

Throughout this book, I have tried to come to terms with the difference in the positions of parents and children that Suzanne Kessler's paired studies present. I have tried to make sense of this difference in an effort to identify and to overcome the ethical problems in a standard of care that has led to physical injury to those with atypical sex anatomies and caused emotional injury not only to those individuals but also to their parents. Reading the recommendations of the Bioethics and Intersex Group through the work of Bergoffen and now through that of Elliott, I think we must confront the difficult possibility that parents who decide in favor of normalizing genital surgery may not be acting for the sake of protecting the vulnerable child, but—consciously or unconsciously—to protect themselves from their own vulnerability. That is to say, the impulse to normalize a child is an effort to secure the confidence that theirs will be a child to whom they will desire to be bound. If this is the case, then the object of the prevailing standard of care—effectively the treatment of the parents through the "reagent" of the child—should be clarified and modified, much as it has been in the cases of children born with other kinds of congenital anomalies.[7]

If this presentation of the problem appears overly focused on parents, I think we have to recall that the most prominent rationale for normalizing genital surgery has been cast in terms of the needs of the parents, most notably in the 2006 Consensus Statement but also in the "human rights" framework in the recommendations by the Bioethics and Intersex Group. While the group places more emphasis than the Consensus Statement on the importance of counseling parents, both take for granted, and at the same time seek to protect, the putative right of parents to make these decisions. Putting the dignity of vulnerability at the center of ethical obligation does not change the important role of what I have argued is parents' "treatment," but it must change our understanding of the consequences of failing to identify vulnerability as the source of our human dignity. Where extending protection of parents' rights to raise their children in the traditions, cultures, and languages of their choosing must be respected as an effort to honor the dignity of parents' vulnerability, I think we may see that normalizing surgery cannot be regarded in this way but, rather, constitutes a violation with respect both to a child and that child's parents.

Unlike the aim of a social scientific study that seeks to provide an account of how things are, the aim of ethical theory is to provide a ground for saying how things should be. It seems to me that another way in which the work of the Bioethics and Intersex Group errs in its analysis is in accepting, and so reproducing, the idea that there is an irreconcilable difference between parents and their children with atypical sex anatomies. When, following Bergoffen's analysis, we reconsider the grounding of human rights in terms of the principle of autonomy we must see that the Bioethics and Intersex Group fails in its refusal to examine the framing of the ethical question it considers, opting instead to respond to the question posed by specialists who support the standard of care, namely, the question of permissibility. This is a serious shortcoming, because the identification of the question determines the possibilities for ethical thinking, and so for action. The group's reproduction of the opposition between (vulnerable) children and (autonomous) parents restricts the question they can ask to the permissibility of parents' consent to normalizing surgery.

If we see instead that parents and children are both vulnerable, and that their dignity as vulnerable bodies is truly shared, then it no longer makes sense to see the ethical question as concerned first or only with respect to the permissibility of surgery and parents' authority to consent to or even to seek surgery on behalf of their child. Instead, we must make obligation the focus of our attention, that is, we must ask how the duty to honor the dignity of the child's vulnerability may be fulfilled. It seems to me that if we ask the question this way, parents of children with atypical sex would not have the experience that Sonja and Elias report having with specialists in the care of children with conditions like Shai's, an experience that in many respects looks much the same as it did twenty, thirty, or even fifty years ago. Instead we would ask how best to secure the connection to their child, that is, how to support parents in their duty to honor the dignity of the child's vulnerability, and to help them to see early in their child's life what most parents will understand only after many years: how the dignity of their child's vulnerability is also their own.

Conclusion
Lessons from Physicians

Perhaps particularly in medicine, discussions of ethics today have become increasingly difficult to distinguish from discussions concerning "legality." Asking about what is right or good can too easily become a question of what is permissible or what constitutes culpability. Returning to ancient and early modern sources of ethics, as I have proposed in the last two chapters, may serve to remind us that, while ethical concepts or frameworks figure prominently in the law, questions concerning what is ethical or moral are not identical with those concerning what is legal. So many practices in which we engage in our lives are matters of rich ethical reflection falling outside the realm of legal regulation.

When I began researching the history of bioethics fifteen years ago, I was surprised by the incongruity between the conception of what was in medicine called "ethics" and the understanding of ethics that I had received in my training in philosophy. Many disciplines have been developed for—and are well suited to—crafting answers to questions. But philosophy is first and foremost a discipline developed to *ask* questions. If we do not ask why we think as we've been taught, or why we do as we've been trained or as we have become accustomed, we will take for granted that what we think is true and what we do is right. Just as important, as Socrates first demonstrated, is asking whether the questions we ask are the right questions. Do they move us to consider or investigate what is important, vital, true, consequential? Are the questions informed questions, themselves grounded in knowledge that is reliable? And, we should ask, why do we ask the questions we ask? For what purpose, to what end, and for whose benefit do we ask them?

What it means for philosophers to consider "the problem" of intersex—that is, to understand the ethical significance of the treatment, both medical and social, of those with atypical sex anatomies—is to consider both what questions are asked and what questions are not asked and why. In retrospect, I think it was my awareness that I didn't know much at all about atypical sex or the experience of those who had been subjected to normalizing interventions that led me to think about how the tools of philosophy could be put to work to understand what has motivated treatment and to clarify the nature of the wrongs that have occurred. The point with which I continued to struggle, and that I had put aside, was the question of change. It was not so clear to me what role philosophy could play in changing the standard of care.

The series of conversations I had with the parents Sonja and Elias directed me to return to the ethical tradition of the ancient Greeks for guidance in thinking about how we might understand the possibilities for change in the care of children with atypical sex anatomies. Through this lens I began to return to some of the conversations I had had with physicians about their practices and began to see that perhaps I had been asking the wrong questions.

When I sought out physicians to learn what was occurring in their clinics, the questions I would ask, as I had assured my university's Institutional Review Board, would be limited to those concerning how parents of children with atypical sex anatomies were counseled in the clinics where they worked. It had not occurred to me that during those conversations any of the physicians would spontaneously offer what I came to recognize as a form of testimony. Their stories revealed awareness of their own fallibility, of the mistakes they had made, or in which they felt implicated as doing harm. But in these stories, too, was a recognition of what I came to understand as the dignity of vulnerability that was so important for understanding the problem of intersex. Rather than ask how philosophy could play a role, then, perhaps the tools of philosophy could be most effective in identifying how ethical reasoning was at work in change that had already begun.

Dr. Spruce's Story

During our conversation about the kind of counseling parents of children with atypical sex anatomies are given today, Dr. Spruce began to think out loud about why he thought change in the prevailing standard of care had proved so difficult. Physicians and medical researchers are not only committed to their work; they are also identified with a line of investigation or innovation that they have inherited from their teachers and will, they hope or expect, project forward as their own legacy. Maybe it is for this reason, he says, that "I don't think they put a lot of energy into exploring the errors in judgment that they have made . . . They can't disconnect from what they have said is right." Admitting error is difficult, he was suggesting, because it was not just about a single mistake but also threatened a whole lineage of work to which one belonged, that was bound up with one's sense of self and of one's value.

Dr. Spruce took his own experience as a case in point. He saw his own error when a teenager seeking to transition to male came to the clinic where Dr. Spruce worked. Reviewing the teenager's record, Dr. Spruce saw that he himself had participated in the decision to reassign the teenager's sex to female as an infant.

"Did the teenager seek you out?" I asked.

"No, it was worse than that," he said. "He didn't know that I had been involved in his care as an infant. And I wound up telling him that." The experience made Dr. Spruce look again at "situation after situation where I . . . declared with a kind of impunity that my assignment of gender was correct. And I can actually remember standing over an infant in a bassinet with a urologist across from me, and saying, 'This kid's phallus is too small for him to ever be a real man. Let's make him a girl.'"

Dr. Spruce is not the first to be made aware of an error in sex assignment in which he participated, nor to be told that the normalizing surgery he recommended had caused harm. But he is one of the few who seems not to have sought to conceal or deny that mistake. At the time of our conversation, I did nothing to prompt the specific revelation of his encounter with the teen and the effect that encounter had had on his view of normalizing surgeries. I had asked to talk to him to better understand how counseling had changed since the publication of the Consensus Statement in 2006; I did not expect him to talk about his experience as he did. I understood that part of what made it possible for him to see his error was timing: between the founding of the Intersex Society of North America in 1993 and the consensus meetings in 2005, there was, as another physician put it, a sea change in general awareness about, and recommended treatment of, atypical sex. This was largely due to ISNA's organizing, which inspired revelations by affected individuals of their experience and the harm they—and sometimes their families—had endured. The powerful critical narratives and analysis these affected individuals, along with academic allies (some of whom were also individuals with atypical sex), produced prompted some physicians to question the medical practices standardized in the mid-1950s. Doubts that this collective work had planted were reinforced and more widely publicized by the revelation of David Reimer's experience just a few years after ISNA's founding. But as marked as these changes have been, the majority of specialists have continued to take normalizing surgery to be in the best interests of children and their families.

Considering the context in which Dr. Spruce remarked on his encounter with the teenager in our conversation, his explanation of his colleagues' resistance to investigating their own mistakes provides insight into why it was that this experience had a significant effect on his understanding. If his colleagues are reluctant to admit error, it may be because they resist disruption of their sense of self, tied as it is to their work, and the connection they understand this work—and themselves—to have, often to the past, and almost always to the future.

In my discussion with him, there was no sense that Dr. Spruce was unsympathetic toward his colleagues; his willingness to admit error was not an assertion of superiority on his part, but it nevertheless acknowledged a difference between himself and those colleagues for whom the admission of error would constitute too great a threat. His sense of self was located not in the sort of legacy attached to discovery or breakthrough, perhaps, but in his sense of mission as a physician, as someone who understands medicine as a practice of caring for others' health and well-being. Such a commitment requires that a mistaken practice be corrected, not denied. The younger Dr. Spruce, who unhesitatingly reassigned sex, might have regarded that standard recommendation as common sense—which for so many physicians, beginning in the late 1960s or early 1970s and continuing through the mid-1990s, it was. The teenager's return to the clinic brought to the seasoned Dr. Spruce undeniable evidence of bad judgment. But I would guess this was not the first experience of "unlearning" he had had in his career or in his life. I don't say this from any intimate knowledge of him but from what I have gathered in the closer study of virtue ethics to which my discussions with physicians like Dr. Spruce have led me.

Foucault's discussion of the work of virtue can help us to understand the changes in Dr. Spruce's thinking. Foucault identifies in Plato's treatment of Alcibiades, a young statesman preparing to lead his fellow citizens, the starting place for a study of the care of the self. Alcibiades's capacity to care for the city depends, Foucault says, on his ability to care for himself. The two directions in which he must "concern [him]self with . . . justice," Foucault reminds us, "appl[y] both to the soul and to the city" (2005 [2001], 174). In the *Alcibiades,* where Foucault locates "the founding of all philosophy" (189), we see the ways that care of the self and care of others are—must be—connected. It is not possible to care properly for others without caring for oneself, and each expression of care also serves the other. Alcibiades must learn that leading his fellow citizens well will allow him to "benefit from the prosperity of all and from the salvation and victory of the city that I have ensured" (176). The *Alcibiades* emblematizes the ancient notion of care of the self in its emphasis on the pedagogical work that promotes self-care: in his insistent and annoying interrogations of himself and of all those around him, Socrates proves the exemplary teacher who insists that we attend to ourselves. Foucault explains that the importance of pedagogy on display in the *Alcibiades* "tends," after Plato, "to give way to other functions" made salient in the work of Stoics like Seneca. Undertaken over the course of a life such as Dr. Spruce's, the incident with his returning patient suggests the operation of these "other functions" in the care of the self. Foucault identifies, first of all, a "critical function": "The practice of the self," he writes, "must enable one to rid oneself of all one's bad habits and all the false opinions one may get from the crowd or from bad teachers, as well as from parents and associates. To 'unlearn' (*de-discere*) is an important task of the culture of the self." In Dr. Spruce's case this unlearning would only be possible with the second function, what Foucault characterizes as the "struggle" that care is understood to involve, and for which one must be equipped not only with weapons but also with courage (495).[1]

The function of struggle is one to which we should devote some attention. Foucault's emphasis on the importance of struggle in the care of the self is echoed in the discussion of "the curling parent" in chapter 7. The cultivation of the virtuous character depends on learning how to navigate obstacles and to overcome difficulties. And yet, as Sonja and Elias experienced, parents faced with decisions about normalizing their child's sex anatomy may be encouraged to neglect this sort of moral education with respect to not only their child's development but also to their own, as parents. In studying virtue ethics we learn that failure to recognize the salience of struggle in moral development is a failure to understand the nature of virtue; indeed, finding ourselves drawn to the "the easy path," we may see any difficulty or challenge as an indication that that course of action is wrong.[2] In Dr. Spruce's account, one may gather that he had taken for granted the idea that normalizing atypical sex was the right thing to do. This confusion is understandable, as one of the continuities between virtue ethics from the ancient Greeks and Romans and utilitarianism is that the end of moral philosophy is *eudaimonia,* the human flourishing we call "happiness." If a course of action does not result in happiness, or what we take to be happiness, we will understand an action to be—or to have been—wrong.

It is possible that one could see Dr. Spruce's experience in utilitarian terms, as a matter of failing to promote happiness. And yet I think he would understand the wrong in which he repeatedly participated, and in which the majority of specialists in DSD continue to participate today, as wrong not only because it resulted finally in unhappiness but also because it constituted a deeper violation than he could have recognized at the time. The problem existed with both his action and his own inability to engage in "reflective scrutiny" (Hursthouse 1999, 166), a capacity that depends on the development of the practical wisdom he would likely characterize as lacking when he was a younger man. Rather than focus on moral actions and their consequences in narrow terms—what I think we should understand as a kind of crude utilitarianism—virtue ethics demands that we focus on the moral agent, and on the development of the moral character of the agent who can exercise the practical wisdom necessary to make sound decisions and reckon with the difficulties and engage in the struggle that life will bring.

The critical functions of care of the self and the struggle in which the moral agent must be engaged over his life, together with the courage these require, are necessary for carrying out what, for Foucault, may turn out to be the signal activity of moral life, namely, telling the truth (*parrhesia*). In Foucault's account, truth-telling, or "speaking freely," is the willingness and the deliberate decision to say what one believes to be true (2005 [2001], 372). But this is not just any truth. It is one that involves criticism, whether of self or of others. Such criticism, Foucault goes on to suggest, entails danger, some form of risk to one's self (2001, 16). One incurs this risk to fulfill a moral duty "to improve or help other people (as well as [one]self)" (19). Admitting error in medical practice poses a considerable legal risk today, one that, as recent articles on the subject indicate, may explain what appears to be an increasing prevalence—or perhaps simply the revelation of a long-standing prevalence—of physicians avoiding telling patients what we might call "the whole truth."[3] In Dr. Spruce's frank account of his experience, we can see the operation of each of the functions of the care of the self that Foucault enumerates, perhaps especially the ways in which his admission exemplifies the third, "curative and therapeutic function" of care of the self. It is fitting that the function of the care of the self (*epimelieia heautou*), promoted by thinkers of later antiquity, is "much closer to the medical model than to the pedagogical model" (Foucault 2005 [2001], 496) of Plato. If it is not clear whether the objects of the curative and therapeutic work that such care of the self performs are those affected in some way by DSD—individuals with DSD or their families, those who have already been or have yet to be treated—or whether it is Dr. Spruce himself, I think it is because, for virtue ethicists, we must consider these as linked. As Dr. Spruce is not only a practicing physician but also a medical educator, the subjects of this therapeutic work must include those patients who have not yet entered the clinic, as well as those physicians he is training now, and for whose development he also takes responsibility. Learning to be a "good" doctor, he demonstrates, involves confronting one's own imperfection. Dr. Spruce's success as a teacher of doctors will not be measured by his students' stubborn unwillingness to admit error or to see decisions in the stark terms as either right or wrong, but by his students' ability to listen to those they treat in their own practice, by their capacity to honor the dignity of their patients' vulnerability that, no longer the arrogant young doctor in his thirties, Dr. Spruce recognizes is also his own.

Dr. Maple's Story

It is easy to see how it could be that Dr. Spruce could experience a sense of responsibility to his patients and to his students, a responsibility that extends also to himself and to his profession. Dr. Spruce's story is easily located in the history of the medical management of atypical sex. This history is usually recounted as a history of those whose bodies, lives, and professions have been directly affected by, or have had a role in, the medical management of atypical sex. Unlike Dr. Spruce, Dr. Maple was not a specialist in DSD care when she began her career; her endocrinological research in the mid-1990s, focused on molecular biology and androgen insensitivity syndrome as a genetic anomaly, provided valuable insight into evolutionary biology. But soon after the publication of her research, a founding member of the fledgling Androgen Insensitivity Syndrome Support Group contacted her to ask if she would attend the inaugural meeting of the North American extension (which would become AISSG-USA) of the group that had started a few years earlier in the United Kingdom.

> We all met in New York City. It was summer, I believe. It was hot, and we were scheduled to meet in a university building. It was a Saturday, so we had to be let in through sort of a back door by a security person, and we surreptitiously made our way up what seemed to me—in my memory anyway—a dark

and winding back stair, into this small, enclosed room that seemed to be very hidden away. There was an air of secrecy and trepidation. As I think back, it seems that the women wanted very intense privacy because of their emotional state about their condition at that time.

We sat there in this quiet, otherwise empty room, maybe twenty people, all women. Most were women with androgen insensitivity syndrome or similar conditions. I think there was one mother. I was the only physician. We sat in a circle on wooden chairs and the women went around, one by one, sharing the stories of their diagnoses and how they had been treated by physicians and sometimes by their parents. They shared how they had eventually come to learn their diagnoses and various aspects of them, including their chromosomes and their history of having had testes removed in childhood or their teenage years, and for some, of having had surgeries performed on their genitalia. For some, the most painful memory was having been examined by multiple people, and for others it was having been lied to by doctors and parents. There were lots of pauses and silences and tears and tissues.

What struck me intensely was how poorly so many of these women had been treated by the medical profession. I felt this great sense of responsibility. And remorse. And in some way guilt, for the harm that had been brought upon them by my colleagues. I felt, from that point forward, a kind of bonding with this group of women and then, by extension, with anyone with these conditions. That experience gave me a sense of needing to make things better for these women—and hopefully for other children and affected individuals in the future—by helping physicians see different ways—hopefully better ways—of treating these individuals.

Aside from a disquieting but routine episode in medical school, when Dr. Maple was one of a number of medical students brought in to see a child with atypical genitalia—an episode she had preferred to forget—she had only limited clinical experience with individuals affected by DSD even during her fellowship in endocrinology. What occurred behind the closed doors of that New York City classroom was unsettling not only because of the anguish to which she now bore witness but also because she felt responsible for it. She had not been consulted in the cases of any of the women in that room. Unlike Dr. Spruce, who had confronted a mistake he had made directly, both in the case of the young man who had returned to the clinic for care and in the other cases much like that young man's, Dr. Maple's work had not been primarily concerned with patient care at all. The responsibility that Dr. Maple felt cannot be explained simply in terms of feeling implicated in the wrong of her profession. She suggests that guilt figured somehow. And yet her account suggests that it was not a sense of culpability so much as it was the attainment of a new knowledge—the truth of what women with AIS experience—that became the source of her feeling of obligation to the women in that room, to the individuals who were not present, and also to her colleagues in the profession.

At the end of the course at Berkeley that took up the question of truth telling or *parrhesia*, Foucault explains that the subject of his lectures had been what he describes as "the problematization of truth" that was at work from the beginning of the period Western philosophers identify as the birth of the discipline of philosophy and that, Foucault believes, must preoccupy us today (2001, 170–171). His investigation into the history of truth telling, he says, is not concerned with people's behavior or even with "ideas in their representative values." Rather than a social history, or a history of ideas, the historical analysis in which Foucault is engaged is intended "to analyze the process of 'problematization'—which means: how and why certain things (behavior, phenomena, processes) become a *problem*" (171; original emphasis). If the history of hermaphroditism in Europe and the United States of the late nineteenth and early twentieth centuries is the story of how and to what effect intersex bodies became a medical problem (Dreger 1998b; Reis 2009) for which normalization would be the answer, I wonder if the stories of Drs. Spruce and Maple, and the "critical attitude" they exemplify, mean that the history of the late twentieth and early twenty-first centuries will come to be understood as the period in which "the problem" of atypical sex began to be recast as a problem not of intersexed bodies, but a problem for "the rest of us."

Dr. Aspen's Story

About halfway through 2011, Dr. Aspen was reflecting on how much had changed in the field. When she started in pediatric surgery, she explained, normalizing surgeries for girls with CAH were not a matter of controversy, and postoperative exams by a surgical team, mostly comprised of men, were routine. Sometimes, she said, it was necessary to force the legs of the girls apart to assess the success of a surgery. The practice may have struck her as out of the ordinary, but she had not challenged it. But then, she remembers, she was asked to make a presentation to a patient organization in place of her supervisor, who was unable to do so that day. In preparing the talk, she read more about the nonsurgical aspects of CAH (including hormone regulation) and collected her slides, including information about standard sorts of surgeries and postoperative treatment with which she was more familiar. She had not expected the immediate criticism that her presentation received. Opposition came not only from the parents and the patient advocates there but also from the pediatric endocrinologist who was in attendance. Turning her head away from me for the first time in our conversation, her face registered pain and renewed surprise at the memory, and after a moment she said, "I really felt like I was slapped in the face." "But," she added, looking directly at me once more, "this is how I learned." What Dr. Aspen learned is that many people condemned the standard of care that she had been trained to uncritically regard as in the best interests of the children she and her team cared for. She also learned from those assembled that it was possible to consider the normalizing surgeries in which she participated in very different terms than she had before. She learned that she had a responsibility at once beyond and attendant to that responsibility to cultivate excellence as a surgeon—namely, a responsibility to engage in reflective judgment—that she had not appreciated in this way before.

In the weeks and months after my conversation with Dr. Aspen, it seemed to me that her response to the incident she described was not only a story about the kind of awareness and understanding that are necessary for physicians like her, and for Drs. Spruce and Maple, to change their own practices and those in the field, but that the story was also an object lesson of another sort. It was the response of an audience at a single presentation that altered the course of Dr. Aspen's thinking and action. Of course, one might say—and judging from my own experience with her, I would agree—that it was entirely consistent with her character that she would take heed of the criticism she received that day. In the wake of that episode she came to understand that even though her intentions were good, the knowledge on which those intentions were based—the conception of the good—was flawed. But for any number of factors—her colleague's schedule conflict or the willingness of that first audience member to voice criticism—Dr. Aspen might not have had the experience she had that day and so might well have continued unquestioningly to regard herself and her colleagues as the experts in care rather than the patients.

Dr. Aspen's is a story that in some important respects is much like that of parents, most often new parents, who believe they have done the right thing by consenting to normalizing surgery on behalf of their children. It seems obvious—until perhaps suddenly it does not—that normalizing surgery and the routinized practices that accompany it, are in the child's best interests. What she describes as the experience of feeling slapped in the face was a confrontation with her assumptions and, eventually, with a sense of responsibility for her failure to recognize and to criticize those assumptions.

In his later work on care of the self, Foucault repeatedly remarks on the affiliation that the ancient Greek philosophical injunction to self-care had with medicine and with it the close association between "self-knowledge" (*gnōthi seuton*)—the "essential condition of philosophical practice" (Foucault 2005 [2001], 170)—and the Socratic injunction to care for the self. For the ancients, the cultivation of self is a lifelong task that is both "a duty and a technique, a fundamental obligation and a set of carefully fashioned ways of behaving" (494). Turning to Foucault's analysis, involving, as it does, readings of mostly neglected primary texts in ancient philosophy, for insight into the revelation of Dr. Aspen's mistake might appear unnecessary or unnecessarily arcane. But I think Foucault's effort to understand ethics as a way of living, and not—as it seems to be regarded by physicians and many bioethicists today—primarily as a tool for problem-solving, provides a means of appreciating what I believe to be the broader significance of Dr. Aspen's experience. Confronting a different understanding and a different knowledge than she possessed, she investigated her own ignorance and found insight that allowed her to change her practice.

The Virtue of Regret and the Ethics of Self-Care

The common thread that runs through the experience of these three physicians is acknowledgment of their own ignorance along with regret for the harm that resulted from that ignorance. I understand much better than I did at the start of this project the extent to which ethical reflection requires recognition of, and tolerance for, untidiness, imperfection, and the mistakes we make. We make mistakes not only in the failure or refusal to engage in moral deliberation—when, history tells us, the worst problems can arise—but also in our unwillingness to reckon with the complexity that this untidiness so often entails.

In the absence of negligence, mistakes do not constitute a moral violation. But that does not mean that mistakes made in ignorance or good faith should not occasion regret. It also does not mean that regret is an appropriate response only to what would be regarded as mistakes, as even decisions that can be described as the "right" decisions can—and in cases that involve the most difficult decisions almost certainly will—entail consequences that are lamentable, unfortunate, or even awful.

In her defense of virtue ethics, contemporary philosopher Rosalind Hursthouse offers a vivid illustration of the moral danger that may result when we "cut ourselves off" from bringing in to moral decision making this kind of regret, or what is called the "remainder" (1999, 47–48). Hursthouse takes doctors as her example.

> Although I am, personally, sympathetic to doctors rather than otherwise, one does hear occasional hair-raising stories about the arrogance and callousness of some. What people often complain about is not whatever decision the doctors made, but the manner in which they delivered it or acted on it. No expressions of regret, no expression of concern over whether anything could be done to make it less likely that such decisions would have to be made in the future; having made (what they take to be) the morally right decision, they seem to think they can review their own conduct with complete satisfaction. But if someone dies, or suffers, or undergoes frightful humiliation as a result of their decision, even supposing it is unquestionably correct, surely regret is called for. (48)

In *On Virtue Ethics,* Hursthouse is concerned with demonstrating the value of the Aristotelian approach for providing direction in moral decision making, but her criticism of approaches such as those dominant in medicine compellingly illustrates how such frameworks can work to restrict the scope of our moral judgment and so our capacity for moral engagement with others in the world.

What distinguishes virtue ethics from the most "influential strands in contemporary Anglo-American bioethics[,] . . . prioritizing logic and abstract rationality, and drawing extensively on the formalism of consequentialist, utilitarian, and rights-based approaches to ethics" (Scully, Shakespeare, and Banks 2006, 760), is its focus on the moral agent, and not solely on the rightness of a given action. The treatment of atypical sex anatomies in children by the German Bioethics and Intersex Group, as I discussed in chapters 7 and 8, provides an example of applied ethical thinking insofar as it illustrates the limitations of casting as primary the principle of (parental) autonomy for identifying the moral questions posed by the medical management of atypical sex anatomies in children. Boiling down the ethical question to assessment of "right action" (in this case the question of where to locate consent), the group cannot provide due consideration to the questions concerning social and familial obligation it has set aside in favor of answering how to respect "parental rights." It is not that the approach of the Bioethics and Intersex Group could not, using the tools of deontology, consider more carefully the importance of the regret that figures centrally in the accounts of Drs. Spruce, Maple, and Aspen. Hursthouse grants that these approaches (with some direction from virtue ethics) could certainly do so. But the work of the Bioethics and Intersex Group is characteristic of a resistance to acknowledge the harm that individuals and their families began to reveal in the mid-1990s; refusing to criticize the imperative of normality, the group cannot examine, and therefore cannot address, the regrettable consequences that have resulted from following the dictates of this imperative.

Promulgations of unsupported theories of the development of gender identity (evidenced in the claim that a typically male child with micropenis could be castrated and raised as a girl, or that shortening or removing a clitoris will ensure a heterosexual orientation in a 46,XX female); early surgical techniques found to be flawed (such as colon vaginoplasties that not only fail but are also prone to cancer); insistence that a normalized anatomy guarantees happiness, or is a condition of its possibility in the face of otherwise certain unhappiness: physicians have maintained that given the limited knowledge available, the decisions to reassign sex; to perform normalizing surgeries; and to conceal from children, and sometimes from their parents, the "truth" about their chromosomes or the anatomies with which children were born were *good* decisions.

It is not that physicians have refused wholesale to acknowledge bad outcomes, however. For example, there has been substantial analysis of what urologists unfortunately call "hypospadias cripples." Hypospadias is a congenital condition affecting genetically typical males in which the urinary meatus, the opening that is typically at the end of the penis, appears on the underside or at its base.[4] The comparatively robust evidence of the success of hypospadias repair has meant that criticism of this intervention has not had as much effect as criticism of other normal-izing interventions for atypical sex anatomies. Despite what has become regarded as the routine character of these surgeries, among those who have undergone re-pair there are also a number of patients who have had repeated and unsuccessful repair, leaving them with significant functional problems.

"Hypospadias cripples" has remained a term of art in the medical literature since its introduction in 1970 by urologists Charles E. Horton and Charles J. Devine (1970). One might expect that its use would have fallen out of favor by now; ap-plied to a whole person, the term "cripple" is offensive, certainly, identifying the individual with a damaged part of one's anatomy. Indeed, it was the awareness of just this problem—that is, the identification of a whole person, "hermaphrodite," with the medical condition (Dreger et al. 2005, 732)—that prompted the change in nomenclature in 2005. However, the retention of the term may be more sur-prising for the way it calls attention to how the medical treatment of atypical sex anatomies can themselves cause—or even be the primary source—of what phy-sicians regard as the serious damage to a sense of self that motivates the repair in the first place.[5] In considering what Hursthouse views as the failure to take re-gret seriously in dominant models of moral reasoning, the continued and appar-ently uncritical reference to hypospadias cripples in the medical literature illus-trates the consequences of this failure. It is not that the mistakes physicians have made—technical mistakes—are unacknowledged or not investigated.[6] But if most physicians who continue to recommend and perform normalizing surgeries see these results as "regrettable," they see the problem in the bodies of those affected. Any regret is not such that it will, as Hursthouse puts it, "mar" the agent whose choices resulted in harm (1999, 74).

The unwillingness to see oneself as damaged by the decisions one makes, es-pecially including what a virtuous agent would regard as the right decisions, given difficult circumstances constituting a dilemma, is understandable. We see how readily Socrates elicited from his interlocutors in the *Protagoras* the claim that we like to see ourselves as "good." Philosopher Alphonso Lingis could be quoting Plato some twenty-five hundred years later when he observes, "We want to see ourselves as ethical persons . . . Our actions are just, honorable. We like to think of ourselves as moral, concerned with standards of behavior based on a sense of right and wrong" (2003, 197). Hursthouse's analysis suggests that our interest in seeing ourselves as good actors may be promoted by the emphasis that dominant ethical theories place on determining the goodness or rightness of acts. This em-phasis, she observes, encourages what she describes as a "tendency to overlook remainder" (1999, 47).

To overlook remainder is to deny the moral complexity that attends living in a world, the imperfection of which, Kant taught us, makes ethics necessary in the first place. Virtue ethics, more than deontology or utilitarianism, helps us to see that the aim of ethical agents is not to have "clean hands" (Hursthouse 1999, 71), if what is meant by having clean hands is the sort of complacency or self-satisfaction that the feeling of making the right decision can bring. For virtue ethics, moral reflection does not begin or end with the judgment of the goodness of an act or the intention that motivated it. It resists "the assumption that, in any case of moral dilemma or conflict, one side must be unqualifiedly morally right and the other plain wrong[, an assumption that] runs very deep in everyday thought" (45). Focusing on the moral agent, Hursthouse's approach is especially well suited for reflection on the objectification of moral challenges we face as embodied subjects in a damaged world, including those challenges posed by our efforts to deny our vulnerability.

Boy *or* Girl: Beyond an Ethics of Right or Wrong

The observations that Hursthouse makes regarding the neat divisions between right and wrong and good and bad, to which we may reflexively turn in everyday thought, also apply to the thinking that has shaped the standard of care and are perhaps especially evident in the responses to calls for change. Recall that after David Reimer's story was told, first in the 1997 article by Milton Diamond and H. Keith Sigmundson, and then in stories in the *New York Times* (Angier 1997) and in *Rolling Stone* (Colapinto 1997), there was some interest among physicians, albeit limited, in questioning the standard of care. Reimer's story was important not only because it marked a failure with respect to the putative evidence of the "optimal-gender theory" that had once supported normalizing atypical sex anatomies but also because it demonstrated so vividly the human stakes involved in such failures. This was a story of twins whose experiences seemed to have led inexorably to the tragic end of their lives, and of parents who endured years of doing what they were told would best support their children only to learn that they had not supported or protected their children as they intended. And it hardly ended there, for the misplaced faith in these devastating interventions, and the intransigence of those who had a vested interest in protecting the legacy of the sex and gender research conducted at Johns Hopkins, had implications far beyond the Reimer family.

In an atmosphere in which doubts about the standard of care are given voice, we can make historical sense of Dr. Spruce's acknowledgment of error and of his experience of regret. His was not, however, the "common sense" of his colleagues. An editorial by pediatric urologist Kenneth Glassberg published in the *Journal of Urology* in 1999 was more representative of specialists in DSD care at the time. While Glassberg, too, found the consequences of Money's most famous experiment regrettable, he condemned the conclusion that surgery—which he conflated with sex assignment—should be stopped. Asking if those who have had "successful assignment" should be "condemned to growing up as what would be inevitably considered freaks by their classmates" (1999, 1309), Glassberg reasserted the imperative of normality that by this time had become the primary rationale for normalizing interventions for atypical sex in children, subsuming the previous concern about the risk to individuals' psychosocial development that "ambiguous sex" was thought to pose. Despite the confidence Glassberg expresses with regard to the "successes" he claims, he nevertheless grants in this same editorial that there was insufficient evidence of those successes to justify that confidence.

Glassberg's response—one that could have been written by any number of specialists over the decade that followed—reflects the shortcomings in moral reflection to which Hursthouse points—that is, the resistance to seeing decisions made with the good intention to spare children shame as "bad decisions" and to viewing those who made decisions resulting in harm as sullied by the actions they took. The candor Glassberg displays in his insistence that without normalizing interventions children with atypical sex will be "inevitably considered freaks" has been, indisputably, the most important motivation shaping the standard of care since physicians began to defend the treatment of atypical sex anatomies in the mid-1990s. This shift explains how atypical sex became figured as a problem of gender.

For those activists and allies who advocate the multiplication or abolition of the categories of gender, and for those physicians and parents who take for granted that children with atypical sex anatomies will be burdened by their stigmatic difference, there is a fervent belief that the most pressing questions we should ask about atypical sex and its management are those concerned with sexual identity. While it is true that a clear and unassailable division of the sexes has been taken to be foundational to social order, it is less clear that this division is important today in quite the way that it has been. The division of the sexes nevertheless remains the primary "structure," the "structuring structure" that orders our social world. I think it was for this reason that—despite many and repeated assertions to the contrary—in its fifteen years of advocacy to change the standard of care, ISNA never sought acceptance of a "third sex," or even, as Anne Fausto-Sterling (1993) proposed, a fourth or fifth sex, a suggestion that she later made clear she had made "with tongue-in-cheek" (2000, 78).

Surely it is a measure of how entrenched the prevailing views of sexual difference remain that the recognition of bodies that do not clearly hew to the standard for male and female could seem to require the creation of new categories or constitute an argument for the abolition of sexual difference itself. When the rules of a rigid system of sex and gender have resulted in so much harm, it may seem that abolition or a "way out" is the best or only means of righting the wrong— the innumerable wrongs—that have occurred. To adults whose bodies bear those scars, or to those who have been brought to consciousness of the damage that has been done, it can seem like the answer is—or can only be, as some second-wave feminists proposed with all of the optimism and earnestness of the age—to create a society free of gender. But utopian visions provide little support or hope for new parents of children with atypical sex anatomies who must envision a future for their children in which parents' own desired connection to, and involvement with, their children makes sense in the here and now. The idea of raising a child with "no gender" implies a life in which their child either has no place or will always be in struggle.

Because the vision of a society free from the restraints of a rigid system of gender has not been realized, and because gender and sexual identity remains for most an essential feature of a sense of self, the "choice" faced by parents of infants and young children with atypical sex anatomies has perhaps not seemed like a choice at all. Presented as a decision of whether to provide the possibility of inclusion or of living a life on the margins, as a decision to do something to ensure one's child a life where it may appear that options and choices are possible, or to do nothing and so guarantee a certain, and certainly miserable, existence, the mapping of right and wrong in the construction of the decision facing parents closely mirrors the construction of the ethical questions we ask when we focus on the question of "which action is right, x or y?" One answer is right, and one is wrong. The construction of the problem in these terms makes the decision to normalize a child's body easy and puts the messy remainder out of sight.

What the construction of the questions also excludes is what has seemed like the obvious question that activists asked from the very beginning of the movement to change the standard of care. What if—as history and as parents like Sarah, Sonja, and Elias show us—children with atypical sex anatomies can be raised as boys or girls without normalizing surgery?

A Way Forward: Affirming Ambiguity

For several years it did not appear that change beyond that modestly outlined in the 2006 Consensus Statement was possible. But the independent 2012 opinions issued by the Swiss National Advisory Commission and the German Ethics Council demonstrate the real and present opportunities for changing the standard of care.[7] Their recommendations do not rely on utopian possibilities, but address the immediate needs of children and their parents. They recognize how past practices have constituted violations of children's rights to autonomy and bodily integrity and impeded the bonds between children and their parents for the sake of which normalizing interventions had been viewed as essential.

Detailing the problems, both in past and in still-current practices, both opinions call for a more nuanced view of medicalization, clarifying, for example, that "a diagnosis does not in itself entail any treatment or other medical measures" (Swiss National Advisory Commission 2012, 11). They echo the calls that for years have been made by ISNA and allied physicians that normalizing interventions on reproductive organs be undertaken only where there is a "danger to life" or the risk of "serious and grave damages to a child's health" (German Ethics Council 2012, 166; also see Consortium on the Management of Disorders of Sex Development 2006a).

Precisely because rationales for normalization in the past have focused on parents, the Swiss and German opinions recognize the importance of the provision of parental support in the care of children with atypical sex anatomies. The recommendations for parental support made by the Swiss go further than formal statements have in the past to propose that such support be regarded as an integral component of treatment for conditions involving atypical sex anatomies in children. Because no provision currently exists for state medical support for treatment of parents, the Swiss opinion also recommends "that a legal basis . . . be established which would provide for a special obligation to cover counseling and support for parents" and that it be provided well beyond infancy (Swiss National Advisory Commission on Bioethics 2012, 17).

It is not that the importance of support for parents of children with DSD was ignored in the 2006 Consensus Statement. In an appendix the statement acknowledges that the "value of peer and parent support for many medical conditions is widely accepted, and DSD, being lifelong conditions that affect developmental tasks at many stages of life, are no exception." Peer support can help individuals and parents and their parents find "a feeling of normalcy" and can help parents "find the best quality care" (Hughes et al. 2006, 562). While the statement acknowledges the importance of such support, in other words, it is regarded as an adjunct to care. The difference between the approach of the Consensus Statement and the Swiss opinion, I propose, is a matter not so much of emphasis but of object. I do not mean to suggest that ultimately the object of care differs between the two: For both, care for the child is central. But apparently taking seriously "the possibility," as Alice Dreger puts it, "that the child is not the wound that needs healing" (2006a, 78), the Swiss opinion signals a change in the object of treatment. Where in the 2006 statement there is no question that the object of treatment is the body of the child with atypical sex anatomy, the Swiss opinion makes clear that in many cases of DSD, the object of treatment must be the parents, for whom education and support are necessary for the child's well-being as well as the parents' own.

The opinion by the Swiss National Advisory Commission also addresses the limitations of prevailing constructions of the ethical questions guiding treatment. For example, they take on the previously insoluble dilemma of where in time to locate a child's interests to establish a basis for decisions regarding sex assignment: is it the present or the child's future that should be most salient? Where that question has proved to stymie moral reasoning, and has even been set aside as unanswerable, the Swiss acknowledge the difficulties the question must entail and assert what should be obvious, namely, that "determination of the child's welfare should be based as far as possible *both* on the current interests of the child and on the anticipated interests of the future adult" (Swiss National Advisory Commission 2012, 12; emphasis added). There is no attempt, in other words, to simplify the questions posed by the medical treatment of atypical sex. They do not set as their task resolution of the problem that atypical sex anatomies in children have been taken to pose. As a result, they avoid the trap of trying to solve—or resolve—an "ambiguity" that cannot be corrected or concealed.

In a dramatic reversal of the logic guiding the prevailing defense of the standard of care, the Swiss emphasize that "if interventions are performed solely with a view to integration of the child into its family and social environment, then they run counter to the child's welfare" (13). Where the problem of intersex has previously been located in the anatomies of children with atypical sex anatomies, the Swiss opinion sees the problem instead as a violation of the obligation of the state and by the families to their vulnerable children. In other words, what guides the opinion is not a determination to provide an answer to what has been posed as a conflict between parents' rights versus children's rights, or between the variety that nature offers and society's insistence on conformity to a norm; instead, it is guided by an effort to recognize the harm that has occurred and to outline the steps necessary to avert that harm in the future.

Forthright acknowledgment of the harm that normalizing surgeries may effect, and have already effected, leads both the Swiss National Advisory Commission on Biomedical Ethics and the German Ethics Council to see these harms as violations of human rights. Both make recommendations for reparation for the harm caused by normalizing interventions "which, given today's knowledge," the German Ethics Council argues, "no longer meet medical standards, and which have caused continuous suffering or a reduced quality of life for those so affected" (German Ethics Council 2012, 164). However, this is not to say that mistakes will not be made in the future. The clarity of the focus on obligation leads the German Ethics Council to take steps to address the harms that cannot be anticipated today and for which reparation may be necessary. Accepting that the decisions we make cannot be perfect, and that knowledge and understanding is never complete, the German Ethics Council recommends that comprehensive documentation of all treatment of children should "remain accessible to all concerned for at least 40 years," and that statutes of limitations be extended in the case of "irreversible impairment of fertility and/or sexual sensitivity" in order to provide the opportunity to recognize harms that have been committed, even with the best of intentions.

The work of the German Ethics Council and Swiss National Advisory Commission demonstrates the promise of the kind of ethical engagement that makes acknowledgment of remainder central to moral reasoning. If we are able to bring that remainder back into view, we will remember to tolerate the imperfection that distinguishes humanity, to affirm the existence of ambiguities in ethics as much as in biology. Recognizing—and valuing—this variability, the "problem" of intersex can no longer make sense as a problem. Atypical sex anatomy is not some exceptional difference, but an ordinary matter of our humanity. Like most human matters, it is not clean, or tidy, or easy, but it is a vital measure of the embodied vulnerability we are obligated to protect. Acknowledging the value of our imperfection lays the groundwork for the ongoing reflection that is the condition of our flourishing.

Notes

Introduction

1. The issue of "incidence" of atypical sex has been a vexed one, as it concerns not only the frequency with which children are born with atypical sex anatomies but also what counts as atypical sex. Early discussions of the varying estimates and questions they raise may be found in Dreger 1998b, 40–42, and in Fausto-Sterling 2000, 51–54. More conservative estimates of 1 in 2,000 (Intersex Society of North America) or 1 in 4,500 (Hughes et al. 2006, 554) (an incidence comparable to cystic fibrosis) refer to cases where sex is unclear at birth. The estimate of 1.7 in 100 at which Fausto-Sterling's team arrived—what she cautioned "should be taken as an order of magnitude estimate rather than a precise count" (2000, 51)—refers to overall incidence of birth in which sex anatomy differs from the norm. This number would include the high, and apparently increasing, incidence of hypospadias (where the urinary meatus that is typically located at the tip of the penis appears elsewhere in children who are usually regarded as unquestionably male) (Center for the Study and Treatment of Hypospadias 2013). Questions of "rarity" can serve to justify extraordinary care in pediatric conditions, including those concerned with atypical sex or gender identity (see, e.g., Feder 2007, 55–56).

2. Like Kessler's article, Eve Kosofsky Sedgwick's 1991 article "How to Bring Your Kids Up Gay" brought attention of the new diagnosis to those outside of psychology. As she points out, the inclusion of gender identity disorder coincided with the removal of the diagnosis of "homosexuality" from the *Diagnostic and Statistical Manual of Mental Disorders*.

3. I would elaborate on this point in *Family Bonds* (Feder 2007, 60–67).

4. McCumber published the book by that same title in 2001. He notes that philosophers were disproportionately targeted by the House Un-American Affairs Committee (HUAC), whose work began in 1949, and argues that the significant changes that occurred at this time shaped the discipline in ways that have gone unremarked upon in the field. "The McCarthy era," McCumber contends, "imposed an important restriction on just what kind of goal philosophers can pursue. It limited them to the pursuit of true sentences (or propositions, or statements)" (2001, xvii–xix).

5. In his famous essay "How Medicine Saved Bioethics," philosopher Stephen Toulmin makes a similar point about the dominant nature of ethical inquiry at this time. However, he argues that bioethics greatly enriched ethical inquiry precisely by bringing "cases," the individual "situation," to the fore. He writes admiringly of the contribution made in the 1950s by Joseph Fletcher, who introduced the phrase "situation ethics." But as Toulmin points out, "Fletcher's use of the term met with harsh criticism" (1982, 740). While Toulmin argues for seeing the ways that bioethics enriched the field of ethical inquiry in philosophy, bioethics itself, as Hilde Lindemann (2006a) has provocatively put it, continues to occupy a "feminized"—that is to say, devalued—position within the discipline of philosophy.

6. Hannah Arendt was one of the notable exceptions in this regard, but lest the rich contemporary engagement with her work lead us to forget, Arendt was herself the target of scorn by American philosophers even in the late 1970s. McCumber recounts in his book how members of the APA working on an accreditation committee for the state of New York described Arendt as "an unproductive drone because her works were not cited in important journals such

as the *Journal of Philosophy* and *Philosophical Review*. Of course, she published regularly in the *New York Review of Books* (no obscure venue), had been on the cover of *Time* magazine, and was one of the most famous political thinkers in the world" (McCumber 2001, 51–52).

7. See, e.g., the discussion of Henry Beecher's article that was eventually published in the *New England Journal of Medicine*, in D. Rothman (1991, 70ff).

8. President Clinton issued the first apology by the government in 1997, addressing the eight remaining survivors and the descendants of the subjects of the study.

9. *The Belmont Report* (1979) was commissioned by Congress to "identify the ethical principles which should underlie the conduct of biomedical and behavioral research with human subjects and develop guidelines that should be followed in such research." The report was the product of the congressional commission formed after the passage of the National Research Act of 1974. The act was prompted by congressional hearings convened after the revelation of the infamous Public Health Service study of untreated syphilis in African American men from 1932 to 1972 and mandated that federally funded research be subject to Institutional Review Board (IRB) approval. According to Jonsen, some guidelines already existed, namely, those produced by the Nuremberg Code (1947) and the Declaration of Helsinki (1962) (see Jonsen 1998, 102). Tellingly, not a single member of the commission was trained as a philosopher, though two of its members held doctoral degrees from departments of religion, thus illustrating the longer history of a claim that philosopher Jorge Gracia made in 1998: "Philosophy has no place in public life. There are no discussions of public policy that include philosophy. Philosophers are generally excluded from policy-making bodies or posts in which they can have serious influence on the development of public policy" (quoted in McCumber 2001, 93).

10. As if it were possible to have an even dimmer view of the existing problems and future prospects for bioethics, in recent years Carl Elliott has sounded an alarm about the state of bioethics. He sees in the shortcomings of bioethics a worrisome problem in medicine that he attributes to the "studied indifference to deeper moral questions" (1999, 7). In this climate, clinical ethics, he writes, "has increasingly become part of the bureaucratic structures whose problems it was intended to correct" (11). Indeed, Laura Stark's recent account of the development of IRB review in *Behind Closed Doors: IRBs and the Making of Ethical Research* suggests that this indifference became entrenched a decade before *The Belmont Report* and continues still. She describes the efforts beginning in the 1960s of NIH leaders whose development of human subject review committees was intended "to avoid getting sued, while also protecting researchers' 'scientific freedom' and continuing to be well funded with taxpayer money" (2012, 138). Stark's account suggests that IRBs were intended and continue to function for the purpose of protecting the institution from liability rather than as a means to safeguard the human rights of the subjects of their research.

11. I would learn directly from Katrina Karkazis, who was at this time beginning work on her dissertation in anthropology, that she was watching the angry exchange provoked by my request with great interest and that, learning from my mistakes, she had better success in soliciting research subjects for the work that would become *Fixing Sex* (2008).

12. Most of these interviews were conducted by phone or via Skype, but some were conducted in person. With the permission of all participants, I recorded these conversations and transcribed them using pseudonyms—the names of trees—and eliminated the locations of the physicians and hospitals in order to protect the identities of any patients who had been in their care.

13. As I discuss in chapter 1, it is clear that a greater number of individuals with atypical sex anatomies became "medicalized" in the late nineteenth century. With the increasing number of specialists in this area of medicine, it may be that the standards of "normal" anatomy have

a wider reach, which is to say that more children with atypical sex anatomies are medicalized today even than they were twenty or thirty years ago. But in the absence of anything more than anecdotal evidence, which would be very hard to come by, it is not possible to substantiate this hypothesis.

14. That is not to say that intracultural conflict is absent. See, e.g., the essays in Parens 1998 and Parens and Asch 2000.

1. The Trouble with Intersex

1. In the 2012 meetings of both the American Association of Clinical Endocrinologists and the Endocrine Society, there was no discussion or substantial call for training of endocrinologists in the management of CAH in adults. Only a handful of specialists have detailed knowledge of adult care for individuals with CAH. I thank Richard Auchus, professor and fellowship program director in the Division of Metabolism, Endocrinology, and Diabetes at the University of Michigan, for his help in clarifying the current state of care for adults.

2. While it was distinctive, it was not unique in this respect. Hermaphroditism shared the dual status of medical curiosity and social threat during this period with other "ills" such as prostitution (see, e.g., Walkowitz 1982) and "racial difference" (see, e.g., Gilman 1985).

3. It is unfortunate that there remain so many gaps in the historical studies that could provide more insight about these developments and the continuities (and discontinuities) between and among them. Dreger's history ends with the work of the Briton William Blair Bell, whose work appears to mark the beginning of what we might call "the age of gender." Blair Bell's contribution resonates powerfully with salient features of the standard of care evident still. As Dreger writes: "If men and women were to be kept distinct, Blair Bell realized, hermaphrodite-sorting would have to be accomplished in such a way as to *quiet sex anomalies,* not accentuate them" (1998b, 166; emphasis added). The ongoing legacy from the Age of Gonads, however, is the insistence that each body be understood as having "a single true sex, and the medical doctor would be the determiner or creator of it" (166).

One can imagine a thread connecting the work of Blair Bell in England to that of Wilkins in the United States. Eder's work is particularly significant in addressing the gap between the end of the period Dreger examines in France and England in the 1910s and the work of John Money and his colleagues in the United States four decades later, but there is a good deal to fill in between the two. There are also no systematic studies of the late nineteenth-century treatment of hermaphroditism in the United States. From Elizabeth Reis's study we may gather that physicians in the States relied upon influential work by British and French physicians (e.g., Arthur Evans and Charles-Marie Debierre) (Reis 2009, 86). More detailed investigation would be particularly illuminating to better understand the significance of the ways that US work in the mid-twentieth century may have radically reversed the geographical flow of influence in the field of medicine, or perhaps especially in this particular field. Understanding, too, the extent to which the treatment of "hermaphroditism" on both sides of the Atlantic mirrored the treatment of other kinds of conditions that provoked social anxiety might also provide further insight into the ways that the medical management of atypical sex was characteristic of medical treatment of its time.

4. The exception may be found in the work of the French surgeon Jean Samuel Pozzi, who was responsible for the "therapeutically important observation that undescended testicles in male pseudohermaphrodites often become cancerous" (Dreger 1998b, 64–65).

5. See also Michel Foucault 2003 [1999], 315–318.

6. Writing of the US context during this period, Elizabeth Reis (2009) suggests how anxieties about perceived violations of sexual borders in cases of both atypical sex and homosexual desire intersect with anxieties about racial "mixing."

7. There are very few cases of males who survived, such that there are today few middle-age and fewer elderly adults with CAH who are not genetically female. The severity of the condition is easy to overlook in public discussion of "intersex." Few are aware that as the result of concerted lobbying by parent groups (most notably the CARES Foundation), most developed countries today have instituted mandatory newborn screening for CAH.

8. Young's autobiography provides insight into the state of medical training during this period. He reports that he received his MD just one year after completing his BA and MA at the University of Virginia in 1893 (where, he admiringly notes, all of his professors had been "officers in the Confederate Army") (H. Young 1940, 40). Having begun the first year of medical school in his last year of completing the requirements for the BA and MA, he finished medical school the following year (44). Having received no surgical training in medical school, he made the decision to go to the Johns Hopkins Hospital, "which, although only five years old, had already risen to the front rank" (48).

9. In his autobiography Young offers this description of the problem of females with CAH, noting that the "literature contains several amazing cases of which these females have lived vigorous masculine lives and had apparently happy wives who were surprised when the true condition was disclosed after death. Since early times the social and legal complications that have arisen among these 'female pseudo-hermaphrodites' have been frequently described." "The only treatment," he continues, "is to attack the offending organ—a greatly enlarged adrenal." His method of surgical extraction, involving the double retractor he devised for this purpose, is illustrated in an accompanying drawing (H. Young 1940, 206–207). This treatment did not result in cure, but rather in exhausting efforts to compensate for the lost function of the glands. As Eder found, "practitioners were driven 'almost crazy in trying to keep these people alive afterwards'" (2012, 72).

10. See, e.g., Elizabeth Sheehan's (1981) discussion of the controversial work of the mid-nineteenth-century British physician Isaak Baker Brown, author of the 1866 book *On the Curability of Certain Forms of Insanity, Epilepsy, Catalepsy, and Hysteria in Females.*

11. Young provides citations for nearly every source on which he draws but attributes the reproductions of art featuring hermaphrodites only to a "Hirschfeld." It is possible—perhaps likely—that Young's reference is to the work of the German Jewish physician Magnus Hirschfeld, who was active before the Second World War in his efforts to repeal laws prohibiting homosexuality, cofounding the *Wissenschafflich-Humanitaeres Komitee* (Scientific-Humanitarian Committee) in Berlin in 1897.

12. From Samuel Loveman, *The Hermaphrodite and Other Poems* (Caldwell, Idaho: Caxton Printers, 1936), quoted in H. Young 1937, 21–22.

13. Howard Jones is at the center of a number of noteworthy medical developments in the second half of the twentieth century. He is best known for his work on in vitro fertilization (IVF) with his wife, Georgeann Jones, a reproductive endocrinologist, with whom he worked to conceive the first baby born in the United States using IVF in 1981. Moreover, he was not only one of the gynecologic surgeons at Johns Hopkins who worked with Wilkins to perform feminizing surgeries in children with atypical sex, but he was also the gynecologist who took the original malignant cells from Henrietta Lacks in 1951 (Skloot 2010, 15–17). As Rebecca Skloot details in *The Immortal Life of Henrietta Lacks,* these cells, known globally as "HeLa," not only launched an industry in human biological materials but also have made, and continue to make, enormous advances in science and medicine possible.

14. Perhaps the best-known claim here is that of the physician Eryximachus in Plato's *Sym-*

posium, who speaks of health as harmony (Plato 1989,187a-e). Polybus, Hippocrates's son-in-law, writes in *On the Nature of Man* that "health is primarily that state in which [its] constituent substances are in the correct proportion to each other, both in strength and quantity, and are well mixed" (Lloyd 1983, 262). In his history of Hippocrates, Jacques Jouanna writes that health "is defined both negatively, by the absence of suffering, and positively, by the balanced mixture of the constitutive elements of man. But insofar as this mixture holds together, the elements do not manifest themselves" (1998, 326). Jouanna sums up the ancient conception of good health as "a precarious and fragile equilibrium" (331) defined by the individual, a conception clearly at odds with the later understanding of "the model man," for which the standard of health is no longer derived from the individual, but externalized as a standard against which individuals are measured.

15. These categories were as follows: "male pseudo-hermaphrodites," "female pseudo-hermaphrodites," and "true hermaphrodites." These categories were based on one's gonads, so a male pseudohermaphrodite would have (likely undescended) testes but a feminine appearance, as would be typical in someone with complete androgen insensitivity, while a female pseudo-hermaphrodite would include a female with CAH with a phallus more closely resembling a penis than a clitoris. A true hermaphrodite would have mixed gonadal tissue, such as ovotestes.

16. Criticizing Preves's work, Heino Meyer-Bahlburg characterizes Tiger's experience as "an extreme example of a past generation of medical patients when compared to current figures as to the number of genital operations per hypospadias patient and their outcomes with current techniques" (2005a, 179). There is evidence that outcomes in hypospadias repair are much improved; however, the question I raise here does not depend on the success of the surgeries so much as the effects of the practice.

17. A 2004 BBC documentary, "Dr. Money and the Boy with No Penis," recounts not only the fate of David but that of his twin brother, Brian, as well. Although it was David who was a patient of Money's, Money encouraged Brian to join in on his "sister's" visits to Money's clinic as a kind of "control." Brian committed suicide two years before David. There is some speculation that Brian's suicide was prompted, in part, by the deception to which he was also subject, as well as by the revelation of what the twins experienced as sexual abuse in Money's clinic. Colapinto published a story on *Slate* following Reimer's suicide in 2004.

18. The composition of the group proposing the change is itself historically noteworthy. Chase is the founder of the Intersex Society of North America, and Dreger is the historian whose work brought her into the forefront of activism and leadership of ISNA with Chase. Sousa, a specialist in internal medicine, is also Dreger's spouse and longtime ally and supporter of ISNA. Grupposo and Frader are both pediatric endocrinologists, contemporaries of Daaboul who had similar training, as well as similar stories of understanding the problems with the standard of care. This group was the first to call for a change in nomenclature. It is not clear why the Consensus Statement settled on "disorders of sex development" rather than Dreger and her colleagues' proposal of "disorders of sexual differentiation."

19. The authors remark in particular on Sousa's experience of having to "calm an adult patient after an internal medicine resident announced to her that she was 'really' a man, because he had found testes in the patient." It is not only "a patient's understanding of her condition [that] will be strongly affected by labels she encounters in her own medical record or in medical journals or texts," they suggest, but also the clinician's understanding of his patient. "What use is there," they ask, "in calling a woman with [complete androgen insensitivity syndrome] a 'male,' when her external phenotype and her gender identity are female?" (Dreger et al. 2005, 732).

20. This problem with the term "disorders of sex development" is also magnified in the translation of the term in Romance languages. In Spanish, for example, the term is "*trastorno de de-*

sarollo sexual," which has the effect of re-invoking the identification of one's "sex" as male or female, man or woman, and "sexuality," with one's object preference ("sexuality"), and to suggest that the "disorder" applies equally not only to one's development of sex but to one's sexual desire as well.

21. A chart prepared by Alice Dreger following the guidelines proposed by Cheryl Chase was posted on the ISNA website (Chase with Dreger 2000).

22. As Dreger and Herndon recount in their contemporary history of intersex, there was also some resistance to the use of DSD in the handbooks to support parents and clinical care that were developed by a collective of individuals with intersex conditions, along with parents and clinicians, and published in 2006 (Consortium on the Management of Disorders of Sex Development 2006a; 2006b): "Several months after publication of the DSD Consortium's handbooks, three participating intersex adults—[David] Cameron, Esther Morris Leidolf, and Peter Trinkl—asked that a one-sentence disclaimer be added noting that, though they support the documents, they do not support the term [DSD]" (Dreger and Herndon 2009, 212).

23. In the field of disability studies there is a well-developed analysis of the ways that bodily differences defined as "disabilities" figure in conceptions of identity (see, e.g., Mitchell and Snyder 1997; Siebers 2008). However, this work has not been invoked in any sustained way in criticisms of the new nomenclature for atypical sex anatomies.

24. There is, however, evidence that at least some specialists maintained this view into the twentieth century. See, e.g., Meyer-Bahlburg's essay "Intersexuality and the Diagnosis of Gender Identity Disorder" (1994).

25. See also, e.g., Dreger 1998b, 8–9; Casper and Muse 2006. And concern with promoting heterosexual orientation appears to have persisted in significant measure. In a 2004 survey of pediatric endocrinologists and urologists, a startling proportion (42 percent and 57 percent, respectively) reported that projected sexual orientation of infants informs decisions on gender assignment (Sandberg et al. 2004, cited in Karkazis 2008, 148).

26. As Karkazis attests, gay activism and queer theory were by no means the only influences; feminist as well as health care and disability activism were also important (2008, 246), but I would suggest a certain priority in the influence of gay rights movements for the reasons I have detailed.

27. The term "intersexuality," first employed by Richard Goldschmidt in 1917, identified atypical sex with homosexual desire. As Dreger recounts in her history, "Before Goldschmidt, some authors had used the term 'intersexuality' to refer to what we would call homosexuality and bisexuality, and even Goldschmidt himself suggested that human homosexuality might be thought of as one form of intersexuality" (1998b, 31).

Morgan Holmes's injunction to "seize the name 'intersexual' as our own and take away its pathologizing power" is the most direct statement of this point (2000, 106). Other moving and provocative examples of this sort of "coming out" and reclamation of "intersex" can be found in the first-person narratives in the collection *Intersex in the Age of Ethics* (Dreger 1999b).

28. In this respect the treatment of those with DSD may be compared with the medical treatment of women through much of the twentieth century, whose difference from men was disregarded in most health research, with the result that medical care provided to women was often inappropriate. For an extended discussion, see Rosser 1994.

29. There is a broad range of individuals diagnosed with DSD who might seek hormone replacement. For some, hormone therapy might not be understood precisely as a "choice," given the serious risks of osteoporosis for those without gonads; others might elect hormone replacement because the function of their gonads is at odds with their gender of assignment.

30. It is obviously not the case that homosexual practices were unrecognized before this time; Katz's claim is that the category of "the homosexual" (and with it, "the heterosexual")

transformed the meaning of sexual desire and divided people along a normal/abnormal axis that the homo-/heterosexual terms consolidated and naturalized.

31. The condition of 5-alpha reductase deficiency affects genetic males whose bodies are, as the name suggests, lacking the enzyme that converts testosterone into dihydrotestosterone. Babies with 5-ARD are usually born appearing typically female (and are raised as female) and become more masculine at puberty, often developing a masculine gender identity. The protagonist in Jeffrey Eugenides's *Middlesex* (2002) had 5-ARD.

32. Even as the preservation of privacy is taken to be paramount in medical management of DSD, we must recall those who have been subjected to photographic sessions for purposes of research, as well as repeated exams by medical residents and their supervisors for educational purposes. It appears that the privacy of the family, rather than the individual patient, is the object of protection. It may also be that it is the public that is being protected from the "revelation" of atypical sex (see, e.g., S. J. Kessler 1998, 32).

2. "In Their Best Interests"

1. This prediction is borne out by the fact that there is no published evidence suggesting any "hazards, biological or otherwise, of having a large clitoris." While men with small penises have reported some medical challenges, published studies have found that, "contrary to conventional wisdom, it is not inevitable that such [men] must 'recognize that [they] are incomplete, physically defective and . . . must live apart.'" See Kipnis and Diamond 1999 [1998], 181.

2. The exception is a single article by Bing and Rudikoff (1970) that juxtaposes the stories of two families, one described as white and upper-middle-class, the other as uneducated and of Mexican descent. According to the authors, rather than partnering with the doctors like the "West" family, the "Torres" family "coped with the intersex problem . . . by accepting the ambiguity of the situation and . . . actively implement[ed] it by giving the baby a neuter name (the name of a warlike tribe)" (80). While the aim of the article is to promote in physicians a sensitivity to cultural differences that will assist them in making recommendations to parents in the best interests of the child, it is also the first documented case of parents' resistance to the standard of care. Discussions of parental resistance in the critical literature remain few, not appearing again until around 1998. The publication of *Intersex in the Age of Ethics* (Dreger 1999b) includes the interview of a parent and grown daughter that told the story of a parent's resistance to surgery (Dreger and Chase 1999). That same year, Helena Harmon-Smith's story of the birth of the son doctors wanted to assign female began to appear. Despite her best attempts to see to her son's best interests, Harmon-Smith was devastated to learn that her consent to the removal of what she had been told was a "cancerous" gonad amounted to the amputation of a healthy testis (Lehrman 1999; Fausto-Sterling 2000, 92).

3. The names of parents and their children have been changed to protect their privacy. The parents from the eight families I interviewed live in nearly every region of the United States, with the exception of one mother, who lives in a Westernized country outside the States. All quotations without citations are taken from transcripts of interviews on file with the author.

4. "Mothering," for Ruddick, describes the distinctive kind of "work out of which a distinctive kind of thinking arises" that is typically associated with women but can be assumed by women or by men (1989, 40). Following Ruddick, I use "mothering" because it captures the specific nature of the ethical responsibility at issue here.

5. Perhaps for this reason, many parents of children with ambiguous genitalia, including many of those who have girl children with CAH, resisted the association of the term "intersex" with their children. As used in the medical literature, however, the term "intersex" (now "dis-

orders of sex development," or DSD) designates any "defect in the normal processes of sexual maturation that results in abnormality in . . . the [sex chromosomes], the internal and external sexual organs, the gonads and the secondary sex characteristics which appear at puberty." See Creighton 2002, 218. Resistance to the term "intersex" can also be understood as an effort by individuals with intersex as well as their parents to deny their difference and fit in or accommodate to the categories given by society. Bourdieu's analysis of habitus makes sense of this resistance.

6. Things have changed since this time, as evidenced by the recent publication of *Disorders of Sex Development: A Guide for Parents*, which ends with a short chapter on the importance of peer support (Wisniewski et al. 2012, 100–104). The work of the guide's authors at Oklahoma's SUCCEED clinic is unique in the support it provides, however, and many specialists in the care of children with atypical sex anatomies remain concerned about the prospect of misinformation as well as perhaps the challenge to their authority that parents' participation in support groups might bring.

7. While Kittay extends the notion of a transparent self as a regulatory ideal intended to discern another's needs, some have rightly cautioned that the concept can be taken to assume that an ideal of transparency is possible and good. I do not think that Kittay's analysis suggests either, but it is a caution that is important to keep in mind.

8. "Clitoroplasty" is a term that can encompass both a cutting of clitoral tissue or what is known as "recession," a procedure that has since fallen out of favor, in which the exterior (visible) portion of the clitoris is concealed. The use of the term "clitorectomy" is controversial. Western doctors beginning in the late twentieth century do not typically use the term, even when their practice involves cutting ("-ectomy"). This may be an effort to distinguish current practices from those that are now decades old, or that are associated with genital-cutting practices in Africa, a point to which I will return in chapter 5.

9. As Kessler documented, penises were deemed inadequate if they were not of sufficient length to penetrate a vagina, something that began to change after 1997. Surgery continues to be the standard of care also in cases of hypospadias, that is, if the position of the urinary meatus will not permit a boy to urinate in a standing position. Similarly, through the 1990s, genital surgery was conducted on those assigned female with an eye not to performance but to appearance. There is some indication that physicians are now more cautious about these surgeries, as I will discuss in chapter 6.

10. Of her examination of approximately one hundred letters written by mothers of children with ambiguous genitalia, Suzanne Kessler notes that parents' accounts of their children's surgery focus "disproportionately on how the genitals look rather than on what the child might be experiencing or how her genitals might function in the future" (1998, 98).

11. See, for example, D. W. Winnicott's discussion of the "good enough" mother (1971, 10–14). There is a strong resonance between the kind of attunement necessary to meet an infant's needs and Kittay's discussion of the "transparent self" in *Love's Labor*.

12. About a decade after I completed these interviews, elective cosmetic genital surgeries for adult women started to become increasingly available. This continuing trend would seem to confirm the extent to which parents value "normalizing" the appearance of their children's genitals.

13. All but one of the parents I interviewed had consented to surgery. One family had adopted a child whose surgery had taken place while she was a ward of the state.

14. La Leche League is an organization whose stated mission is "to help mothers worldwide to breastfeed through mother-to-mother support, encouragement, information, and education and to promote a better understanding of breastfeeding as an important element in the healthy development of the baby and mother." See www.lalecheleague.org.

15. It wasn't so long ago that diapers were sold in packages marked "boy" and "girl." The last generation of such diapers were designed with extra absorption in different locations and were correspondingly decorated with designs and colors associated with each sex.

16. If Robin's body had not responded to testosterone, doctors would have strongly recommended that he be assigned female and castrated, his penis refashioned to resemble a clitoris, with a vaginoplasty performed then or, more likely, at some projected point. One doctor told Sarah that he thought it best to reassign Robin in any case, but the idea seemed too preposterous to her to consider seriously.

17. See, e.g., essays by Martha Coventry, Howard Devore, David Cameron, Kim, Tamara Alexander, Hale Hawbecker, and Angela Moreno in *Intersex in the Age of Ethics* (1999, 71–81, 90–116, 137–140).

18. On its face it would appear that 18 U.S.C. § 116, a federal law prohibiting "Female Genital Mutilation" (1996), would apply to normalizing genital surgeries performed on children. The law states that "whoever knowingly circumcises, excises, or infibulates the whole or any part of the labia majora or labia minora or clitoris of another person who has not attained the age of 18 years shall be fined under this title or imprisoned not more than 5 years, or both." An exception is noted, however: "A surgical operation is not a violation of this section if the operation is . . . *necessary to the health of the person on whom it is performed,* and is performed by a person licensed in the place of its performance as a medical practitioner." In applying this exception, a further subsection of the law clarifies that "no account shall be taken of the effect on the person on whom the operation is to be performed of any *belief on the part of that person, or any other person, that the operation is required as a matter of custom or ritual*" (emphases added). That the very conventions of gender (as understood by Money and his colleagues) that explicitly motivate the surgeries could themselves be understood as "a matter of custom or ritual" is elided by the health exception written into the law. I return to the comparison between normalizing genital surgeries in the developed world and ritual circumcision in chapter 5.

3. Tilting the Ethical Lens

1. The definition of intersex conditions—characterized as "disorders of sex development" following the 2005 European and U.S. Consensus Statement—is "congenital conditions in which development of chromosomal, gonadal, or anatomical sex is atypical" (Hughes et al. 2006, 554).

2. To appreciate the significance of the sample size in Money's dissertation, consider that no study since has involved a number of individuals close to this one.

3. Nietzsche consistently uses the French term "ressentiment" to describe an unrelenting kind of hatred—to which is joined an unacknowledged envy—that has no equivalent in his native German. English translations follow suit, because the English cognate, "resentment," does not carry the nuances that Nietzsche develops in his account.

4. A particularly illustrative example of monster ethics may be found in bioethicist Yechiel Michael Barilan's discussion of the principle of autonomy, which, he explains, cannot apply in the exemplary case of conjoined twins:

> As respect for personal autonomy is a fundamental aspect of ethics, it necessitates a clear distinction between the voice representing the autonomy (or wellbeing) of a given person, and all other persons and voices that are required to respect the autonomy and privacy in question . . . Conjoined twins are a case in point . . . If one conjoined twin wishes to consult a certain doctor, while the other twin prefers a different physician, neither doctor may treat either of the twins. This simplistic [!] example illustrates that a single conjoined twin cannot be regarded as a patient in the full sense of the word.

If the autonomous (or self-directed) conduct of one person typically and unavoidably encroaches upon or dispossesses the privacy or autonomy of another person, neither may be separately considered beneficiaries of rights. (2012, 221)

An extended and persuasive criticism of this view and the assumptions that motivate it may be found in *One of Us: Conjoined Twins and the Future of Normal* (Dreger 2004).

5. As I will clarify, I do not literally mean that everyone has this ressentiment, but I do mean to call attention to the representation of the universality of disgust—the apparent "obviousness" of the monstrosity it connotes.

6. Another physician, Dr. P., similarly remarks, "These girls [with enlarged clitorises] don't look right. It's unsettling. It's repulsive" (Karkazis 2008, 147).

7. See, e.g., Kipnis and Diamond 1999, 188; Howe 1999, 211–212; Dreger 2002; Systma 2002, 5; Dreger 2006b, 254–255. For attributions to physicians of good intentions by people with DSD, see also, e.g., Nicholson 1999, 20.

8. See, e.g., Minto et al. 2003; Schützmann et al. 2009.

9. Such photographic displays of atypical genitalia, as Shelley Wall, a specialist in biomedical communication argues, carry what she characterizes as "latent" content that conveys their abnormality and the attitudes that such abnormality should provoke in the viewer (2010, 80). Images such as these are not "neutral" in their presentation (81). Furthermore, she argues, the conventional depiction of dimorphic genitalia allots to atypical anatomy "no place in the space of representation" (82). An interesting counterexample of such representation may be found in Robert Latou Dickinson's 1949 *Atlas of Human Sex Anatomy,* whose detailed pen-and-ink drawings of typical and atypical genitalia convey something more like a sense of the spectrum of variety.

10. These are derived from the bioethical principles enumerated to guide clinical practice: autonomy, beneficence and non-maleficence, and justice (see, e.g., Beauchamp and Childress 2001). For two discussions that take up bioethical principles with specific regard to the treatment of intersex, see Dreger 1999a, 16–17, and Systma 2002.

11. We should recall Nietzsche's tart comment in *Twilight of the Idols* that "the will to a system is a lack of integrity" (2009 [1889], 1.26).

12. It bears remembering that the sorts of guidelines I argue doctors should (but don't) follow may themselves be characterized as expressions of a slave morality; for Nietzsche, all systems we would recognize by the name "ethical" are products of slave morality. The bioethical imperative of informed consent, for example, can be traced to the idea that all persons deserve equal respect. My aim here is not to propose replacement of the existing bioethical framework with one that might be cast as Nietzschean, but to make use of Nietzsche's intervention to examine and make sense of the failure in the treatment of DSD to apply accepted ethical principles to medical practice.

13. The important exception here is Suzanne Kessler's 1990 article "The Medical Construction of Gender: Case Management of Intersex Infants," which is reprinted in her book as chapter 2, "The Medical Construction of Gender" (1998). But since this chapter, critical work on intersex has largely focused on the experience of those with atypical sex. Karkazis's *Fixing Sex* (2008) is a departure in this regard, for it focuses equally on the experience of parents and physicians.

14. I primarily draw on Nussbaum's analysis in *From Disgust to Humanity: Sexual Orientation and Constitutional Law* (2010), a concise argument drawn in part from her longer book, *Hiding from Humanity: Disgust, Shame, and the Law* (2004). Nussbaum's discussions of primary-object disgust are grounded in the extensive empirical research of Paul Rozin and his colleagues, who use the term "core disgust"—i.e., disgust from which they find all other instances of disgust to

originate. But Nussbaum's concept of "projective disgust" ultimately departs from the frame-work offered by Rozin and his colleagues, for her aim is to highlight the ethical consequences of projective disgust. See Rozin et al. 2008 for an overview of this work.

15. But, one might object, if Nietzsche identified ressentiment with "the Jews," how can it be that the projective disgust directed at Jews constitutes an instance of ressentiment? Recall that Nietzsche's account is something like a speculative history, describing a transformation in the framework of moral values first organized around the distinction between "good and bad" resulting in a reversal or inversion, that itself resulted in the organization of moral value around the terms of "evil and good." In other words, those lesser mortals who had previously occupied the position of "the [merely] bad" in the old system, "became good" (a shift that en-tailed a transformation of the meaning of "good"), and those values associated with what had previously been taken to be good became *evil*. Nietzsche's account attempts to describe the ori-gins of the reversal of value that results not in rendering "good" Jews or Judaism, but rather the values that are associated with Christianity. The long and largely—if not entirely—discredited identification of Nietzsche's views as anti-Semitic appear to account for a persistent confusion on this point, though scholars continue to discuss the issue of Nietzsche's thinking about the Jews. See, e.g., essays in Golomb 1997.

16. Consider, for example, the now comically lambasted response people have to uttering or hearing the word "vagina." See also Rodriguez and Schonfeld"s "The Organ-That-Must-Not-Be-Named: Female Genitals and Generalized References" (2012).

17. I address this point in greater detail in chapter 5.

18. It appears that this is something that may grow increasingly rare in the current climate of access to internet photos of genitalia. There is some evidence that the proliferation of such photos is promoting a desire for labiaplasty in girls with typical genitals, as physician Lenore Tiefer (2008) has discussed in what could be taken for a direct response to a question Kessler posed ten years earlier regarding what seemed like an outrageous question: "What will hap-pen if it becomes fashionable to alter one's genitals?" (S. J. Kessler 1998, 119).

19. Karkazis (2008, 269–289) details both the acknowledgment by many physicians of long-term damage, physical and psychological, and how physicians have resisted yet begun to re-spond to these revelations, most saliently with the U.S. and European endocrinological socie-ties' consensus meeting in 2005 (Hughes et al. 2006). It remains to be seen the extent to which the separate opinions issued by the Swiss National Advisory Commission and by the German Ethics Council in 2012, as well as the 2013 United Nations "Report of the Special Rapporteur on Torture and Other Cruel, Inhuman, or Degrading Treatment or Punishment," will have on medical practice (Méndez 2013).

20. Alice Dreger and April Herndon similarly criticize the instrumental "use" of intersex to "sit around debating nature versus nurture" without consideration of how these very theo-ries have caused injury to "real people with intersex" (2009, 216). Dreger and Herndon's criti-cism implies that such discussions themselves participate in, or reproduce, the sorts of inves-tigations that motivated Money's Psychohormonal Research Unit at Johns Hopkins University, founded, as Money wrote, to examine "all the different types of hermaphroditism in order to discover the principles of psychosexual differentiation and development they would illumi-nate" (Money 1986, 10, cited in Karkazis 2008, 51).

21. For a discussion of Freud's declarations that he had "never" read Nietzsche, see Wester-ink 2009.

22. Flax writes that "polysexual" is preferable to "bisexual," "because 'bisexual' implies that there are two fixed, stable poles between which a singular identity shifts. 'Polysexual' conveys the sense of a complex, unstable range of possibilities, of sites with varying attributes in mul-tiple mixtures and forms" (Flax 2004, 58). We might add that "polysexual" provides a better

translation of Freud's claim, as to our ears "bisexual" may indicate object choice more than gender expression or sexual identity.

23. If there is something that can unite the disparate waves of feminist activism, it is this: to lay bare the injustice of these sacrifices, exposing the social and historically specific understandings that naturalize them.

24. Following the significant strides toward marriage equality made in the 2012 elections and then the 2013 U.S. Supreme Court decision *United States* v. *Windsor,* Flax's point begins to look like it could someday become a historical example of projective disgust.

25. "—These weak ones—someday they too want to be the strong ones, there is no doubt, someday their 'kingdom' too shall come—among them it is called 'the kingdom of God' pure and simple, as was noticed: they are of course so humble in all things! Even to experience that they need to live long, beyond death—indeed they need eternal life so that in the 'kingdom of God' they can also recover eternally the losses incurred during that earth-life 'in faith, in love, in hope'" (Nietzsche 1998 [1887], I:15).

26. To engage in this analysis, it is necessary to set aside the way that Scheler, contra Nietzsche, understands the answer to ressentiment to lie in a "true" Christianity. While Scheler's argument distorts the central contribution of Nietzsche's analysis, Scheler's psychologization of ressentiment is nevertheless illuminating and resonates with Melanie Klein's important work on envy, to which I turn.

27. "There is in the infant's mind a phantasy of an inexhaustible breast which is his greatest desire . . . [but] envy arises even if the baby is adequately fed. The infant's feelings seem to be that when the breast deprives him, it becomes bad because it keeps the milk, love, and care associated with the good breast all to itself. He hates and envies what he feels to be the mean and grudging breast" (Klein 1975 [1957], 183).

28. A detailed account of the operation of adult envy and its social consequences may be found in Kittay's "Womb Envy: An Explanatory Concept" (1983).

29. Recognizing the harms that the objectification of children with DSD can suffer from their parents as well as physicians, the *Clinical Guidelines* prepared by the Consortium on the Management of Disorders of Sex Development (2006a) remarks repeatedly on the importance of physicians discussing "your" child with parents of children newly diagnosed with DSD. Such objectification is not limited to children with intersex conditions. Argentine psychologist Gabriela Planas recounts the story of a mother whose one-year-old child suffered sudden hearing loss. Planas (2006) notes the discursive change in the mother's account that occurs as she relates her memory of "*my* child" before the onset of his deafness and "*the* child" she brings through doctor's offices in pursuit of cochlear implants.

30. In making this claim it is important to note that Diprose does not propose parent-child relationships as a model for corporeal generosity; the relationship between parent and child is not one typically understood to be concerned with the kind of alterity that Diprose seeks to overcome. There is, however, at least one point in the text that suggests Diprose herself takes for granted that parent-child relationships are generally understood to share an intimacy that could be described in terms of corporeal generosity (see Diprose 2002, 107).

31. A radio program produced by the BBC featured a woman who recounted the devastating effects of surgery to reduce the size of her enlarged clitoris. On the heels of her testimony, a prominent surgeon explained that "this [ambiguous genitalia] is very distressing to the family, and surgery is available to make that appearance more acceptable." "Intersex Conditions" radio broadcast on the BBC, December 11, 2001.

32. In her essay (one of many created by the working group that published the original position piece), Adrienne Asch offers a counterargument, that non-consenting surgery undermines a child's feeling of "loveableness" (2006, 229). In response to an urge to fix, she urges par-

ents to cultivate instead an empathic appreciation of the child's difference (237ff). Disgust or contempt is at odds with the development of this empathy—which resonates powerfully with Diprose's concept of "corporeal generosity" and bears important echoes of Klein's discussion of gratitude.

4. Reassigning Ambiguity

1. A German study of psychological distress in individuals with DSD conducted soon after the Consensus Statement was published demonstrated alarmingly high rates of "self-harming behavior and suicidal tendencies" among those in the study, "comparable to the traumatized comparison groups of women with physical or sexual abuse" (Schützmann et al. 2009, 16). Previous studies, as the authors noted, had been restricted mainly to outcomes relating to "psychosocial development" or successful gender assignment.

2. Laura Hermer (2002) points to the work of Slijper et al. (1998) to suggest that parents who have consented to normalizing surgery for their children have not been satisfied, though she concludes that surgery may be in children's best interest to secure parents' love (cited in Tamar-Mattis 2006, 90n226). Anne Tamar-Mattis points to the 2005 report of the San Francisco Human Rights Commission's finding that "parents of intersex children report feeling shame, fear, horror, humiliation, regrets, and ongoing doubt about the choices they may have made for their children" (Arana 2005, 22). There is as much room for debate about parents' "satisfaction" as that of affected individuals' satisfaction. Just as no adults have come forward in support of genital surgery, no parents of grown children have come forward. It may be that parents have not come forward because they believe that doing so could compromise the privacy of their grown children. Such concerns could be addressed by a properly conducted study, however, and, I would argue, such evidence should also figure in parents' informed consent to the extent that in this case they are not only providing proxy consent but are also, in the treatment of atypical sex, themselves regarded as objects of medical care. Remarkably, the recent opinion provided by the Swiss National Advisory Commission on Biomedical Ethics, "On the Management of Differences of Sex Development: Ethical Issues Relating to 'Intersexuality'" (2012), is especially noteworthy for its recognition of this very problem.

3. The revelation of the clitoral sensitivity exams performed by pediatric urologist Dix Poppas (Dreger and Feder 2010) was perhaps especially appalling in light of the profession's recognition of the substantial risk of harm that unnecessary and repeated genital exams carry.

4. See, e.g., narratives in Dreger 1999b, Preves 2003, and Karkazis 2008.

5. Elizabeth Grosz argues that "since the inception of [Western] philosophy as a separate and self-contained discipline in ancient Greece, philosophy has established itself on the foundations of a profound somatophobia" (1994, 5).

6. In closed adoptions, records that include information concerning birth parent(s) are sealed. It was long thought in Western Europe and the United States that maintaining the secret of adoption was a benefit not only to the parents, who had an interest in concealing the shame of infertility, but also to the child, who would otherwise feel she had been abandoned by birth parents or did not truly belong to her adopted family.

7. This point is one that scholars of Merleau-Ponty's work are exploring further and that merits more elaboration than I can pursue here. See, e.g., essays by Jorella Andrews (2006) and Lawrence Hass (2008).

8. For example, "In females with classic 21-OHD CAH who are virilized at birth, feminizing genitoplasty may be performed to remove the redundant erectile tissue while preserving the sexually sensitive glans clitoris and to provide a normal vaginal orifice that functions ade-

quately for menstruation, intromission, and delivery. Clitoroplasty is typically performed in early childhood (preferably at age 6–18 months)" (New and Nimkarn 2006 [2002], 12). More recent recommendations indicate that surgery between three and six months is preferable. See Cornell University's description of normalizing genital surgery at http://www.cornellurology .com/uro/cornell/pediatrics/genitoplasty.shtml#technique (Weill Cornell Medical Center 2010).

9. Interestingly, in following the reading of Henri Wallon, whose work predates Lacan's, Merleau-Ponty emphasizes the role of the other in this stage, but in the form of the father (see Merleau-Ponty 1964 [1960], 127–128).

10. The notion of alienation, taken up in existentialist-psychoanalytic terms, carries a different valence in Merleau-Ponty's work, which casts "alienation" as an integral moment of intersubjectivity. In "The Child's Relation with Others," Merleau-Ponty writes that it "is this transfer of my intentions to the other's body and of his intentions to my own, my alienation of the other and his alienation of me, that makes possible the perception of others" (1964 [1960], 118).

11. African American musician Ysaye Maria Barnwell's celebration of her grandmother in "There Were No Mirrors in my Nana's House" (1993) comes to mind. When she sings, "The beauty that I saw in everything . . . was in her eyes / So I never knew that my skin was too Black . . . that my nose was too flat . . . that my clothes didn't fit," she acknowledges the affirmative "mirroring" that also protected her from racist denigrations of her body, of her self. For an extended and insightful discussion of the "social constitution" of identity described here, see Linda Martín Alcoff's *Visible Identities: Race, Gender, and the Self* (2006).

12. Merleau-Ponty might characterize Jim's as a kind of "latent knowledge" (1962 [1945], 238).

13. In his treatment of individuation at the mirror stage, Merleau-Ponty similarly observes that this "process . . . is never completely finished" (1964 [1960], 119).

14. Cornell's gloss on Lacan here resonates with that of another analyst, D. W. Winnicott, whose analysis of "the mirror" focuses on what he regards as the "precursor of the mirror," namely, the mother's face (Winnicott 1971, 111). Rather than see "recognition" as "misrecognition," as Lacan does, Winnicott's account emphasizes an embodied and intersubjective model of development that may provide a better ground from which to consider ethical responses of the sort I explore in chapters 7 and 8.

15. Complete gonadectomy such as Jim had undergone, renders one's bone health vulnerable to the extreme, and makes hormone replacement a medical necessity. Those ignorant of their diagnosis are not only misinformed, but they are also prevented from caring for themselves adequately.

16. There is some—likely intended—irony in the physician's pronouncement, as the decisions to medicalize Jim's atypical anatomy would result in the necessity of continued care, but the pronouncement that he is "demedicalized" might be read as an assertion of the reversal of one important dimension of the damage to his health.

17. Some might ask, not unreasonably, whether Jim was going "back" to an original identity when he began to live as a man. A phenomenological analysis would recast that question in terms of the somatic experience and the "sense" (*sens*) of which it is made in the world. The experience of injecting testosterone, for example, supplies a somatic experience, the available meaning for which is marked as masculine in our world, one that cannot be disentangled from history and culture. We should recall Merleau-Ponty's claim that "it is impossible to establish a cleavage between what will be 'natural' . . . and what . . . acquired. In reality the two orders are not distinct; they are part and parcel of a global phenomenon" (1964 [1960], 108). For a contemporary treatment of the cleavage between "natural . . . and acquired" that draws explicitly on the case of intersex, see Rosario 2009.

18. Karkazis describes the persistent myth that those who have not had surgery will be suicidal. Many of the affected adults with whom she spoke had contemplated suicide. These indi-

viduals attributed these thoughts not to any diagnosis, but to their treatment by parents and physicians. "Some claimed to have suicidal thoughts not because surgery had not been performed but because it had. This is not necessarily because results were poor, though for many they were, but because the surgical decision formed part of a series of decisions and actions that led the child to feel there was something horribly wrong about her or his body and condition and hence self" (2008, 193).

19. For a fascinating account of the imperative of concealment and the measures taken to ensure concealment in early twentieth-century Britain, see "Other People's Bastards," in *Family Secrets: Shame and Privacy in Modern Britain* (Cohen 2013, 124ff).

20. Kimberly Leighton raises important questions about this putative "right" and the assumptions that ground it. While acknowledging that having access to information concerning one's biological or genetic origins may be important to individuals, it is not clear that there is a necessary harm in "not knowing." Claims that this lack of knowledge (of the identity of a gamete donor, for example) is equivalent to the active withholding of knowledge (such as the fact of one's adoption or that one's conception involved gamete donation) are ungrounded at best and, according to Leighton (2012), may in fact promote the suffering they purport to identify.

21. They also appear to motivate secrecy maintained in donor insemination in heterosexual couples, a case when it is felt that shame (or social stigma) of a spouse's infertility must be concealed (see, e.g., Turner and Coyle 2000, 2042).

22. Safer archly notes that "'siblings' does not appear in the 404-page index to the twenty-three-volume *Standard Edition* of Freud—but 'Siberia' does. The founder of psychoanalysis symbolically relegated his own seven siblings there and set the precedent for his followers to ignore the influence of their own and their patients' closest kin to this day" (2002, 29–30).

23. See the collected essays in Meyer 2009 and the Sibling Support Project at http://www.siblingsupport.org/sibshops.

5. A Question of Ethics as/or a Question of Culture

1. There is some debate about the extent to which physicians have historically believed in or acknowledged the importance of the clitoris in women's "sexual function," a question that hinges on how one defines women's sexual function. On the one hand there is the "evidence" by Hampson (1955) and Gulliver (by way of "personal communication of personal data" in 1958), cited by Gross, Randolph, and Crigler, that "a clitoris is not necessary" for sexual function (1966, 300). Eder cites the work of Lawson Wilkins, who recommended complete clitorectomy in cases of female infants with CAH because he thought an enlarged clitoris would prove "a source of extreme embarrassment and erotic stimulation" (Wilkins 1950, 274, cited in Eder 2012, 73). Research by medical historian Sarah (Webber) Rodriguez is clarifying for its powerful demonstration of the contradictions in the research that reveal a finer understanding of "the function" of the clitoris in women's sexuality than has been understood (Webber 2005).

2. Because the disorder is autosomal recessive—that is, requires two copies of a gene (one from each parent) for expression of a condition or disease—it is concentrated in particular ethnic groups, as other, better known disorders are, such as Tay-Sachs disease or sickle cell anemia. There are identifiable concentrations in Yupik Eskimos and in Ashkenazic Jews, and perhaps also in those of Filipino and Mexican descent. One might expect many more published analyses of the effects and cultural impact of the disorder, but, in the clinical literature at least, the disorder generally remains "individualized." For evidence of the "ethnic-specific" distribution of CAH, see, e.g., Therell 2001 and R. Wilson et al. 2007.

3. The accomplishment of universal newborn screening in the United States in 2008 stems

from the work of the CARES Foundation, which advocates for children and families affected by CAH. In 2010 the Endocrine Society published guidelines reaffirming the value of universal screen for CAH (Speiser et al. 2010). The National Newborn Screening and Genetics Resource (NNSGR) Center reports that between 1991 and 2000, when little more than half of states had instituted mandatory testing, 774 cases were reported. In the latest available report of cumulative cases through 2010, the total number of cases exceeded 3,000. My thanks to Dr. Bradley Therrell at NNSGR for his assistance in gaining access to this data.

4. Clitoral recession did not become common until the 1970s but was effectively replaced as a standard procedure after the 1980s by the "nerve-sparing clitoroplasties" practiced today. For a report on the poor outcomes associated with clitoral recession, see Minto et al. 2003.

5. It is clear that the prevention of lesbianism is one of the primary reasons motivating the prenatal administration of dexamethasone, which until 2010 was regarded as standard of care (see Speiser et al. 2010) and continues to be promoted by some in the field, such as pediatric endocrinologist Maria New and psychologist Heino Meyer-Bahlburg (see Dreger, Feder, and Tamar-Mattis 2012).

6. Richard Hurwitz's historical review of feminizing treatment relates that clitoral amputation was the standard of care during these years and was "common until the mid-1970s and persisted even into the early 1980s." A relatively small number of clitoral recessions were performed beginning in 1958, and the technique was refined around 1965, but at least one textbook of urologic surgery from that era recommending amputation represented clitoral recession as well as the glans-preserving surgery that removed the shaft of the clitoris while attempting to preserve sensation as "newer unproven techniques" (Hurwitz 2011, 167). There was obviously no uniform opinion or practice, so treatments could vary a great deal from one physician to another. There remain differences in practice today, but there is comparatively more consistency in treatment.

7. The medical notation is something of a mystery and disturbed her pediatrician, who informed me in no uncertain terms that Andie had *not* been circumcised. Nevertheless, this is the term used in the record and may refer to a trimming of the clitoral hood.

8. Citing Torah and the Talmud, bioethicist Yechiel Michael Barilan explains, "In Judaism, Imago Dei [i.e., the notion that man is made in the image of God] is related to the human body— especially its external appearance. The violation of the human body . . . by disfiguration, directly offends the dignity of God and God's love toward man . . . External disfiguration . . . is considered a more serious offense than meddling with internal organs" (2012, 41).

9. Here my own ignorance is evident: There are different traditions of Orthodox Judaism, and the tradition with which I have any familiarity is that associated with Ashkenazic Judaism. I have since learned that other Jewish traditions—albeit traditions that are in the minority— have different commitments. These would include the Gur Hasidic community, which is not concerned with the sort of pleasure that belongs to mortal life here and now, but with a spiritual life that transcends this one. For an ethnographic treatment of women from this community, see Tamar El-Or 1994.

10. My hunch could find some ground, as I would learn that thinkers such as Fred Rosner have argued for the identification of medicine and religion in the history of Jewish tradition, where at one time, "the priest and the physician were one and the same person." Rosner's brief history traces the contemporary articulation of this identification to a doctoral thesis titled "Jewish Medical Ethics," submitted by Rabbi Lord Immanuel Jakobivits to London University, and published in New York in 1959 (Rosner 2007, 109).

11. DES was prescribed to stunt the growth of girls beginning in the 1950s and was extended years after the U.S. Food and Drug Administration (FDA) issued a safety warning following the revelation of a correlation between DES exposure and clear-cell adenocarcinoma in 1971

(Cohen and Cosgrove 2009, 46–47). Though there is now greater societal acceptance of taller girls, journalists Susan Cohen and Christine Cosgrove reported in the *Lancet* that "some tall girls are still prescribed oestrogens to stunt height, especially when parents insist" (2010, 454).

12. One of the most cited claims to this effect comes from renowned pediatric urologist Ian Aaronson, who wrote that a moratorium on normalizing surgeries would "signify a return to the 'dark ages' of intersex management, which has given rise to a host of psychological cripples" (1999, 119).

13. Warne's would be an explicit case of what Erik Parens describes as an unwarranted understanding of the goal of medicine to intervene when some condition or state falls out of the realm of "*normal* or *species-typical* functioning." As Parens dryly remarks, it "would be lovely if we could look to nature and discern the line . . . between disease and health. That way it wouldn't be our ethical responsibility to decide, based on our understanding of the facts and our values, whether to intervene. We'd just point to nature." But as Parens points out, this notion—presented as one based on natural science rather than any judgment—is not only ethically suspect but also not supported by natural scientists who specialize in the etiology of disease (2011, 4; original emphasis). There is, nevertheless, a tradition of "naturalistic" ethical approaches to which Warne's work may be linked (see, e.g., Lenman 2008).

14. In her invited response to the Public Policy Advisory Network on Female Genital Surgeries in Africa, gynecologist Nawal M. Nour points to the lack of substantiation for a number of the claims made by the network. These include the assertion that a "high percentage of [circumcised] women have rich sexual lives" and the purported safety regarding "the vast majority of genital surgeries in Africa" (2012, 31). The lack of evidence for the positive claims on behalf of genital cutting in Africa to which Nour points is mirrored in the unsubstantiated claims of safety and "success" of normalizing genital interventions for atypical sex, though there is far more support for sexual responsiveness of African women who have been circumcised (see, e.g., Hernlund and Shell-Duncan 2007, 30–32).

15. An alternative reading would follow from the psychoanalytic discussion of the assumption of sex in chapter 3. In those terms we could see the sacrifice made by the Kono and that described by Jane Flax as a sacrifice that all unambiguously sexed individuals would make, though only in the former society would surgical modification of genitalia be required. Following this analysis, the surgical modification of children with atypical sex anatomies in the West do not mark a "sacrifice," but, as I proposed in chapter 1, a punishment.

16. Ahmadu discusses how legal prohibitions can paradoxically serve to exacerbate the vulnerability of the indigenous and immigrant women such laws seek to protect—for example, fear of revealing their excision in the context of seeking health care, particularly during pregnancy, has prompted some to delay or put off seeking necessary care (Shweder 2009, 15).

17. The legislation introduced in the mid-1990s in Australia is nearly identical to the 1996 federal law prohibiting "Female Genital Mutilation" in the United States, 18 USC § 116.

18. Iain Morland has provocatively suggested that interventions are, in his words, "traumatic by design" (2011, 148).

19. See also Public Policy Advisory Network on Female Genital Surgeries in Africa 2012, 23. Cheryl Chase makes this same point in her own comparison of the experiences of African and American women who had had clitorectomies. Following her interviews with these women, Chase reflects that "African mothers, no less than American surgeons, act from a desire to care for their daughters." She adds, "American surgeons, no less than African mothers, are misguided when they direct a knife at a child's clitoris" (1999, 152).

20. This was the model that was reported to have been successful in Senegal (Mackie 2000). A 2011 article in the *New York Times* described the efforts of *Tostan* ("breakthrough" in Wolof) to end genital cutting "in more than 5,000 villages" (Dugger 2011). Legal scholar L. Amede

Obiora discusses the importance of the representation of women's power in resisting circumcision in the 2004 film *Moolade* (2007, 70–71).

21. The most common form of this claim—one frequently made, if not in print, in conversation—is exemplified in remarks made by pediatric urologist Larry Baskin to a *New York Times* reporter in 2006, the same year the Consensus Statement was published: "There haven't been any studies that would support doing nothing . . . That would be an experiment: don't do anything and see what happens when the kid's a teenager. That could be good, and that could also be worse than trying some intervention" (quoted in Weil 2006).

6. Neutralizing Morality

1. In *One of Us*, Alice Dreger reminds us that "in the 1920s and '30s, the United States led the world in scientifically advanced ideas on reducing the incidence of inborn mental and physical 'deformities' in the general population. Many Americans, liberal as well as conservatives, saw eugenics . . . as both just and scientific" (2004, 117–118).

2. For an excellent overview of the moral questions raised by such enhancement, see the essays collected in *Enhancing Human Traits: Ethical and Social Implications* (Parens 1998). A more recent discussion may be found in Mills 2011, 11–34.

3. Caplan addresses head-on what others do not, namely, the way that the emergence of more widely available genetic counseling "was inextricably intertwined with the issue of abortion. The only option available to women or parents in almost all situations where congenital anomalies were discovered prenatally was abortion. Abortion was and remains a subject that generates enormous moral conflict . . . Genetic counselors could not be accused of favoring or promoting abortion if they adhered to a strict ethic of value neutrality" (Caplan 1993, 162). A Hastings Center project that explored the relationship among prenatal testing, selective abortion, and attitudes regarding disability resulted in the collection *Prenatal Testing and Disability Rights* (Parens and Asch 2000).

4. We can look also to the role that nondirective counseling is playing in cancer treatment. See, e.g., Simonoff and Step 2005.

5. As we know from individual narratives, there were exceptions, whether because a doctor—generally outside of a major metropolitan area—quietly thought otherwise, or because the rare parent resisted normalizing surgery or sex reassignment: As one mother told me of her now middle-age son, "you don't castrate a boy and make him a girl"; Bing and Rudikoff noted that one family refused normalizing surgery from a religious conviction that a child's appearance is "God's will" (1970, 80). Some other children escaped surgery because their health was too fragile for their physicians to consider normalization. It is not at all clear, however, how many individuals have atypical sex anatomies that have not been "medicalized," a point on which little persuasive or effective argument (to physicians) can rest, because there is little hope for collecting the evidence that could ground it.

6. As I noted in the introduction, the names of the physicians I interviewed for the work are pseudonyms.

7. The surgeon who specialized in adolescent gynecology did recount one case in which a young, sexually active woman had sought surgery following discomfort in certain kinds of athletic activity. The young woman sought normalizing surgery with full knowledge, and follow-up reports provided by the gynecologist were positive.

8. The problem of continuity of care has been raised in other contexts and seems especially critical in DSD care, for which few adult specialists in endocrinology and gynecology, particularly, are trained.

9. Karkazis discusses the question of outcome studies and the contradictory commitment to evidence in this area of medicine in some detail. She documents how outcome studies of vaginoplasties appearing as late as 1998, for example, did not investigate the preservation of erotic sensation; instead, they made use of rates of marriage or frequency of sex to determine success. All others, from the late 1970s through the late 1990s, organized their research questions around "sexual activity," mostly focusing on frequency of intercourse as the marker of success; questions about women's satisfaction or the pleasure they might have experienced went unasked (165–166). Perhaps the most famous series of studies since 2000 was undertaken by a British team lead by female doctors and has raised significant questions about the successes, purported and assumed, of cosmetic genital surgeries (166–167). These studies document poor outcomes with respect to preservation of erotic sensation and call attention to the open secret that many of these cosmetic procedures needed to be repeated or required repair. But, Karkazis remarks, "many physicians regard these studies as suspect for what is purported to be their bias 'toward poor outcomes'" (2008, 168). More recently, a team in Germany undertook a review of existing research on outcomes concerning those with 46,XY DSD, observing that existing studies are inadequate for a variety of reasons, but concluded that "overall, all [existing studies] indicate that [sexual quality of life] is impaired, particular[ly] with regard to sexual dysfunctions and satisfaction" (Schönbucher et al. 2010, 193).

10. Nor do we have significant information at this time about what is occurring in Europe as far as the increase or decrease in surgical procedures is concerned. The 2010 analysis based on the polling of European endocrinologists reports significant changes in policy and wide adoption of and compliance with 2006 recommendations (Pasteriski et al. 2010), but the 2006 Consensus Statement offered strong recommendations against surgery *only* in the case of reassignment of boys with micropenis; in addition, it advised that when surgery was performed, only qualified surgeons undertake it. Work by a French team of urologists suggests that in France there is no less surgery overall. It cautions that hypospadias repair—that is, surgery aiming to normalize a penis in which the urinary meatus appears on the underside or base of the penis—may present far more complications than is generally acknowledged, including a "number of disasters" many physicians see as a problem of the past (Vidal et al. 2010, 318). In our conversation, Dr. Elm remarked that he has noticed far more caution when it comes to reducing the size of a girl's clitoris, but has noted no hesitation whatsoever in surgeons' strong recommendations for hypospadias repair, for which evidence of long-term success has continued to raise some questions.

11. See chapter 1 for a discussion of Lawson Wilkins's discovery of cortisone's effectiveness in treating the symptoms of CAH. It is important to acknowledge that so much is known about the regulation of cortisol thanks to families like Ruby's. The severity of their CAH helped research physicians to understand and refine treatment in children.

12. Specialists also seem to think that prenatal interventions such as the use of dexamethasone are in children's best interests. While the issue of prenatal counseling with respect to DSD has been almost entirely limited to the prenatal treatment of pregnant women with dexamethasone (see Dreger et al. 2012), there is some indication that prenatal management of DSD will become more prominent, as a European group predicts (Chitty et al. 2012).

13. And it may not be prudent for doctors to make enthusiastic recommendations of surgery to parents who might eventually sue them; hence Dr. Pine's observation of a difference between his discussions with parents (who are more often of color and of lower socioeconomic class) as compared with those of a colleague of his who works in a university hospital (whose patients are more likely to come to him having done extensive research). "He tells parents, 'I don't want to do this unless you want me to do it. If you want me to do it, I'll do a good job, I'm happy to do it.'" The differences between the treatment of parents working within different systems of

health care is an interesting one and merits further study. At this point it seems that the differences are present but may not significantly affect care.

14. The recognition of the time it takes for parents to absorb information and make truly informed decisions in cases of DSD led the Supreme Court of Colombia to establish a new standard for informed consent in 1999 (see Greenberg 2012, 36–37). Ten years later, however, research indicates that despite the court's decisions mandating significant changes in standards for consent, the decisions have not had any measurable impact on medical care for children with DSD in Colombia (Bocanete 2009).

7. Practicing Virtue

1. There are now many accounts of adults who have undergone such surgeries and express the wish that they had not. By contrast, as Dreger notes, "*not a single person with intersex has come forward publicly to say she or he thinks her or his infant genital surgeries were a good idea*" (2006a, 89; original emphasis). There is also wide agreement that follow-up studies have not provided good evidence of the "success" of such surgeries, though there is some indication that not all children subjected to normalizing surgeries are doing poorly. In his response to a 2010 study reporting comparatively positive outcomes of masculinizing genitoplasty, pediatric urologist Richard Hurwitz, a proponent of the standard of care, expresses skepticism about the value of the results reported; he wonders whether some of the better outcomes recorded may be attributed not to good surgeries, but to enhanced psychosocial care (2010, 831). "It may be," he concludes, "that long-term psychological support is of equal or superior importance to the anatomical result" of surgery (832).

2. Since the publication of the *Belmont Report* in 1979, serious efforts have been made within medicine to put into practice the principles of respect and justice through elevation of the principle of autonomy, what boils down in bioethical practice to the right of patients or their proxies to make informed and uncoerced decisions (see, e.g., Faden and Beauchamp 1986, 15). Although the principles of autonomy and informed consent originated in the special concerns for the vulnerability of human research subjects, these principles soon became extended to guide decision making in clinical medicine more broadly (see, e.g., Schermer 2002, 24).

3. In "Gift Not Commodity?: Lay People Deliberating Social Sex Selection," Jackie Leach Scully, Tom Shakespeare, and Sarah Banks similarly argue that a view of parenting in terms of virtue challenges what they describe as the focus on "parental autonomy" dominant in bioethics (2006, 756–757).

4. In making this observation, I follow the criticism made by contemporary philosopher Rosalind Hursthouse regarding what she sees as the risk of deontological reasoning to simplify the problem of moral judgment. See Hursthouse 1999, 47. I do not think the reductive approach is a necessary problem in Kant's work itself; however, I agree that a robust account of moral decision making must avoid too narrow a focus on moral action apart from reflection on the moral agent, or what we might describe as "situated moral agency." I return to this point in the conclusion.

5. In a history of the ethical interventions of the standard of care, notable moments would include the special issues of the journals *Chrysalis* (Chase and Coventry 1997) and the *Journal of Clinical Ethics* (Dreger 1998c), which were dedicated to intersex and appeared in 1997 and 1998, respectively; the collection *Intersex in the Age of Ethics*, which combined selected contributions of these two collections in a single volume (Dreger 1999b); and the collected essays in *Surgically Shaping Children* (Parens 2006). What must be counted as the first thoroughgoing effort to craft an ethical approach to care should be located in the two handbooks published

under the name of the Consortium on the Management of Disorders of Sex Development: the *Clinical Guidelines for the Management of Disorders of Sex Development in Childhood* (2006a) and the *Handbook for Parents* (2006b). Separate opinions issued in 2012 by the German Ethics Council and by the Swiss National Advisory Commission on Biomedical Ethics mark the possibility of genuine change. Also notable is the 2013 report by the United Nations Special Rapporteur on Torture and Other Cruel, Inhuman, or Degrading Treatment or Punishment. The report argues that "irreversible sex assignment, involuntary sterilization, [and] involuntary genital normalizing surgery" performed in the absence of genuine medical necessity (Méndez 2013, 19) may "constitute torture or ill-treatment when enforced or administered without the free and informed consent of the person" (7).

6. The sixteen members of the working group include individuals from "patient support groups (persons with DSD/intersex and/or parents); bioethicists; specialists in pediatrics and adolescent medicine, surgery, urology, obstetrics and gynecology, endocrinology; a psychologist and a psychotherapist; a specialist in medical law; and a medical sociologist" (Wiesemann et al. 2010, 672). A fourth author of the main report is Ute Thyen, a prominent member of the German Network DSD/Intersex but apparently not part of the Bioethics and Intersex working group.

7. The North American Task Force on Intersexuality (NATFI) was convened by pediatric urologist Ian Aaronson in early 2000 to address challenges to the standard of care and to try to coordinate efforts to collect meaningful outcome data (see Chase and Aaronson 2000). While it does not appear that any work was completed under the immediate auspices of NATFI, the 2006 Consensus Statement (in which many of the members of NATFI were present) as well as projects under way at major medical centers—including the SUCCEED clinic at Children's Hospital at Oklahoma University Medical Center, UCLA, and the University of Michigan—arguably have roots in the formation of the Task Force; NATFI was the first formal group in which physicians came together to respond to questions raised by the Intersex Society of North America.

8. Wiesemann and her colleagues acknowledge the earlier ethical statement by a Hastings Center group (of which I was a member) that "called for a multidisciplinary approach to the management of DSD, the child's right to know and rigorous follow-up studies but," the authors claim, *"avoided tackling the contentious issue of decision making in early childhood"* (Wiesemann et al. 2010, 672; emphasis added). Among the conclusions reached by the Hastings Center group, however, appears the following: "None of the appearance-altering surgery need be done urgently. Surgery to normalize appearance without the consent of the patient lacks ethical justification, in most cases." It is not clear how the claim that surgery lacks an ethical justification constitutes "avoidance" of the issue of parental consent. Rather than locate the primary ethical problem of surgical normalization in the issue of parental decision making, as Wiesemann and her colleagues do, the Hastings Center group criticized problems in the standard of care intended to shed light on the assumptions that these researchers continue to take for granted. For example, in our statement, we observed that

> when health care professionals . . . inappropriately communicate an urgent need to undertake a surgical "fix," they wrongly substitute these interventions for focusing on the families' discomfort, guilt, and/or sense of shame. All should understand that *a decision to raise an infant as a boy or girl in no way depends on surgery per se.* (Frader et al. 2004, 426; emphasis added)

Rather than present any evidence to the contrary, physicians have followed the response of pediatric endocrinologist Erica Eugster, who was invited to respond to the Hastings Center group's commentary. She writes that even though "historical claims that formation of a stable gender identity requires [the appearance of] concordant genitalia . . . have legitimately been questioned and rejected by many," the health and well-being of a child depends on "an individual family's ability to accept and unconditionally love their child" (2004, 428). Eugster's conclusions that the decision to pursue surgery rests with the parents and "does not present an ethical dilemma, since in our society all major decisions regarding minor children are traditionally made by parents" (429), does not differ substantially from the conclusions of Wiesemann and her colleagues, but they are qualified in the addendum authored by the working group as a whole. The recommendations detailed there are substantially more consistent with those of the Hastings Center group. Criticizing the standard of care does not, however, appear to be the aim of the German Network DSD/Intersex working group.

9. One suspects a willful ignorance in the authors' failure to engage the substance of significant ethical arguments in the literature. The authors do not cite the groundbreaking essay published by Dreger in the *Hastings Center Report* (1998a), which contains most of the points that Kipnis and Diamond enumerate, as well as the major monographs by Kessler (1998) and Fausto-Sterling (2000), each of which echoes the earlier arguments made by Dreger and Kipnis and Diamond. Notably, not one of these works frames the argument against surgery in the terms that Wiesemann and her colleagues employ in their summary treatment of objections to the standard of care.

10. We can see how Warne and Bhatia's work in their 2006 essay is an attempt to address this point, but doing so from a "cross-cultural perspective" as they have cannot provide the evidence they seek, since, as Kipnis and Diamond suggest, the comparison group for outcome studies must be "like those" considering surgery—particularly, one might add, a surgery performed, as all acknowledge, not from medical necessity, but from what parents and physicians understand, and assert, as cultural necessity. That is to say, the disparate cultural and economic conditions that characterize the lifeworlds of the populations Warne and Bhatia study in "the east" cannot provide meaningful data for those residing in "the west."

11. In this way, current practice has been able to set aside the second recommendation that Kipnis and Diamond make in their article. The second recommendation proposes that the moratorium described in the first recommendation remain in place until retrospective outcome studies of past practices have been completed. The third recommendation, "that efforts be made to undo the effects of past deception by physicians" (1999 [1998], 406), has gone almost entirely unheeded. Nevertheless, there has been one case of an apology by a physician to a former patient arranged in 2010 by Advocates for Informed Choice. See Guterman 2012. http://www .soros.org/voices/why-are-doctors-still-performing-genital-surgery-on-infants

12. In reflections on the question of "dependency" with regard to recipients of state welfare, Iris Marion Young provides an excellent discussion of what she calls "the ideology" of autonomy that, she argues, serves to devalue recipients of state welfare. But critical as she is of the ideology of autonomy in that regard, Young writes that this ideology "is convincing partly because it relies . . . on a core value we ought to affirm: autonomy" (2002, 45). She argues that the structure of welfare deprives recipients of autonomy and that we should be aware of the ways that the rhetoric of welfare works against respecting, and furthermore supporting, individuals' capacity to make their own decisions and be contributing members of their families and communities. Young argues that we should affirm the value of autonomy with the understanding that "a need for aid or support" is not at odds with autonomy, but grounds what she casts as a claim to a *right* to autonomy: "Everyone should have the right to be autonomous; a condition of the realization of such autonomy for most people, at least at some times in their lives, is that they receive some resources and/or interpersonal support and assistance from others. Certain forms of dependence and interdependence, that is, should be understood as *normal* conditions for being autonomous" (2002, 47; original emphasis).

13. In his treatment of duty in the *Groundwork of the Metaphysics of Morals*, Kant distinguishes between "perfect" duties and "imperfect" duties. Perfect duties are those that allow "no exception" (1964 [1785], 89) in the obligation they command—for example, truth-telling. Duties such as beneficence or the cultivation of one's talents are imperfect in the sense that one's inclination can figure in one's fulfillment of them without wholly compromising their "moral worth." If one is especially talented in playing a particular instrument, for example, but despises the sound, or feels disproportionate discomfort in the playing, one may cultivate one's talents in another way and still fulfill this duty.

14. In the *Apology*, Socrates proposes to those beseeching him to flee his death sentence that they should instead "let no day pass without discussing [virtue] and all the other subjects about which you hear me talking and examining both myself and others [for this] is really the very best thing that a man can do . . . life without this sort of examination is not worth living" (Plato 1961b, 38a).

15. Foucault says this is a complicated matter for Christianity, since "achieving one's salvation is also a way of caring for oneself" (1997 [1984], 285). This is a point that we also find in Nietzsche's notion of the ascetic in the *Genealogy of Morality* and the possibilities for "overcoming" in ways that can affirm (or deny) the kind of self-possession of which Foucault speaks.

16. Such worries are hardly new, as we should recall from Rousseau's churlish remarks to the mothers to whom he directed his *Emile*. In Book I, Rousseau castigates mothers for swaddling their newborns: "You thwart [your children] at birth. The first gifts they receive from you are chains. The first treatment they experience is torment . . . They cry because you are hurting them" (1979 [1762], 43). But women's failure in particular aspects of child rearing appears to be a symptom of a greater problem, namely, women's increasing resistance to assume their natural role as child bearers. At stake, he writes, is "the impending fate of Europe. The sciences, the arts, the philosophy, and the morals . . . will not be long in making a desert of it" (44–45).

8. Protecting Vulnerability

1. "Crimes against humanity" are defined in Article 6 of the first volume of the *Nuremberg Trial Proceedings* as "murder, extermination, enslavement, deportation, and other inhumane acts committed against any civilian population, before or during the war; or persecutions on political, racial or religious grounds in execution of or in connection with any crime within the jurisdiction of the Tribunal, whether or not in violation of the domestic law of the country where perpetrated" (International Military Tribunal 1947–1949).

2. This understanding has also framed current conflicts over the status of individuals with cognitive disabilities, as is evident in Eva Kittay's criticism of the work of Jeff McMahan and Peter Singer in "The Ethics of Philosophizing: Ideal Theory and the Exclusion of People with Severe Disabilities." McMahan argues that those with "congenital severe cognitive impairments fall below the threshold of capacities needed for personhood and thus are not subject to the claims of justice" (Kittay 2009, 134). But if, following O'Neill, we should understand moral theory to be focused on articulating "duties" rather than "rights," then we should be concerned not with whether anyone falls "below the threshold of capacities needed for personhood," but instead with identifying the obligations owed to those with cognitive disabilities. The salient moral issue is not personhood, then, but obligation. Focusing on obligation, we should not fall prey to what Kittay rightly identifies as the "moral dangers of drawing lines among human beings" (135).

3. Kant is admittedly inconsistent in his identification of dignity with autonomy, however, and certainly one finds an identification of dignity with "man."

4. Von der Pfordten's analysis of the appearance of the term "dignity" in the third formulation of the categorical imperative and not in the second formula (of the "end-in-itself") substantiates O'Neill's contention that autonomy is not a property of individuals (see Von der Pfordten 2009, 377).

5. The Southbury Training School is a facility for children and adults with cognitive impairments. There is no indication in the film that Heinemann is cognitively impaired, and the film does not remark on the fact that his residency could have been damaging not only because he had no contact with his family but also because, at the very least, the education he would have received there would not have been appropriate for a child with typically developing cognitive capacity.

6. Even in those cases when the deployment of a given technology would appear to make one stand apart, specifically to become abnormal (the case of apotemnophilia, "the attraction to the idea of being an amputee" [Elliott 2003, 209] being the most notorious), the desire to fit in, Elliott argues, plays a central role.

7. Pediatric specialist Walter Miller makes this point with regard to the prenatal administration of dexamethasone, a steroid intended to reduce the masculinization of genitalia in 46,XX females with congenital adrenal hyperplasia. In correspondence with Alice Dreger, he wrote, "It seems to me that the main point of prenatal therapy is to allay parental anxiety. In that construct, one must question the ethics of using the fetus as a reagent to treat the parent, especially when the risks are non-trivial" (see Dreger 2010a). Following the authors of the Consensus Statement, it seems to me that we could make exactly the same observation about many of the practices associated with normalizing atypical sex.

Conclusion

1. For readers who are physicians and medical students, I will add that it should be clear that the ancient philosophical "care of the self" to which Foucault refers is a far more encompassing and demanding notion that shares little with the increasing emphasis on "self-care" that medical schools have integrated into their curricula. These latter are more concerned that medical students attend to getting enough sleep and exercise to manage the stress and anxiety associated with the demanding nature of a medical education (see, e.g., Kushner, Kessler, and McGaghie 2011).

2. On the other hand, any parent who has survived toddlerhood knows—because she has learned—in the words of a parent I admire, that "the easy way is not the easy way": giving in to the tyrannical child with desires to be disruptive or disrespectful or refuse healthy food or watch more TV, and so on, is an invitation to more of the same.

3. In 2012 Lisa I. Iezzoni and her colleagues from the Mongon Institute for Health Policy at Massachusetts General Hospital published findings from a 2009 survey that indicated a disturbing, if unsurprising, admission by a large proportion of the nearly two thousand practitioners surveyed: physicians do not always tell their patients the truth, disclose what many would consider conflicts of interests (e.g., financial ties to a pharmaceutical company), or provide full information about a disease, prognosis, or medical error (see Iezzoni et al. 2012; see also the article appearing in the *New York Times* reporting on the survey [Chen 2012]). But the fact that the avoidance of "paternalism" is one of the fundamental principles of bioethics suggests that its routine violation has long been recognized.

4. Because the sex of assignment is generally not in question in cases of children with hypospadias, there has been some dispute over its inclusion as an "intersex" condition. This dispute may be owing to urologists' resistance to seeing the standard of care for hypospadias as a

part of the standard pertaining to the normalization of other DSD—that is, other conditions involving atypical sex anatomy—that have been subjected to far less thorough testing. The phenomenon certainly is more common than other DSD: the Center for the Study and Treatment of Hypospadias at the University of California–San Francisco describes it as "one of the most common congenital anomalies," and is reported to occur in 1 in 250–300 births. Moreover, its incidence has increased substantially, as reported in Europe and in the United States (Center for the Study and Treatment of Hypospadias 2013). But because hypospadias is regarded as the result of an incomplete development of the penis, its inclusion as a "disorder of sex development," or DSD, seems nonetheless appropriate.

5. Indeed, intersex activists beginning with Cheryl Chase have claimed that if there is something like "an intersex identity," it is the product of a medical treatment. In its effort to normalize the bodies of those with atypical sex anatomy, this treatment has itself "fixed"—that is, produced—the stigmatic difference these interventions are meant to conceal. Argentine activist and scholar Mauro Cabral made this same point in his testimony before the Inter-American Commission on Human Rights in Washington, D.C., in March 2013.

6. A search of Pubmed, the U.S. National Library of Medicine index of biomedical literature, yields multiple citations for the term "hypospadias cripple" through 2012.

7. The Swiss report was immediately available in English, but as of this writing the German report has not been translated, though a summary was disseminated in a press release issued the day the opinion was published. I am indebted to Andrea Tschemplik for her assistance with and translation of the German text.

References

18 U.S.C. § 116. 1996. Female Genital Mutilation.

Aaronson, Ian A. 1999. "When and How to Screen? Editorial Comment on 'The Child with Ambiguous Genitalia.'" *Infectious Urology* 12(4): 113–119.

Aaronson, Ian A., and Alistair J. Aaronson. 2010. "How Should We Classify Intersex Disorders?" *Journal of Pediatric Urology* 6(5): 443–446.

Abramson, Paul R., and Steven D. Pinkerton. 1995. *With Pleasure: Thoughts on the Nature of Human Sexuality*. New York: Oxford University Press.

Abusharaf, Rogia Mustafa. 2001. "Virtuous Cuts: Female Genital Circumcision in an African Ontology." *Differences: A Journal of Feminist Cultural Studies* 12(1): 112–140.

Ahmadu, Fuambai. 2000. "Rites and Wrongs: An Insider/Outsider Reflects on Power and Excision." In Shell-Duncan and Hernlund, *Female Circumcision in Africa*, 283–312.

Alcoff, Linda Martín. 2006. *Visible Identities: Race, Gender, and the Self.* New York: Oxford University Press.

Alderson, Priscilla. 2006. "Who Should Decide and How?" In Parens, *Surgically Shaping Children*, 157–175.

Alexander, Tamara. 1999 [1998]. "Silence=Death." In Dreger, *Intersex in the Age of Ethics*, 103–109.

Ali, Kecia. 2006. *Sexual Ethics and Islam: Feminist Reflections on Qur'an, Hadith, and Jurisprudence*. Oxford, U.K.: Oneworld Press.

Allison, David B. 2001. *Reading the New Nietzsche: The Birth of Tragedy, Thus Spoke Zarathustra, On the Genealogy of Morals*. Lanham, Md.: Rowman and Littlefield.

Alsop, Peter. 1997. "It's Only a Wee Wee, So What's the Big Deal." In *Professional Laughter Series: Songs about Sex and Sexuality*. Moose School Records.

American Academy of Pediatrics. 2000. "Evaluation of Newborn with Developmental Anomalies of the External Genitalia." *Pediatrics* 106(1): 138–142.

Anderson, V. Elving. 2003. "Sheldon Reed, Ph.D. (November 7, 1910-February 1, 2003): Genetic Counseling, Behavioral Genetics." *American Journal of Human Genetics* 73(1): 1–4.

Andrews, Jorella. 2006. "Vision, Violence, and the Other: A Merleau-Pontean Ethics." In *Feminist Interpretations of Maurice Merleau-Ponty*, edited by Dorothea Olkowski and Gail Weiss. University Park: Pennsylvania State University Press, 167–182.

Angier, Natalie. 1997. "Sexual Identity Not Pliable After All, Report Says." *New York Times*, March 14.

Annas, George J. 1987. "Siamese Twins: Killing One to Save the Other." *Hastings Center Report* 17(2): 27–29.

Arana, Marcus de María. 2005. "A Human Rights Investigation into the Medical 'Normalization' of Intersex People: A Report of a Public Hearing by the Human Rights Commission of the City and County of San Francisco." San Francisco: Human

Rights Commission. http://www.sf-hrc.org/ftp/uploadedfiles/sfhumanrights
/Committee_Meetings/Lesbian_Gay_Bisexual_Transgender/SFHRC%20Inter-
sex%20Report(1).pdf, accessed July 10, 2012.

Arendt, Hannah. 1994 [1963]. *Eichmann in Jerusalem: A Report on the Banality of Evil.*
New York: Penguin Books.

Aristotle. 1984. *Aristotle's Nicomachean Ethics.* Translated by Hippocrates G. Apostle.
Grinnell, Iowa: Peripatetic Press.

Asch, Adrienne. 2006. "Appearance-Altering Surgery, Children's Sense of Self, and Parental Love." In Parens, *Surgically Shaping Children,* 227–252.

Aspinall, Cassandra. 2006. "Do I Make You Uncomfortable?: Reflections on Using Surgery to Reduce the Stress of Others." In Parens, *Surgically Shaping Children,* 13–28.

Baecheler, Marie-Noëlle. 2006. Letter to the Editor. *Archives of Disease in Childhood.*
http://www.adc.bmj.com/cgi/eletters/91/7/554#2562, accessed July 10, 2012.

Baran, Annette, and Ruben Pannor. 1990. "Open Adoption." In *The Psychology of Adoption,* edited by David M. Brodzinsky and Marshall D. Schechter. New York: Oxford University Press, 316–331.

Barilan, Yechiel Michael. 2012. *Human Dignity, Human Rights, and Responsibility: The
New Language of Global Bioethics and Biolaw.* Cambridge: MIT Press.

Barnwell, Ysaye Maria. 1993. "There Were No Mirrors in My Nana's House." Sweet
Honey in the Rock. In *Still on the Journey.* Redway, Calif.: EarthBeat! Records.

Bayer, Ronald. 1987. *Homosexuality and American Psychiatry: The Politics of Diagnosis.*
Princeton, N.J.: Princeton University Press.

BBC Radio. 2001. "Intersex Conditions." *BBC Woman's Hour,* December 11. http://www
.bbc.co.uk/radio4/womanshour/2001_50_tue_01.shtml, access July 3, 2012.

BBC TV. 2004. "Dr. Money and the Boy with No Penis." London: British Broadcasting
Corporation.

Beauchamp, Tom L., and James F. Childress. 2001. *Principles of Biomedical Ethics,* 5th
ed. New York: Oxford University Press.

Belmont Report. 1979. "Ethical Principles and Guidelines for the Protection of Human
Subjects of Research." Washington, D.C.: Department of Health, Education, and
Welfare. http://www.hhs.gov/ohrp/humansubjects/guidance/belmont.html, ac-
cessed July 9, 2012.

Bergoffen, Debra B. 2012. *Contesting the Politics of Genocidal Rape: Affirming the Dignity of the Vulnerable Body.* New York: Routledge.

Bernhardt, Barbara A. 1997. "Empirical Evidence That Genetic Counseling Is Directive:
Where Do We Go from Here?" *American Journal of Human Genetics* 60: 17–20.

Biale, Rachel. 1984. *Women and Jewish Law: The Essential Texts, Their History, and Their
Relevance for Today.* New York: Schocken Books.

Biddle, Jennifer. 1997. "Shame." *Australian Feminist Studies* 12(26): 227–239.

Bing, Elizabeth, and Evelyn Rudikoff. 1970. "Divergent Ways of Dealing with Hermaphrodite Children." *Medical Aspects of Human Sexuality,* December: 77.

"Biological Imperative." 1973. *Time,* January 8: 44–46.

Bocanete, Andrea Castillo. 2009. "¿Qué es doctor, niño o niña?: prácticas médicas en
torno a la intersexualidad." PhD diss., Facultad de Ciencias Sociales, Departa-
mento de Antropología, Pontificia Universidad Javeriana.

Boddy, Janice. 2007. "Gender Crusades: The Female Circumcision Controversy in Cultural Perspective." In Hernlund and Shell-Duncan, *Transcultural Bodies,* 46–66.

Bourdieu, Pierre. 1990 [1980]. *The Logic of Practice.* Translated by Richard Nice. Stanford, Calif.: Stanford University Press.

Bradley, S. J., G. D. Oliver, A. B. Chernick, and K. J. Zucker. 1998. "Experiment of Nurture: Ablatio Penis at 2 Months, Sex Reassignment at 7 Months, and a Psychosexual Follow-up in Young Adulthood." *Pediatrics* 102(1): e9.

Bredimus, Kate. 2001. "No Dream Too Big, No Dreamer Too Small." *Richmond.com.* http://www2.richmond.com/entertainment/2001/apr/27/no-dream-too-big-no-dreamer-too-small-ar-607826/, accessed March 17, 2012.

Butler, Judith. 1990. *Gender Trouble: Feminism and the Subversion of Identity.* New York: Routledge.

———. 1997. *The Psychic Life of Power: Theories in Subjection.* Palo Alto, Calif.: Stanford University Press.

———. 2005. "Merleau-Ponty and the Touch of Malebranche." In *The Cambridge Companion to Merleau-Ponty,* edited by Taylor Carman and Mark B. N. Hansen. New York: Cambridge University Press, 181–205.

Callahan, Daniel. 1970. "Institute of Society, Ethics, and the Life Sciences: A Survey of Goals, Plans, and Budgetary Needs." Rockefeller Brothers Fund, Rockefeller Archives. In folder ISELS: 1.

———. 1973. "Bioethics as a Discipline." *Hastings Center Studies* 1: 66–73.

———. 1996. "Calling Scientific Ideology to Account." *Society* 33(4): 14–19.

Cameron, David. 1999. "Caught Between: An Essay on Intersexuality." In Dreger, *Intersex in the Age of Ethics,* 90–96.

———. 2006. Letter to the Editor. *Archives of Disease in Childhood.* http://www.adc.bmj.com/cgi/eletters/91/7/554#2479, accessed July 10, 2012.

Canguilhem, Georges. 1991 [1966]. *The Normal and the Pathological.* Translated by Carolyn R. Fawcett with Robert S. Cohen. New York: Zone Books.

Caplan, Arthur L. 1993. "Neutrality Is Not Morality: The Ethics of Genetic Counseling." In *Prescribing Our Future: Ethical Challenges in Genetic Counseling,* edited by Dianne M. Bartels, Bonnie S. LeRoy, and Arthur L. Caplan. New York: Aldine de Gruyter, 149–165.

Carman, Taylor. 1999. "The Body in Husserl and Merleau-Ponty." *Philosophical Topics* 27(2): 205–226.

Casper, Monica J., and Courtney Muse. 2006. "Genital Fixations." San Francisco: Center for Research and Education on Gender and Sexuality, March 16. http://cregs.sfsu.edu/article/genital_fixations_intersex, accessed July 10, 2012.

Center for the Study and Treatment of Hypospadias. 2013. "Mission Statement." http://www.urology.ucsf.edu/research/children/center-study-treatment-hypospadias, accessed March 26, 2013.

Chase, Cheryl. 1993. Letter to the Editor. *The Sciences,* July/August: 3.

———. 1996. *Hermaphrodites Speak!* Rohnert Park, Calif.: Intersex Society of North America.

———. 1999. "Surgical Progress Is Not the Answer." In Dreger, *Intersex in the Age of Ethics,* 146–159.

———. 2003. "What Is the Agenda of the Intersex Patient Advocacy Movement?" *The Endocrinologist* 13(3): 240–242.

———. 2006. "Disorders of Sex Development Similar to More Familiar Disorders." *Archives of Disease in Childhood.* http://adc.bmj.com/cgi/eletters/91/7/554, accessed July 11, 2012.

Chase, Cheryl, and Ian Aaronson. 2000. "North American Task Force on Intersex Formed." Intersex Society of North America, February 23. http://www.isna.org /node/153, accessed July 6, 2012.

Chase, Cheryl, and Martha Coventry, eds. 1997. "Intersex Awakening." Special issue, *Chrysalis: The Journal of Transgressive Identities* 2(5).

Chase, Cheryl, with Alice Dreger. 2000. "Shifting the Paradigm of Intersex Treatment." Intersex Society of North America. http://www.isna.org/pdf/compare.pdf, accessed July 5, 2012.

Chen, Pauline W. 2012. "When Doctors Don't Tell the Truth." *New York Times,* March 1. http://well.blogs.nytimes.com/2012/03/01/when-doctors-dont-tell-the-truth/, accessed March 31, 2012.

Chitty, Lyn S., Pierre Chatelain, Katja P. Wolffenbuttel, and Yves Aigrain. 2012. "Prenatal Management of Disorders of Sex Development." *Journal of Pediatric Urology* 8(6): 576–84.

Cohen, Deborah. 2013. *Family Secrets: Shame and Privacy in Modern Britain.* New York: Oxford University Press.

Cohen, Susan, and Christina Cosgrove. 2009. *Normal at Any Cost: Tall Girls, Short Boys, and the Medical Industry's Quest to Manipulate Height.* New York: Penguin.

———. 2010. "The Art of Medicine: Too Tall, Too Small? The Temptation to Tinker with a Child's Height." *Lancet* 375: 454–455.

Colapinto, John. 1997. "The True Story of John/Joan." *Rolling Stone,* December 11: 54–97.

———. 2000. *As Nature Made Him: The Boy Who Was Raised as a Girl.* New York: Harper-Collins.

———. 2004. "What Were the Real Reasons David Reimer Committed Suicide?" *Slate,* June 3. http://www.slate.com/articles/health_and_science/medical_examiner /2004/06/gender_gap.html, accessed June 18, 2012.

Consortium on the Management of Disorders of Sex Development. 2006a. *Clinical Guidelines for the Management of Disorders of Sex Development in Childhood.* Whitehouse Station, N.J.: Accord Alliance. http://www.accordalliance.org /dsdguidelines/clinical.pdf, accessed July 6, 2012.

———. 2006b. *Handbook for Parents.* Whitehouse Station, N.J.: Accord Alliance. http:// www.accordalliance.org/dsdguidelines/parents.pdf, accessed July 6, 2012.

Cooley, Charles Horton. 1964 [1902]. *Human Nature and Social Order.* New York: Charles Scribner's Sons.

Cornell, Drucilla. 1995. *The Imaginary Domain: Abortion, Pornography, and Sexual Harassment.* New York: Routledge.

Coventry, Martha. 1999. "Finding the Words." In Dreger, *Intersex in the Age of Ethics,* 71–78.

Creighton, Sarah. 2002. "Surgery for Intersex." *Journal of the Royal Society of Medicine* 94: 218–220.

Daaboul, Jorge J. 2000. "Does the Study of History Affect Clinical Practice? Intersex as a Case Study: The Physician's View." Paper presented at the annual meeting of American Association for the History of Medicine, Bethesda, Maryland. http:// www.isna.org/articles/daaboul_history, accessed July 9, 2012.

Dayner, Jennifer, Peter A. Lee, and Christopher P. Houk. 2004. "Medical Treatment of Intersex: Parental Perspectives." *Journal of Urology* 172: 1762–1765.

Devore, Howard. 1999. "Growing Up in the Surgical Maelstrom." In Dreger, *Intersex in the Age of Ethics,* 78–81.

Diamond, Milton, and Hazel G. Beh. 2006. Letter to the Editor. *Archives of Disease in Childhood.* http://www.adc.bmj.com/cgi/eletters/91/7/554#2460, accessed July 10, 2012.

Diamond, Milton, and Keith Sigmundson. 1997. "Sex Reassignment at Birth: Long-term Review and Clinical Application." *Archives of Pediatric and Adolescent Medicine* 15(11): 298–304.

Dickinson, Robert Latou. 1949. *Atlas of Human Sex Anatomy,* 2nd ed. Baltimore: Williams and Wilkins.

Diprose, Rosalyn. 2002. *Corporeal Generosity: On Giving with Nietzsche, Merleau-Ponty, and Levinas.* Albany: SUNY Press.

Dreger, Alice Domurat. 1996. "Hermaphrodites in Love: The Truth of the Gonads." In *Science and Homosexualities,* edited by Vernon Rosario, New York: Routledge, 46–66.

———. 1998a. "Ambiguous Sex"—or Ambivalent Medicine? *Hastings Center Report* 28(3): 24–35.

———. 1998b. *Hermaphrodites and the Medical Invention of Sex.* Cambridge, Mass.: Harvard University Press.

———. 1998c. "Intersexuality." Special issue, *Journal of Clinical Ethics* 9(4).

———. 1999a. "A History of Intersex: From the Age of the Gonads to the Age of Consent." In Dreger, *Intersex in the Age of Ethics,* 5–22.

———, ed. 1999b. *Intersex in the Age of Ethics.* Hagerstown, Md.: University Publishing Group.

———. 2000. "Jarring Bodies: Thoughts on the Display of Unusual Anatomies." *Perspectives in Biology and Medicine* 43(2): 151–172.

———. 2002. "Intersex." *FatherMag.com,* July 23. http://www.fathermag.com/206/intersex/, accessed March 14, 2010.

———. 2004. *One of Us: Conjoined Twins and the Future of Normal.* Cambridge, Mass.: Harvard University Press.

———. 2006a. "Intersex and Human Rights: The Long View." In Sytsma, *Ethics and Intersex,* 73–86.

———. 2006b. "What to Expect When You Have the Child You Weren't Expecting." In Parens, *Surgically Shaping Children,* 253–266.

———. 2010a. "Issue: Reasonable Experiment?" Fetaldex.org. http://www.fetaldex.org/experimentation.html, accessed April 27, 2012.

———. 2010b. "To Have Is to Hold." *Psychology Today* Blog. http://www.psychologytoday.com/blog/fetishes-i-dont-get/201006/have-is-hold-0, accessed March 5, 2012.

———. 2011. "Are Children Dying for an Inch or Two? The Ethics and Dangers of Treating Children with Height-boosting Drugs." *Chicago Tribune,* March 20. http://articles.chicagotribune.com/2011-03-20/news/ct-perspec-0320-height-20110320_1_growth-hormone-hgh-drug-companies, accessed July 5, 2012.

Dreger, Alice Domurat, and Cheryl Chase. 1999. "A Mother's Care: An Interview with 'Sue' and 'Margaret.'" In Dreger, *Intersex in the Age of Ethics,* 83–89.

Dreger, A. D., C. Chase, A. Sousa, P. A. Gruppuso, and J. Frader. 2005. "Changing the Nomenclature/Taxonomy for Intersex: A Scientific and Clinical Rationale." *Journal of Pediatric Endocrinology and Metabolism* 18(8): 729–733.

Dreger, Alice, and Ellen K. Feder. 2010. "Bad Vibrations." *Bioethics Forum,* June 16. http://www.thehastingscenter.org/Bioethicsforum/Post.aspx?id=4730, accessed July 3, 2012.

Dreger, Alice, Ellen K. Feder, and Anne Tamar-Mattis. 2012. "Prenatal Dexamethasone for Congenital Adrenal Hyperplasia: An Ethics Canary in the Modern Medical Mine." *Journal of Bioethical Inquiry* 9(3): 277–294.

Dreger, Alice D., and April M. Herndon. 2009. "Progress and Politics in the Intersex Rights Movement: Feminist Theory in Action." *GLQ: A Journal of Lesbian and Gay Studies* 15(2): 199–224.

Dugger, Celia W. 2011. "Senegal Curbs a Bloody Rite for Girls and Women." *New York Times,* October 15.

Eder, Sandra. 2010. "The Volatility of Sex: Intersexuality, Gender and Clinical Practice in the 1950s." *Gender and History* 22(3): 692–707.

———. 2012. "From 'Following the Push of Nature' to 'Restoring One's Proper Sex'—Cortisone and Sex at Johns Hopkins's Pediatric Endocrinology Clinic." *Endeavor* 36(2): 69–76.

Elliott, Carl. 1999. *A Philosophical Disease: Bioethics, Culture, and Identity.* New York: Routledge.

———. 2003. *Better Than Well: American Medicine Meets the American Dream.* New York: W. W. Norton.

El-Or, Tamar. 1994. *Educated and Ignorant: Ultraorthodox Jewish Women and Their World.* Translated by Haim Watzman. Boulder, Colo.: Lynne Rienner.

Elwyn, Glyn, Jonathan Gray, and Angus Clarke. 2000. "Shared Decision Making and Non-directiveness in Genetic Counseling." *Journal of Medical Genetics* 37: 135–138.

Eugenides, Jeffrey. 2002. *Middlesex: A Novel.* New York: Farrar, Strauss, and Giroux.

Eugster, Erica A. 2004. "Reality vs. Recommendations in the Care of Infants with Intersex Conditions." *Archives of Pediatric Medicine* 158: 428–429.

Faden, Ruth R., and Tom L. Beauchamp. 1986. *A History and Theory of Informed Consent.* New York: Oxford University Press.

Fausto-Sterling, Anne. 1993. "The Five Sexes." *The Sciences* (March/April): 20–24.

———. 2000. *Sexing the Body: Gender Politics and the Construction of Sexuality.* New York: Basic Books.

Feder, Ellen K. 2007. *Family Bonds: Genealogies of Race and Gender.* New York: Oxford University Press.

Fineman, Martha. 1995. *The Neutered Mother, the Sexual Family, and Other Twentieth-Century Tragedies.* New York: Routledge.

FitzGerald, Eileen. 2004. "Lesson on Dwarfism Touches Studies." *Danbury News-Times,* November 30. http://www.newstimes.com/news/article/Lesson-on-dwarfism-touches-students-89129.php, accessed July 6, 2012.

Flax, Jane. 2004. "The Scandal of Desire: Psychoanalysis and Disruptions of Gender." *Contemporary Psychoanalysis* 40(1): 47–68.

Foucault, Michel. 1979 [1975]. *Discipline and Punish: The Birth of the Prison.* Translated by Alan Sheridan. New York: Vintage.

———. 1988 [1984]. *The History of Sexuality,* vol. 3: *The Care of the Self.* Translated by Robert Hurley. New York: Vintage.

———. 1990 [1976]. *The History of Sexuality,* vol. 1: *An Introduction.* Translated by Robert Hurley. New York: Vintage.

———. 1994 [1963]. *The Birth of the Clinic: An Archaeology of Medical Perception.* Translated by A. M. Sheridan Smith. New York: Vintage.

———. 1996. "The Social Extension of the Norm," interview by T. Warner. In *Foucault*

Live: Collected Interviews, 1961–1984, 2nd ed., edited by Silvère Lotringer, translated by Lysa Hochroth and John Johnston. New York: Semiotext(e), 196–199.

———. 1997 [1984]. "The Ethics of the Concern for Self as a Practice of Freedom." In *Michel Foucault: Ethics, Subjectivity and Truth*, edited by Paul Rabinow, 281–301.

———. 2001. *Fearless Speech*. Edited by Joseph Pearson. New York: Semiotexte.

———. 2003 [1999]. *Abnormal: Lectures at the College de France, 1974–75*. Edited by Valerio Marchetti and Antonella Salomoni. Translated by Graham Burchell. New York: Picador.

———. 2005 [2001]. *The Hermeneutics of the Subject: Lectures at the Collège de France 1981–1982*. Edited by Frédéric Gros. Translated by Graham Burchell. New York: Picador.

Frader, Joel, et al. 2004. "Health Care Professionals and Intersex Conditions." *Archives of Pediatric Medicine* 158: 426–428.

Freud, Sigmund. 2005 [1930]. *Civilization and Its Discontents*. Translated by James Strachey. New York: W. W. Norton.

German Ethics Council. 2012. "Intersexualität: Stellungnahme." *Deutscher Ethikrat* 23 (February). http://www.ethikrat.org/dateien/pdf/stellungnahme-intersexualitaet .pdf, accessed March 28, 2013.

Germon, Jennifer. 2009. *Gender: A Genealogy of an Idea*. New York: Palgrave MacMillan.

Gilman, Sander L. 1985. *Difference and Pathology: Stereotypes of Sexuality, Race, and Madness*. Ithaca, N.Y.: Cornell University Press.

Glassberg, Kenneth. 1999. "Gender Assignment and the Pediatric Urologist." *Journal of Urology* 161 (April): 1308–1310.

Goffman, Erving. 1963. *Stigma: Notes on the Management of Spoiled Identity*. Englewood Cliffs, N.J.: Prentice-Hall.

Golomb, Jacob, ed. 1997. *Nietzsche and Jewish Culture*. New York: Routledge.

Gough, Brendan, Nicky Weyman, Julie Alderson, Gary Butler, and Mandy Stoner. 2008. "'They Did Not Have a Word': The Parental Quest to Locate a 'True Sex' for Their Intersex Children." *Psychology and Health* 23(4): 493–507.

Gray, Hillel. 2012. "Not Judging by Appearances: The Role of Genotype in Jewish Law on Intersexuality." *Shofar: An Interdisciplinary Journal of Jewish Studies* 30(4): 126–149.

Greenberg, Julie A. 2012. *Intersexuality and the Law: Why Sex Matters*. New York: New York University Press.

Gross, Robert E., Judson Randolph, and John F. Crigler. 1966. "Clitorectomy for Sexual Abnormalities: Indications and Technique." *Pediatric Surgery* 59(2): 300–308.

Grosz, Elizabeth. 1994. *Volatile Bodies: Toward a Corporeal Feminism*. Bloomington: Indiana University Press.

Guterman, Lydia. 2012. "Why Are Doctors Still Performing Genital Surgery on Infants?" *Open Society Foundations*, January 30. http://www.soros.org/voices/why-are -doctors-still-performing-genital-surgery-on-infants, accessed June 14, 2012.

Hacking, Ian. 1986. "Making Up People." In *Reconstructing Individualism: Autonomy, Individuality, and the Self in Western Thought*, edited by Thomas C. Heller, Morton Sosna, and David E. Wellbery with Arnold I. Davidson, Ann Swidler, and Ian Watt. Stanford, Calif.: Stanford University Press, 222–236.

Hampson, Joan G. 1955. "Hermaphroditic Genital Appearance, Rearing and Eroticism in Hyperandrenocortism." *Bulletin of the Johns Hopkins Hospital* 96(6): 265–273.

Hampson, John L., and Joan G. Hampson. 1961. "The Ontogenesis of Sexual Behavior in Man." In *Sex and Internal Secretion*, edited by W. C. Young and G. W. Corner. Baltimore: Williams and Wilkins, 1401–1432.

Hass, Lawrence. 2008. "Elemental Alterity: Levinas and Merleau-Ponty." In *Intertwinings: Interdisciplinary Encounters with Merleau-Ponty*, edited by Gail Weiss. Albany: SUNY Press, 31–44.

Hawbecker, Hale. 1999. "Who Did This to You?" In Dreger, *Intersex in the Age of Ethics*, 111–113.

Hedley, Lisa Abelow. 2001. *Dwarfs: Not a Fairy Tale*. America Undercover Series. HBO Studios.

Hermer, Laura. 2002. "Paradigms Revised: Intersex Children, Bioethics and the Law." *Annals of Health Law* 11: 195–236.

Hernlund, Ylva, and Bettina Shell-Duncan. 2007. "Transcultural Positions: Negotiating Rights and Culture." In Hernlund and Shell-Duncan, *Transcultural Bodies*, 1–45.

Hester, J. David. 2006. "Intersex and the Rhetorics of Healing." In Sytsma, *Ethics and Intersex*, 47–72.

Holmes, Morgan. 2000. "Queer Cut Bodies." In *Queer Frontiers: Millennial Geographies, Genders, and Generations*, edited by Joseph A. Boone, Debra Silverman, Cindy Sarver, Karin Quimby, Martin Dupuis, Martin Meeker, and Rosemary Weatherston. Madison: University of Wisconsin Press, 84–110.

———. 2008. *Intersex: A Perilous Difference*. Selinsgrove, PA: Susquehanna University Press.

Hoopes, Janet L. 1990. "Adoption and Identity Formation." In *The Psychology of Adoption*, edited by David M. Brodzinsky and Marshall D. Schechter. New York: Oxford University Press, 144–166.

Horton, Charles E., and Charles J. Devine. 1970. "A One-stage Repair for Hypospadias Cripples." *Plastic and Reconstructive Surgery* 45(5): 425–430.

Houtzager, Bregje A., Frans J. Oort, Josette E. H. M. Hoekstra-Weebers, Huib N. Caron, Martha A. Grootenhuis, and Bob F. Last. 2004. "Coping and Family Functioning Predict Longitudinal Psychological Adaptation of Siblings of Childhood Cancer Patients." *Journal of Pediatric Psychology* 29(8): 591–605.

Howe, Edmund G. 1998. "Intersexuality: What Should Care Providers Do Now?" *Journal of Clinical Ethics* 9(4): 337–344.

———. 1999. "Intersexuality: What Should Care Providers Do Now?" In Dreger, *Intersex in the Age of Ethics*, 211–223.

Howell, Brian M., and Jenell Williams Paris. 2011. *Introducing Cultural Anthropology: A Christian Perspective*. Grand Rapids, Mich.: Baker Academic.

Hughes, I. A., C. Houk, S. F. Ahmed, and P. A. Lee. 2006. "Consensus Statement on Management of Intersex Conditions." *Archives of Disease in Childhood* 91(7): 554–563.

Hursthouse, Rosalind. 1999. *On Virtue Ethics*. Oxford, U.K.: Oxford University Press.

Hurwitz, Richard S. 2010. "Long-Term Outcomes in Male Patients with Sex Development Disorders—How Are We Doing and How Can We Improve?" *Journal of Urology* 184(3): 831–832.

———. 2011. "Feminizing Surgery for Disorders of Sex Development: Evolution, Complications, and Outcomes." *Current Urology Reports* 12:166–172.

Iezzoni, Lisa I., Sowmya R. Rao, Catherine M. DesRoches, Christine Vogeli, and Eric

G. Campbell. 2012. "Survey Shows That at Least Some Physicians Are Not Always Open or Honest with Patients." *Health Affairs* 31(2): 383–391.

Imperato-McGinley, J., R. E. Peterson, R. Stoller, and W. E. Goodwin. 1979. "Male Pseudohermaphroditism Secondary to 17 Beta-Hydroxysteroid Dehydrogenase Deficiency: Gender Role Change with Puberty." *Journal of Clinical Endocrinology and Metabolism* 49: 391–395.

International Military Tribunal. 1947–1949. *Trial of the Major War Criminals before the International Military Tribunal, Nuremberg, 14 November 1945–1 October 1946.* Nuremberg, Germany: Secretariat of the International Military Tribunal. http://www.loc.gov/rr/frd/Military_Law/NT_major-war-criminals.html, accessed July 10, 2012.

Intersex Society of North America. Nd. *How Common Is Intersex?* http://www.isna.org/faq/frequency, accessed March 29, 2013.

Irigaray, Luce. 1993 [1984]. *An Ethics of Sexual Difference.* Translated by Carolyn Burke and Gillian C. Gill. Ithaca, N.Y.: Cornell University Press.

Johnsdotter, Sara. 2007. "Persistence of Tradition or Reassessment of Cultural Practices in Exile?: Discourses on Female Circumcision among and about Swedish Somalis." In Hernlund and Shell-Duncan, *Transcultural Bodies,* 107–134.

Johnson, Michelle C. 2007. "Making Mandinga or Making Muslims?: Debating Female Circumcision, Ethnicity, and Islam in Guinea-Bissau and Portugal." In Hernlund and Shell-Duncan, *Transcultural Bodies,* 202–223.

Jones, Howard W., and William Wallace Scott. 1958. *Hermaphroditism, Genital Anomalies, and Related Endocrine Disorders.* Baltimore: Williams and Wilkins.

Jones, James H. 1993. *Bad Blood: The Tuskegee Syphilis Experiment,* revised ed. New York: Free Press.

Jonsen, Albert R. 1998. *The Birth of Bioethics.* New York: Oxford University Press.

Jouanna, Jacques. 1998. *Hippocrates.* Translated by Malcolm B. DeBevoise. Baltimore: Johns Hopkins University Press.

Kant, Immanuel. 1964 [1785]. *Groundwork of the Metaphysic of Morals.* Translated by H. J. Paton. New York: Harper and Row.

———. 1996 [1797]. *The Metaphysics of Morals.* Translated and edited by Mary Gregor. Cambridge, U.K.: Cambridge University Press.

Karkazis, Katrina. 2005. "Beyond Treatment: Broadening Debates over Genital Surgery for Intersex Infants." American Psychological Association Annual Meeting, Washington, DC, August 18.

———. 2008. *Fixing Sex: Intersex, Medical Authority, and Lived Experience.* Durham, N.C.: Duke University Press.

Karkazis, Katrina, and Wilma C. Rossi. 2010. "Ethics for the Pediatrician: Disorders of Sex Development: Optimizing Care." *Pediatrics in Review* 31: e82–e85. http://pedsinreview.aapublications.org/cgi/content/full/31/11/e82, accessed March 22, 2013.

Karkazis, Katrina, Anne Tamar-Mattis, and Alexander A. Kon. 2010. "Genital Surgery for Disorders of Sex Development: Implementing a Shared Decision-Making Approach." *Journal of Pediatric Endocrinology and Metabolism* 23: 789–806.

Katz, Jonathan Ned. 1995. *The Invention of Heterosexuality.* New York: Dutton.

Kenen, Stephanie Hope. 1998. "Scientific Studies of Human Sexual Difference in Interwar America." PhD diss., University of California, Berkeley.

Kessler, Seymour. 1997. "Genetic Counseling Is Directive? Look Again." Letter to the Editor. *American Journal of Human Genetics* 61: 466–467.

Kessler, Suzanne J. 1990. "The Medical Construction of Gender: Case Management of Intersexed Infants." *Signs: Journal of Women in Culture and Society* 16(1): 3–26.

———. 1998. *Lessons from the Intersexed.* New Brunswick, N.J.: Rutgers University Press.

Kim. 1999. "As Is." In Dreger, *Intersex in the Age of Ethics,* 91.

Kipnis, Kenneth, and Milton Diamond. 1999 [1998]. "Pediatric Ethics and the Surgical Assignment of Sex." In Dreger, *Intersex in the Age of Ethics,* 172–193.

Kittay, Eva Feder. 1983. "Womb Envy: An Explanatory Concept." In *Mothering: Essays in Feminist Theory,* edited by Joyce Trebilcot. Totowa, N.J.: Rowman and Allanheld, 94–128.

———. 1999. *Love's Labor: Essays on Women, Equality and Dependency.* New York: Routledge.

———. 2006. "Thoughts on the Desire for Normality." In Parens, *Surgically Shaping Children,* 90–110.

———. 2009. "The Ethics of Philosophizing: Ideal Theory and the Exclusion of People with Severe Cognitive Disabilities." *Feminist Ethics and Social Political Philosophy* 2: 121–146.

Klein, Melanie. 1975 [1957]. "Envy and Gratitude." In *Envy and Gratitude and Other Works 1946–1963.* New York: New Press, 176–235.

Kushner, Robert F., Sheila Kessler, and William C. McGaghie. 2011. "Using Behavior Change Plans to Improve Medical Student Self-Care." *Academic Medicine* 86(7): 901–906.

La Leche League International. Nd. "Mission Statement." http://lalecheleague.org/, accessed July 3, 2012.

Lacan, Jacques. 1977 [1966]. "The Mirror Stage as Formative of the Function of the I." In *Écrits: A Selection.* Translated by Alan Sheridan. New York: W. W. Norton, 1–7.

Laqueur, Thomas. 1990. *Making Sex: Body and Gender from the Greeks to Freud.* Cambridge, Mass.: Harvard University Press.

Lee, Peter A., and Christopher P. Houk. 2010. "The Role of Support Groups, Advocacy Groups, and Other Interested Parties in Improving the Care of Patients with Congenital Adrenal Hyperplasia: Pleas and Warnings." *International Journal of Pediatric Endocrinology.* http://www.ncbi.nlm.nih.gov/pmc/articles/PMC2905711/, accessed July 3, 20012.

Lehrman, Sally. 1999. "Sex Police." *Salon.com,* April 5. http://www.salon.com/health/feature/1999/04/05/sex_police/pring.html, accessed April 5, 2011.

Leighton, Kimberly. 2012. "Addressing the Harms of Not Knowing One's Heredity: Lessons from Genealogical Bewilderment." *Adoption and Culture* 3: 63–107.

Lenman, James. 2008. "Moral Naturalism." In *The Stanford Encyclopedia of Philosophy* (Winter 2008 Edition), edited by Edward N. Zalta. http://plato.stanford.edu/archives/win2008/entries/naturalism-moral/, accessed January 12, 2013.

Leslie, Jeffrey A., Mark Patrick Cain, and Richard Carlos Rink. 2009. "Feminizing Genital Reconstruction in Congenital Adrenal Hyperplasia." *Indian Journal of Urology* 25(1): 17–26.

Lindemann, Hilde. 2006a. "Bioethics' Gender." *American Journal of Bioethics* 6(2): W15–W19.

———. 2006b. "The Power of Parents and the Agency of Children." In Parens, *Surgically Shaping Children,* 176–188.

Lindemann, Hilde, Ellen K. Feder, and Alice Dreger. 2010. "Fetal Cosmetology." *Bioethics Forum,* February 8. http://www.thehastingscenter.org/Bioethicsforum/Post .aspx?id=4470, accessed July 6, 2012.

Lingis, Alphonso. 2003. "The Immoralist." In *The Ethical,* edited by Edith Wyschogrod and Gerald P. McKenny. Oxford, U.K.: Blackwell, 197–216.

Lloyd, G. E. R., ed. 1983. *Hippocratic Writings.* Translated by J. Chadwick. New York: Penguin.

Loveman, Samuel. 1936. *The Hermaphrodite and Other Poems.* Caldwell, Idaho: Caxton Printers.

Mackie, Gerry. 1996. "Ending Footbinding and Infibulation: A Convention Account." *American Sociological Review* 61(6): 999–1017.

———. 2000. "Female Genital Cutting: The Beginning of the End." In Shell-Duncan and Hernlund, *Female Circumcision in Africa,* 253–281.

Malmqvist, Erik, and Kristin Zeiler. 2010. "Cultural Norms, the Phenomenology of Incorporation, and the Experience of Having a Child Born with Ambiguous Sex." *Social Theory and Practice* 36(1): 133–156.

Marks, J. H. 1993. "The Training of Genetic Counselors: Origins of a Psychosocial Model." In *Prescribing Our Future: Ethical Challenges in Genetic Counseling,* edited by D. M. Bartels, B. S. LeRoy, and A. L. Caplan. New York: Aldine de Gruyter, 15–24.

Marsh, Jeffrey L. 2006. "To Cut or Not to Cut? A Surgeon's Perspective on Surgically Shaping Children." In Parens, *Surgically Shaping Children,* 113–124.

McCumber, John. 1996. "Time in the Ditch: American Philosophy and the McCarthy Era." *Diacritics* 26(1): 33–49.

———. 2001. *Time in the Ditch: American Philosophy and the McCarthy Era.* Chicago: Northwestern University Press.

Méndez, Juan E. 2013. "Report of the Special Rapporteur on Torture and Other Cruel, Inhuman, or Degrading Treatment or Punishment. Human Rights Council." United Nations General Assembly. 22nd session, February 1. http://www.ohchr .org/Documents/HRBodies/HRCouncil/RegularSession/Session22/A.HRC.22.53 _English.pdf, accessed March 22, 2013.

Menvielle, Edgardo. 1998. "Gender Identity Disorder." Letter to the Editor. *Journal of the American Academy of Child and Adolescent Psychiatry* 37(3): 243–244.

Merleau-Ponty, Maurice. 1962 [1945]. *Phenomenology of Perception.* Translated by Colin Smith. New York: Humanities Press.

———. 1964 [1960]. "The Child's Relation with Others." In *The Primacy of Perception,* translated by William Cobb, edited by James M. Edie. Evanston, Ill.: Northwestern University Press, 96–155.

———. 2001 [1968]. *The Incarnate Subject: Malebranche, Biran, and Bergson on the Union of Body and Soul.* Translated by Paul B. Milan, eds. Andrew G. Bjelland Jr. and Patrick Burke. Amherst, N.Y.: Humanity Books.

Meyer, Don, ed. 2009. *Thicker Than Water: Essays by Adult Siblings of People with Disabilities.* Bethesda, Md.: Woodbine House.

Meyer-Bahlburg, Heino F. L. 1994. "Intersexuality and the Diagnosis of Gender Identity Disorder." *Archives of Sexual Behavior* 23(1): 21–40.

———. 1999. "Gender Assignment and Reassignment in 46,XY Pseudohermaphroditism and Related Conditions." *Journal of Clinical Endocrinology and Metabolism* 84(10): 3455–3458.

——. 2005a. "Intersex—Fact or Fiction?" *Journal of Sex Research* 42(2): 177–180.

——. 2005b. "Gender Identity Outcome in Female-Raised 46,XY Persons with Penile Agenisis, Cloacal Exstophy of the Bladder, or Penile Ablation." *Archives of Sexual Behavior* 34(4): 423–438.

Meyer-Bahlburg, Heino F. L., C. J. Migeon, G. D. Berkowitz, J. P. Gearhart, C. Dolezal, and A. B. Wisniewski. 2004. "Attitudes of Adult 46 XY Intersex Persons to Clinical Management Policies." *Journal of Urology* 171(4): 1615–19.

Mill, John Stuart. 2001 [1861]. *Utilitarianism,* 2nd ed. Indianapolis: Hackett.

Miller, William Ian. 1997. *The Anatomy of Disgust.* Cambridge, Mass.: Harvard University Press.

Mills, Catherine. 2011. *Futures of Reproduction: Bioethics and Biopolitics.* New York: Springer.

Minto, Catherine L., Lih-Mei Liao, Christopher R. J. Woodhouse, Philip G. Ransley, and Sarah M. Creighton. 2003. "The Effects of Clitoral Surgery on Sexual Outcome in Individuals Who Have Intersex Conditions with Ambiguous Genitalia: A Cross-Sectional Study." *Lancet* 361:1252–1257.

Mitchell, David T., and Sharon L. Snyder. 1997. "Introduction: Disability Studies and the Double Bind of Representation." In *The Body and Physical Difference: Discourses of Disability,* edited by David T. Mitchell and Sharon L. Snyder. Ann Arbor: University of Michigan Press.

Mom Enough. 2011. "Do You Feel Pulled Hither and Thither by Each New Bit of Parenting Advice That Comes Your Way?" Podcast. *Mom Enough,* July 4. http://momenough.com/?p=1549, accessed February 2, 2012.

Money, John. 1952. "Hermaphroditism: An Inquiry into the Nature of a Human Paradox." PhD diss., Cambridge, Mass.: Harvard University.

——. 1955. "Hermaphroditism, Gender, and Precocity in Hyperadrenocorticism: Psychological Findings." *Bulletin of the Johns Hopkins Hospital* 96(6): 253–264.

——. 1986. *Venuses Penises: Sexology, Sexosophy, and Exigency Theory.* Buffalo, N.Y.: Prometheus Press.

Money, John, and Anke A. Ehrhardt. 1982. *Man and Woman, Boy and Girl.* Baltimore: Johns Hopkins University Press.

Money, John, Joan G. Hampson, and John L. Hampson. 1955. "Hermaphroditism: Recommendations Concerning Assignment of Sex, Change of Sex, and Psychologic Management." *Bulletin of the Johns Hopkins Hospital* 97(4): 284–300.

Moreno, Angela. 1999. "In Amerika They Call Us Hermaphrodites." In Dreger, *Intersex in the Age of Ethics,* 137–140.

Morland, Iain. 2011. "Intersex Treatment and the Promise of Trauma." In *Gender and the Science of Difference: Cultural Politics of Contemporary Science and Medicine,* edited by Jill A. Fisher. New Brunswick, N.J.: Rutgers University Press, 147–163.

Morris, Sherri G. 2006. "Twisted Lies: My Journey in an Imperfect Body." In Parens, *Surgically Shaping Children,* 3–12.

Mouradian, Wendy E. 2006. "What's Special about the Surgical Context?" In Parens, *Surgically Shaping Children,* 125–140.

Mouradian, Wendy E., Todd C. Edwards, Tari D. Topolski, Nichola Rumsey, and Donald L. Patrick. 2006. "Are We Helping Children? Outcome Assessments in Craniofacial Care." In Parens, *Surgically Shaping Children,* 141–156.

New, Maria I., and Saroj Nimkarn. 2006 [2002]. "21-Hydroxylase-Deficient Congenital Adrenal Hyperplasia." *GeneReviews.* Seattle: University of Washington.

Nicholson, Sven. 1999. "Take charge! A Guide to Home Auto-Catheterization." In Dreger, *Intersex in the Age of Ethics*, 201–210.

Nietzsche, Friedrich. 1967 [1872]. *Birth of Tragedy and the Case of Wagner.* Translated by Walter Kaufmann. New York: Vintage Books.

———. 1973 [1886]. *Beyond Good and Evil: Prelude to a Philosophy of the Future.* Translated by R. J. Hollingdale. New York: Penguin Classics.

———. 1974 [1887]. *The Gay Science.* Translated by Walter Kaufmann. New York: Vintage Books.

———. 1998 [1887]. *On the Genealogy of Morality.* Translated by Maudemarie Clark and Alan J. Swensen. Indianapolis: Hackett.

———. 2009 [1889]. *Twilight of the Idols: or How to Philosophize with a Hammer.* Translated by Duncan Large. New York: Oxford University Press.

Nour, Nawal M. 2012. "Using Facts to Moderate the Message." *Hastings Center Report* 24(6): 30–31.

Nussbaum, Martha. 2004. *Hiding from Humanity: Disgust, Shame, and the Law.* Princeton, N.J.: Princeton University Press.

———. 2010. *From Disgust to Humanity: Sexual Orientation and Constitutional Law.* New York: Oxford University Press.

Obiora, L. Amede. 2007. "A Refuse from Tradition and the Refuge of Tradition: On Anticircumcision Paradigms." In Hernlund and Shell-Duncan, *Transcultural Bodies,* 67–90.

Oduncu, Fuat S. 2002. "The Role of Non-Directiveness in Genetic Counseling." *Medicine, Health Care, and Philosophy* 5: 53–63.

O'Neill, Onora. 2002. *Autonomy and Trust in Bioethics: The Gifford Lectures, University of Edinburgh, 2001.* Cambridge, U.K.: Cambridge University Press.

Parens, Erik, ed. 1998. *Enhancing Human Traits: Ethical and Social Implications.* Washington, D.C.: Georgetown University Press.

———. 2006. "Introduction: Thinking about Surgically Shaping Children." In *Surgically Shaping Children: Technology, Ethics, and the Pursuit of Normality, edited by* Erik Parens. Baltimore: Johns Hopkins University Press, xiii–xxx.

———. 2011. "On Good and Bad Forms of Medicalization." *Bioethics.* 27(1): 28–35.

Parens, Erik, and Adrienne Asch, eds. 2000. *Prenatal Testing and Disability Rights.* Washington, DC: Georgetown University Press.

Parisi, Melissa A., Linda Ramsdell, Mark Burns, Michael Carr, Richard Grady, Daniel Gunther, Gadi Kletter, Elizabeth McCauley, Michael Mitchell, Kent Opheim, Catherine Pihoker, Gail Richards, Michael Soules, and Roberta Pagon. 2007. "A Gender Assignment Team: Experience with 250 Patients over a Period of 25 Years." *Genetics and Medicine* 9(6): 348–357.

Pasterski, V. P. Prentice, and I. A. Hughes. 2010. "Consequences of the Chicago Consensus on Disorders of Sex Development (DSD): Current Practices in Europe." *Archives of Disease in Childhood* 95(8): 618–623.

Pateman, Carole. 1988. *The Sexual Contract.* Stanford, Calif.: Stanford University Press.

Phornputkul, Chanika, Anne Fausto-Sterling, and Philip A. Gruppuso. 1998. "Gender Reassignment at Birth: Three Cases of Reassignment/Ambiguity at or Beyond Adolescence." *Pediatric Research* 43(4): 82.

———. 2000. "Gender Self-Reassignment in an XY Adolescent Female Born with Ambiguous Genitalia." *Pediatrics* 106(1): 135–137.

Planas, Gabriela. 2006. "Filiación del Sordo." *Pagina 12*, October 26. http://www.pagina12
.com.ar/diario/psicologia/9-75122-2006-11-01.html, accessed March 14, 2010.

Plato. 1961a. "Protagoras," translated by W. K. C. Guthrie. In *Plato: The Collected Dialogues*, edited by Edith Hamilton and Huntington Cairns. Princeton, N.J.: Princeton University Press, 308–352.

———. 1961b. "Socrates Defense (Apology)," translated by Hugh Tedennick. In *Plato: The Collected Dialogues*, edited by Edith Hamilton and Huntington Cairns. Princeton, N.J.: Princeton University Press, 3–26.

———. 1989. *Symposium*. Translated by Alexander Nehamas and Paul Woodruff. Indianapolis: Hackett.

Preves, Sharon E. 2003. *Intersex and Identity: The Contested Self*. New Brunswick, N.J.: Rutgers University Press.

Probyn, Elspeth. 2005. *Blush: Faces of Shame*. Minneapolis: University of Minnesota Press.

Public Policy Advisory Network on Female Genital Surgeries in Africa. 2012. "Seven Things to Know about Female Genital Surgeries in Africa." *Hastings Center Report* 42(6):19–27.

Rebelo, Ethelywn, Christopher P. Szabo, and Grame Pitcher. 2008. "Gender Assignment Surgery on Children with Disorders of Sex Development: A Case Report and Discussion from South Africa." *Journal of Child Health Care* 12(1): 49–59.

Redick, Alison. 2005. "What Happened at Hopkins: The Creation of the Intersex Management Protocols." *Cardozo Journal of Law and Gender* 12(1): 289–296.

Reed, Sheldon C. 1970. "A Short History of Genetic Counseling." *Social Biology* 21(4): 332–339.

Reiner, William G. 1996. "Case Study: Sex Reassignment in a Teenage Girl." *Journal of the American Academy of Child and Adolescent Psychiatry* 35(6): 799–803.

———. 1997. "Sex Assignment in the Neonate with Intersex or Inadequate Genitalia." *Archives of Pediatrics and Adolescent Medicine* 151(10): 1044–1045.

———. 2006. "Prenatal Gender Imprinting and Medical Decision-Making: Genetic Male Neonates with Severely Inadequate Penises." In Sytsma, *Ethics and Intersex*, 153–163.

Reis, Elizabeth. 2007. "Divergence or Disorder? The Politics of Naming Intersex." *Perspectives in Biology and Medicine* 50: 535–543.

———. 2009. *Bodies in Doubt: An American History of Intersex*. Baltimore: Johns Hopkins University Press.

Reverby, Susan M. 2009. *Examining Tuskegee: The Infamous Syphilis Study and Its Legacy*. Chapel Hill: University of North Carolina Press.

Rodriguez, Sarah B., and Toby L. Schonfeld. 2012. "The Organ-That-Must-Not-Be-Named: Female Genitals and Generalized References." *Hastings Center Report* 42(3): 19–21.

Roen, Katrina. 2009. "Clinical Intervention and Embodied Subjectivity: Atypically Sexed Children and their Parents." In *Critical Intersex*, edited by Morgan Holmes. Surrey, U.K.: Ashgate, 15–40.

Rosario, Vernon. 2009. "Quantum Sex: Intersex and the Molecular Deconstruction of Sex." *GLQ: Intersex and After* 15(2): 267–284.

Rosner, Fred. 2007. "Judaism and Medicine: Jewish Medical Ethics." In *Principles of Health Care Ethics*, 2nd ed., edited by Richard E. Ashcroft, Angus Dawson,

Heather Draper, and John R. McMillan. West Sussex, England: John Wiley and Sons, 109–115.

Rosser, Sue. V. 1994. *Women's Health—Missing from U.S. Medicine.* Bloomington: Indiana University Press.

Rothman, David J. 1991. *Strangers at the Bedside: A History of How Law and Bioethics Transformed Medical Decision Making.* New York: Basic Books.

Rothman, Sheila. 1994. *Living in the Shadows of Death: Tuberculosis and the Social Experience of Illness in American History.* Baltimore: Johns Hopkins University Press.

Rousseau, Jean-Jacques. 1979 [1762]. *Emile, or On Education.* Translated by Allan Bloom. New York: Basic Books.

Rozin, Paul, Jonathan Haidt, and Clark R. McCauley. 2008. "Disgust." In *Handbook of Emotions,* 3rd ed., edited by Michael D. Lewis, Jeanette M. Haviland-Jones, and Lisa Feldman Barrett. New York: Guilford Press, 757–756.

Ruddick, Sara. 1989. *Maternal Thinking: Toward a Politics of Peace.* New York: Beacon Press.

Safer, Jeanne. 2002. *The Normal One: Life with a Difficult or Damaged Sibling.* New York: Free Press.

Sandberg, D. E., S. A. Berenbaum, L. Cuttler, B. Kogan, and P. A. Lee. 2004. "Intersexuality: A Survey of Clinical Practice." *Pediatric Research* 55(4): abstract 869.

Scheler, Max. 2007 [1915]. *Ressentiment.* Translated by Lewis B. Coser and William W. Holdheim. Milwaukee, Wisc.: Marquette University Press.

Schermer, Maartje. 2002. *The Difference Faces of Autonomy: Patient Autonomy in Ethical Theory.* Dordrecht, The Netherlands: Kluwer Academic.

Schober, Justine. 2006. "Feminization (Surgical Aspects)." In *Pediatric Surgery and Urology: Long-Term Outcomes,* 2nd ed., edited by Mark D. Stringer, Keith T. Oldham, and Pierre D. E. Mouriquand. Cambridge, U.K.: Cambridge University Press, 595–609.

Schönbucher, Verena, Katinka Schweizer, and Hertha Richter-Appelt. 2010. "Sexual Quality of Life of Individuals with Disorders of Sex Development and a 46, XY Karyotype: A Review of the International Research." *Journal of Sex and Marital Therapy* 36: 193–215.

Schützmann, Karsten, Lisa Brinkmann, Melanie Schacht, and Hertha Richter-Appelt. 2009. "Psychological Distress, Self-Harming Behavior, and Suicidal Tendencies in Adults with Disorders of Sex Development." *Archives of Sexual Behavior* 38:16–33.

Scully, Jackie Leach, Tom Shakespeare, and Sarah Banks. 2006. "Gift Not Commodity?: Lay People Deliberating Social Sex Selection." *Sociology of Health and Illness* 28(6): 749–767.

Sedgwick, Eve Kosofsky. 1991. "How to Bring Your Kids Up Gay." *Social Text* 29:18–27.

Sedgwick, Eve Kosofsky, and Adam Frank, eds. 1995. *Shame and Its Sisters: A Silvan Tomkins Reader.* Durham, N.C.: Duke University Press.

Sheehan, Elizabeth. 1981. "Victorian Clitoridectomy: Isaac Baker Brown and His Harmless Operative Procedure." *Medical Anthropology Newsletter* 12(4): 9–15.

Shell-Duncan, Bettina, and Ylva Herlund, eds. 2000. *Female Circumcision in Africa: Culture, Controversy, and Change.* Boulder: Lynne Rienner.

Shiloh, Shoshana, Liora Gerad, and Boleslav Goldman. 2006. "Patients' Information Needs and Decision-Making Processes: What Can Be Learned from Genetic Counselees?" *Health Psychology* 25(2): 311–219.

Shweder, Richard A. 2009. "Disputing the Myth of the Sexual Dysfunction of Circumcised Women: An Interview with Fuambai S. Ahmadu." *Anthropology Today* 25(6): 14–17.

Sibling Support Project. n.d. http://www.siblingsupport.org/sibshops, accessed August 23, 2013.

Siebers, Tobin. 2008. *Disability Theory.* Ann Arbor: University of Michigan Press.

Siminoff, L. A., and M. M. Step. 2005. "A Communication Model of Shared Decision Making: Accounting for Cancer Treatment Decisions." *Health Psychology* 24(4): S99–S105.

Skloot, Rebecca. 2010. *The Immortal Life of Henrietta Lacks.* New York: Crown.

Skoog, Steven J., and A. Barry Belman. 1989. "Aphallia: Its Classification and Management." *Journal of Urology* 141(3): 589–592.

Slijper, Froukje M. E., Stenvert L. S. Drop, Jan C. Molenaar, and Sabine M.P.F. de Muinck Keizer-Schrama. 1998. "Long-Term Psychological Evaluation of Intersex Children." *Archives of Sexual Behavior* 27: 125–144.

Speiser, Phyllis W., Ricardo Azzis, Laurence S. Baskin, Lucia Ghizzohi, Terry W. Hensle, Deborah P. Merke, Heino F. L. Meyer-Bahlburg, Walter L. Miller, Victor M. Montori, Sharon E. Oberfield, Martin Ritzen, and Perrin C. White. 2010. "Congenital Adrenal Hyperplasia due to Steroid 21-Hydroxylase Deficiency: Endocrine Society Clinical Practice Guideline." *Journal of Endocrinology and Metabolism* 95: 4133–4160.

Stark, Laura. 2012. *Behind Closed Doors: IRBs and the Making of Ethical Research.* Chicago: University of Chicago Press.

Stawarska, Beata. 2006. "From the Body Proper to Flesh: Merleau-Ponty on Intersubjectivity." In *Feminist Interpretations of Merleau-Ponty,* edited by Dorothea Olkowski and Gail Weiss. University Park: Pennsylvania State University Press, 91–106.

Stephens, Martha. 2002. *The Treatment: The Story of Those Who Died in the Cincinnati Radiation Tests.* Chapel Hill, N.C.: Duke University Press.

Stevens, M. L. Tina. 2000. *Bioethics in America: Origins and Cultural Politics.* Baltimore: Johns Hopkins University Press.

Sullivan, Nikki. 2007. "'The Price to Pay for our Common Good': Genital Modification and the Somatechnologies of Cultural (In)Difference." *Social Semiotics* 17(3): 395–409.

Swiss National Advisory Commission on Biomedical Ethics. 2012. *On the Management of Differences of Sex Development: Ethical Issues Relating to "Intersexuality."* Opinion No. 20/2012. Berne, Switzerland.

Sytsma, Sharon. 2002. "Surgical Treatment of Intersexuality: Business as Usual?" *Dialogues in Pediatric Urology* 25(6): 5–7.

———, ed.. 2006. *Ethics and Intersex.* Dordrecht, The Netherlands: Springer.

Tamar-Mattis, Anne. 2006. "Exceptions to the Rule: Curing the Law's Failure to Protect Intersex Infants." *Berkeley Journal of Gender, Law and Justice* 21: 59–110.

Terry, Jennifer. 1995. "Anxious Slippages Between 'Us' and 'Them': A Brief History of the Scientific Search For Homosexual Bodies." In *Deviant Bodies: Critical Perspectives on Difference in Science and Popular Culture,* edited by Jennifer Terry and Jacqueline Urla. Indianapolis: Indiana University Press, 129–169.

Therrell, Bradley L. 2001. "Newborn Screening for Congenital Adrenal Hyperplasia." *Endocrinology and Metabolic Clinic of North America* 30(1):15–30.

Thomas, Lynn. 2000. "'*Ngaitana* (I Will Circumcise Myself)': Lessons from Colonia Campaigns to Ban Excision in Meru, Kenya." In Shell-Duncan and Herlund, *Female Circumcision in Africa*, 129–150.

Tiefer, Lenore. 2008. "Female Genital Cosmetic Surgery: Freakish or Inevitable?: Analysis from Medical Marketing, Bioethics, and Feminist Theory." *Feminism and Psychology* 18(4): 466–479.

Toulmin, Stephen. 1982. "How Medicine Saved the Life of Ethics." *Perspectives in Biology and Medicine* 25: 736–750.

Turner, Amanda J., and Adrian Coyle. 2000. "What Does it Mean to Be a Donor Offspring? The Identity and Experiences of Adults Conceived by Donor Insemination and the Implications for Counseling and Therapy." *Human Reproduction* 15: 2041–2051.

United States v. *Windsor*. 570 U.S._____ (2013).

Vidal, Isabelle, Daniela Brindusa Gorduza, Elodie Haraux, Claire-Lise Gay, Pierre Chatelain, Mark Nicolino, Pierre-Yves Mure, and Pierre Mouriquand. 2010. "Surgical Options in Disorders of Sex Development (DSD) with Ambiguous Genitalia." *Best Practice and Research Clinical Endocrinology and Metabolism* 24: 311–324.

Von der Pfordten, Dietmar. 2009. On the Dignity of Man in Kant. *Philosophy* 84: 371–391.

Walcutt, Heidi. 1999. "Time for a Change." In Dreger, *Intersex in the Age of Ethics*, 197–200.

Walkowitz, Judith. 1982. *Prostitution and Victorian Society: Women, Class, and the State*. Cambridge, U.K.: Cambridge University Press.

Wall, Shelley. 2010. "Humane Images: Visual Rhetoric in Depictions of Atypical Genital Anatomy and Sex Differentiation." *Medical Humanities* 36(2): 80–83.

Warne, Garry L., and Vijayalkshmi Bhatia. 2006. "Intersex East and West." In Sytsma, *Ethics and Intersex*, 183–205.

Warne, Garry L., and Annabelle Mann. 2011. "Ethical and Legal Aspects of Management for Disorders of Sex Development." *Journal of Paediatrics and Child Health* 47: 661–663.

Warne, Garry L., and Jamal Raza. 2008. "Disorders of Sex Development (DSDs), their Presentation and Management in Different Cultures." *Reviews in Endocrine and Metabolic Disorders* 9: 227–236.

Webber, Sarah. 2005. "The 'Unnecessary' Organ: A History of Female Circumcision and Clitoridectomy in the United States, 1865–1995." PhD diss., University of Nebraska Medical Center.

Weil, Elizabeth. 2006. "What If It's (Sort of) a Boy and (Sort of) a Girl?" *New York Times Magazine,* September 24. http://www.nytimes.com/2006/09/24/magazine /24intersexkids.html?pagewanted=all, accessed July 5, 2012.

Weill Cornell Medical Center. 2010. "Surgical Management of Congenital Adrenal Hyperplasia. The Institute for Pediatric Urology, Genitoplasty Surgery." http://www.cornellurology.com/uro/cornell/pediatrics/genitoplasty.shtml#technique, accessed July 3, 2012.

Weiss, Gail. 1999. *Body Images: Embodiment as Intercorporeality*. New York: Routledge.

———. 2008. *Refiguring the Ordinary*. Bloomington: Indiana University Press.

Wesson, Miley B. 1947. "Obituary of Hugh Hampton Young, 1870–1945." *Journal of Urology* 57(2): 203–208.

Westerink, Herman. 2009. *A Dark Trace: Sigmund Freud on the Sense of Guilt*. Leuven, Belgium: Leuven University Press.

White, Mary Terrell. 1999. "Making Responsible Decisions: An Interpretive Ethic for Genetic Decisionmaking." *Hastings Center Report* 29(1): 14–21.

Wiesemann, Claudia. 2010. "Ethical Guidelines for the Clinical Management of Intersex." *Sexual Development:* 1–4. http://www.aissg.org/PDFs/Wiesemann-Ethical-Guidelines-2010.pdf, accessed July 6, 2012.

Wiesemann, Claudia, Susanne Ude-Koeller, Gernot H. G. Sinnecker, and Ute Thyen. 2010. "Ethical Principles and Recommendations for the Medical Management of Differences of Sex Development (DSD)/Intersex in Children and Adolescents." *European Journal of Pediatrics* 169(6): 671–679.

Wilkins, Lawson. 1950. *The Diagnosis and Treatment of Endocrine Disorders in Childhood and Adolescence.* Springfield, Ill.: Thomas.

Williams, Phoebe Dauz. 1997. "Siblings and Pediatric Chronic Illness: A Review of the Literature." *International Journal of Nursing Studies* 34(4): 312–323.

Wilson, Bruce E., and William G. Reiner. 1998. "Management of Intersex: A Shifting Paradigm." *Journal of Clinical Ethics* 9(4): 360–370.

Wilson, Robert C., Saroj Nimkarn, Miro Dumic, Jihad Obeid, Maryam Razzaghy Azar, Hossein Najmabadi, Fatemeh Saffari, and Maria I. New. 2007. "Ethnic-Specific Distribution of Mutations in 716 Patients with Congenital Adrenal Hyperplasia Owing to 21-Hydroxylase Deficiency." *Molecular Genetics and Metabolism* 90(4):414–421.

Winnicott, D. W. 1971. *Playing and Reality.* New York: Routledge.

Wisniewski, Amy B., Steven D. Chernausek, and Bradley P. Kropp. 2012. *Disorders of Sex Development: A Guide for Parents and Physicians.* Baltimore: Johns Hopkins University Press.

Young, Hugh Hampton. 1937. *Genital Abnormalities, Hermaphroditism and Related Adrenal Diseases.* Baltimore: Williams and Wilkins.

———. 1940. *Hugh Young: A Surgeon's Autobiography.* New York: Harcourt, Brace, and Company.

Young, Iris Marion. 2002. "Autonomy, Welfare Reform, and Meaningful Work." In *The Subject of Care: Feminist Perspectives on Dependency,* edited by Eva Feder Kittay and Ellen K. Feder. Lanham, Md.: Rowman and Littlefield, 40–60.

———. 2005 [1980]. "Throwing Like a Girl: A Phenomenology of Feminine Body Comportment, Motility, and Spatiality." In *On Female Body Experience: "Throwing Like a Girl" and Other Essays.* Oxford, U.K.: Oxford University Press, 27–45.

Zeiler, Kristin, and Anette Wickström. 2009. "Why Do 'We' Perform Surgery on Newborn Intersexed Children?" *Feminist Theory* 10(3): 359–377.

Index

siblings: affected by medical treatment, 91–92, 103–106, 137; invisibility of, 107; as "normal ones," 106; potential of harm to "unaffected," 95, 103–106

Sigmundson, Keith, 36, 205

Skloot, Rebecca, 214n13

Socrates, 10, 168–169, 193, 204, 233n14. *See also* Plato

Sousa, Aron, 39, 215nn18–19

Southbury Training School, 188, 234n5

spoiling, 81, 83–84, 88, 93

Stark, Laura, 212n10

stigma: attached to atypical anatomies, 43, 145, 153, 166, 174, 189, 206; attached to parents of children with atypical anatomies, 85, 189; as motivating normalizing interventions, 153, 174, 190; "natural" and "social," 123, 136, 225n21; and "the problem" of intersex, 15, 66–67; produced by medicalization of atypical sex anatomies, 73, 129, 235n5

SUCCEED clinic, 218n6, 231n7

Sullivan, Nikki, 128, 130

support groups, 48, 52, 218n6; ISNA as originating as, 41; recognition of importance of, 208, 218n6. *See also* Androgen Insensitivity Syndrome Support Group

Swiss National Advisory Commission, 207–209, 223n2

Terry, Jennifer, 41

Tomkins, Silvan, 73

Toulmin, Stephen, 211n5

trauma: acknowledgement by 2006 Consensus Statement, 89, 158; comparison between medical management of atypical sex and sexual abuse, 223n1; early surgery supposed to produce less, 44, 62; resulting from medical management of atypical sex anatomies, 15, 17, 63, 66, 89–90, 114

Trinkl, Peter, 216n22

tuberculosis, 42–43

Tuskegee Syphilis Experiment, 7

vaginoplasty, 17, 90, 98–99, 145, 148, 203, 219n16

virtue, 165, 168, 170; Aristotle's conception of, 155, 164; in Foucault's work, 174, 196–198; in Kantian ethics, 164, 185. *See also* virtue ethics

virtue ethics, 18, 155–156, 174, 196–197, 202–205. *See also* virtue

Von der Pfordten, Dietmar, 184–186

vulnerability: of bond between parents and children, 1, 176, 188; of caregivers, 10, 45, 51, 54–55; children's, 1, 11, 54, 96, 174, 176, 187–188, 191–192, 209; as condition of intimate relationship, 181, 188; dignity of embodied, 18, 176–182, 184, 187, 191, 194, 210; human, 18, 24, 50, 54, 104, 177–185, 192, 198; of immigrant or indigenous women who have had genital surgery, 227n16; of objects of envy, 79, 86; of parents, 11–12, 45, 50–51, 176, 180, 188, 190–191; of research subjects, 7–8, 230n2

Wallon, Henri, 224n9

Warne, Garry, 121–125, 131, 157–158, 232n10

Weiss, Gail, 87, 108, 173

Wilkins, Lawson: association with John Money, 19–20, 24, 26, 37, 66; and concern with normalization, 21, 26–27, 31–33, 35, 225n1; and Harriet Lane Home, 24, 29; influence/legacy of, 19–24, 30–31, 38, 40, 66, 112, 128, 213n3; relationship with Hugh Hampton Young, 27–29; and research/innovation in treatment of CAH, 21, 24–25, 25–27, 31; view of health, 25–27, 31. *See also* Johns Hopkins University

Wilson, Bruce, 38, 133

Winnicott, D. W., 218n11, 224n14

Wollstonecraft, Mary, 81

Young, Hugh Hampton, 23, 27–31

Young, Iris Marion, 92–93

ELLEN K. FEDER teaches philosophy at American University. She lives in Washington, D.C., with her family.

WITHDRAWN

CPSIA information can be obtained at www.ICGtesting.com
Printed in the USA
BVOW04s0852030414

349637BV00001B/1/P